Pregnancy

All-in-One

for **dummies®**

A Wiley Brand

by Joanne Stone, MD; Keith Eddleman, MD; Catherine Cram, MS; Tara Gidus Collingwood, MS, RDN, CSSD; Rachel Gurevich; Matthew M. F. Miller; Sharon Perkins, RN; Tere Stouffer; and Carol Vannais, RN

for **dummies®**

A Wiley Brand

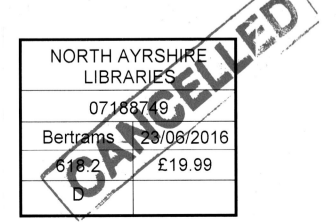

Pregnancy All-in-One For Dummies®

Published by: **John Wiley & Sons, Inc.,** 111 River Street, Hoboken, NJ 07030-5774, www.wiley.com

Copyright © 2016 by John Wiley & Sons, Inc., Hoboken, New Jersey

Published simultaneously in Canada

For general information on our other products and services, please contact our Customer Care Department within the U.S. at 877-762-2974, outside the U.S. at 317-572-3993, or fax 317-572-4002. For technical support, please visit www.wiley.com/techsupport.

Wiley publishes in a variety of print and electronic formats and by print-on-demand. Some material included with standard print versions of this book may not be included in e-books or in print-on-demand. If this book refers to media such as a CD or DVD that is not included in the version you purchased, you may download this material at http://booksupport.wiley.com. For more information about Wiley products, visit www.wiley.com.

Library of Congress Control Number: 2016934262

ISBN 978-1-119-23549-1 (pbk); ISBN 978-1-119-23551-4 (ebk); ISBN 978-1-119-23550-7 (ebk)

Manufactured in the United States of America

10 9 8 7 6 5 4 3 2 1

Contents at a Glance

Table of Contents

Introduction

Prospective parents are truly curious about everything related to pregnancy, from when the baby's heart is formed to whether eating sushi or dyeing your hair is okay. If this describes you, you've come to the right place. In one helpful reference guide, *Pregnancy All-in-One For Dummies* offers the answers to many of your pregnancy-related questions, from fetal development to workouts for moms-to-be to healthy weight gain and more.

About This Book

Pregnancy should be a joy, not a worry. Yet pregnant women are, by nature, already anxious about whether anything they do or eat may hurt the baby. The source of all this anxiety? Often it's information on pregnancy — in print, online, or from the mouths of well-meaning but clueless friends and family — that is outdated, lacks scientific basis, or is exaggerated for shock effect. The result is that many pregnant women and their partners end up incredibly worried about something they've read or heard.

This comprehensive, scientifically correct guide presents the facts of pregnancy based on real scientific data, and it answers many commonly asked questions — all while encouraging the humor and light-heartedness that are part of the miraculous process of having a baby. A big part of the philosophy behind this book is to reassure pregnant women instead of adding to the unnecessary worries they already have.

Prospective parents also want to know about the medical aspects of pregnancy. When are fingers developed? Which blood tests should be done, and why? What options are available for detecting various problems? This book addresses these topics, too, creating what is essentially a medical text on obstetrics for the layperson.

This book provides a lot of factual information, but it isn't gospel. Many of the topics discussed apply to pregnancy in general, but your particular situation may have unique aspects that warrant different or extra consideration, so use this book as a companion to regular medical care.

Sidebars (boxes of text) in this book give you a more in-depth look at a certain topic. Although they further illuminate a particular point, these sidebars aren't crucial to understanding the rest of the book. Feel free to read them or skip them. You can pass over the text that accompanies the Technical Stuff icon as well. The text associated with this icon gives some interesting details about pregnancy, but if you don't read it, you can still come away with the information you need.

Within this book, you may note that some web addresses break across two lines of text. If you're reading this book in print and want to visit one of these web pages, simply key in the web address exactly as it's noted in the text, pretending the line break doesn't exist. If you're reading this as an e-book, you've got it easy — just click the web address to be taken directly to the web page.

Foolish Assumptions

We made some assumptions about you and what you want out of a pregnancy book:

>> You may be a woman who is considering pregnancy, planning to have a baby, or already pregnant.

>> You may be the partner of the mother-to-be.

>> You may know and love someone who is or plans to become pregnant.

>> You want to find out more about pregnancy but have no interest in becoming an expert on the topic.

>> You want reliable information on a variety of topics related to pregnancy, from information on the development of the fetus to how to stay fit as your body changes, whether and how to breastfeed, and more.

If you fit any of these criteria, then *Pregnancy All-in-One For Dummies* gives you the information you're looking for.

Icons Used in This Book

Like other *For Dummies* books, this one uses icons to guide you through the information.

TECHNICAL
STUFF

This icon signals information that delves a little deeper than usual into a medical explanation.

REMEMBER

This icon flags information that's particularly worth keeping in mind.

TIP

This icon marks bits of advice about handling minor discomforts and other challenges you encounter during pregnancy.

WARNING

This icon points out situations and actions that a pregnant woman clearly should avoid.

Beyond the Book

In addition to the material in the print or e-book you're reading right now, this product comes with some access-anywhere goodies on the web. Check out the free Cheat Sheet for info on what to expect when you're admitted to the hospital, how you can avoid some of the maladies that plague pregnant women (like heartburn), and strategies that can help you find time for fitness and motherhood. To get this Cheat Sheet, simply go to www.dummies.com and search for "*Pregnancy All-in-One For Dummies* Cheat Sheet" in the Search box.

Where to Go from Here

If you're the particularly thorough type, go ahead and read this book from cover to cover. If you just want to find specific information and then close the book, take a look at the table of contents or at the index. Dog-ear or bookmark the pages that are especially interesting or relevant to you. Add comments or write little notes in the margins. Have fun, and most of all, enjoy your pregnancy!

1

Getting Started with Your Pregnancy Preparation

Contents at a Glance

IN THIS CHAPTER

Knowing what symptoms to look for

Getting the answer to that all-important question: Are you pregnant?

Knowing what to expect as your pregnancy progresses

Scheduling doctor appointments and routine tests

Chapter 1

Seeing Double (Lines): And So It Begins

So you think you may be pregnant! Or maybe you're hoping to become pregnant soon. Either way, it's important to know what to look for so that you can find out whether you're pregnant as early as possible. This chapter takes a look at some of the most common signals that your body sends you in the first weeks of pregnancy and offers advice for confirming your pregnancy and getting it off to a great start.

Seeing Signs — of Pregnancy, That Is

So assume it has happened: A budding embryo has nestled itself into your womb's soft lining. How and when do you find out that you're pregnant? Quite often, the first sign is a missed period. But your body sends many other signals — sometimes even sooner than that first missed period — that typically become more noticeable with each passing week.

>> **Honey, I'm late!** You may suspect that you're pregnant if your period hasn't arrived as expected. By the time you notice you're late, a pregnancy test will probably yield a positive result (see the next section for more on pregnancy tests). Sometimes, though, you may experience one or two days of light bleeding, which is known as *implantation bleeding*, because the embryo is attaching itself to your uterus's lining.

>> **You notice new food cravings and aversions.** What you've heard about a pregnant woman's appetite is true. You may become ravenous for pickles, pasta, and other particular foods yet turn up your nose at foods you normally love to eat. No one knows for sure why these changes in appetite occur, but experts suspect that these changes are, at least partly, nature's way of ensuring that you get the proper nutrients. You may find that you crave bread, potatoes, and other starchy foods, and perhaps eating those foods in the early days is actually helping you store energy for later in pregnancy, when the baby does most of its growing. As with any other time in life, though, be careful not to overeat. You may also be very thirsty early in pregnancy, and the extra water you drink is useful for increasing your body's supply of blood and other fluids.

>> **Your breasts become tender and bigger.** Don't be surprised if you notice that your breasts become larger during the first portion of your pregnancy. In fact, large and tender breasts are often the first symptom of pregnancy that you feel because very early in pregnancy, levels of estrogen and progesterone rise, causing immediate changes in your breasts.

Determining Whether You're Pregnant

Well, are you or aren't you? These days, you don't need to wait to get to your practitioner's office to find out whether you're pregnant. You can opt instead for self-testing. Home tests are urine tests that give simply a positive result (often showing two lines) or negative result (showing only one line); some use little plus (positive) and minus (negative) signs. These tests are very accurate for most people. Your practitioner, on the other hand, may perform either a urine test similar to the one you took at home or a blood test to confirm that you're pregnant.

Getting an answer at home

Suppose you notice some bloating or food cravings, or you miss your period by a day or two. You want to know whether you're pregnant, but you aren't ready to go to a doctor yet. The easiest, fastest way to find out is to go to the drugstore and pick up a home pregnancy test. These tests are basically simplified chemistry sets, designed to check for the presence of *human chorionic gonadotropin* (hCG, the hormone produced by the developing placenta) in your urine. Although these kits aren't as precise as laboratory tests that look for hCG in blood, in many cases, they can provide positive results very quickly — by the day you miss your period, or about two weeks after conception.

REMEMBER

The results of home pregnancy tests aren't a sure thing. If your test comes out negative but you still think you're pregnant, retest in another week or make an appointment with your doctor. A urine test is positive at a level of about 20–50 IU/L, while a blood test is positive at a level of 5–10 IU/L, depending on the test. So a blood test will be positive a little earlier than a urine test. An ultrasensitive blood test can even detect an hCG level of about 1–2 IU/L.

Going to your practitioner for answers

Even if you had a positive home pregnancy test, most practitioners want to confirm this test in their office before beginning your prenatal care. Your practitioner may decide to simply repeat a urine pregnancy test or to use a blood pregnancy test instead.

REACTING WHEN YOUR PARTNER BREAKS THE NEWS

When your partner tells you the big news, try to mirror her reaction, at least outwardly. If her reaction is "Oh . . . heck," you can go along in that vein also, at least for a minute or two. Remember, though, that she's gauging your reaction to the news, and if you act like having a baby is a huge imposition in your life, she'll be really upset, even if it *is* going to be a huge imposition and even if she just said the same thing five minutes before. Try to throw in a few encouraging statements about how you wanted kids eventually, how having a baby will be fun in the winter when there's nothing else to do, or whatever encouraging babble you can come up with at a stressful time.

Some women get very creative with their announcements, from filling the living room with balloons to baking a cake with a pair of booties inside. Just try not to choke on one, literally or figuratively. If she's gone all out to break the news, you can safely bet that she's really excited, so make sure to be as supportive as possible.

Even if you've been trying to conceive forever, an initial reaction of fear isn't uncommon. Remember that your partner may also be feeling some sudden doubts and fears, and allow her to express them. Under no circumstances is "We spent $20,000 for fertility treatments and now you're not sure this is the right time?!" the right response to her concerns.

A blood pregnancy test checks for hCG in your blood. This test can be either qualitative (a simple positive or negative result) or quantitative (an actual measurement of the amount of hCG in your blood). The test your practitioner chooses depends on your history and your current symptoms and on her own individual preference. Blood tests can be positive even when urine tests are negative.

Calculating your due date

Only 1 in 20 women actually delivers on her due date — most women deliver anywhere from three weeks early to two weeks late. Nonetheless, it's important to pinpoint the due date as precisely as possible to ensure that the tests you need along the way are performed at the right times. Knowing how far along you are also makes it easier for your doctor to see that the baby is growing properly.

The average pregnancy lasts 280 days — 40 weeks — counting from the first day of the last menstrual period. This day is used to calculate your due date.

TIP

If your cycles are 28 days long, you can use a shortcut to determine your due date. Simply subtract three months from your last menstrual period and add seven days. If your last period started on June 3, for example, your due date would be March (subtract three months) 10 (add seven days). If your periods don't follow 28-day cycles, don't worry. You can establish your due date in other ways. If you've been tracking ovulation and can pinpoint the approximate date of conception, add 266 days to that date (the average time between the first day of your last menstrual period and ovulation is about 14 days, or 2 weeks).

If you're unsure of the date of conception or the date your last period started, an ultrasound exam during the first three months can give you a good idea of your due date. A first-trimester ultrasound predicts your due date more accurately than an ultrasound done in the second or third trimester.

TIP

You can also use a pregnancy wheel to calculate how far along you are. To use this handy tool, line up the arrow with the date of your last menstrual period and then look for today's date. Just below the date, you see the number of weeks and days that have gone by. (If you know the date of conception rather than your last period, there's a line on the wheel corresponding to this, too.) You can find online wheels as well as apps that you can download to calculate your due date.

A Week-by-Week Overview of Pregnancy

As indicated throughout this book, pregnancy is usually referred to as a 40-week enterprise, which is a tad misleading. The pregnancy starts at conception, which — with a normal 28-day cycle — is two weeks after the first day of your last menstrual period. So if you start at conception, pregnancy is only 38 weeks, but obstetricians use 40 weeks because most women don't know when they conceive but do remember when their last period was.

REMEMBER

Here are a few things to remember as you read this week-by-week guide:

>> Many of the things discussed in a particular week may still be important at other times throughout the pregnancy. So just because the ultrasound is mentioned at 20 weeks doesn't mean it can't be done at any other time.

>> Some things included in this chapter are optional and may not be necessary for everyone.

>> The week/weeks assigned to prenatal tests or pregnancy events are an approximation. Don't be overly alarmed if, in your pregnancy, they are off by a week or so.

OVERCOMING YOUR FEARS OF BEING A FATHER

You have a lot of time to get used to the idea of being a dad, so don't worry if you have a lot of fears at first. Even if you aren't sure you're ready to become a father, you'll be surprised how quickly you come around to the idea. Besides, the baby will be here before you know it, ready or not.

It's important, however, to use this time to confront your fears about parenting. Spend time with the male role models from your past (and present) and use them as learning tools. Ask them what they did right, what they would change, and what advice they have for you when raising your own child. You may feel like you're the first father ever, but you don't need to reinvent the wheel when it comes to parenting. If you admire other people's skills, monitor and mimic their behaviors.

Working on overcoming your fatherhood fears is doubly important if the father in your life wasn't the best role model for the type of dad you want to be to your son or daughter. To attempt to come to terms with any wrongdoings your father may have committed, talk with a counselor or therapist, or even a trusted friend, about your relationship with your father and try to identify the mistakes you don't want to repeat. Talking about your experience with your own father can also help heal some of the emotional wounds. Being a father is hard work, and you don't want to wait until after the baby arrives to start overcoming your fears or past traumas.

Weeks 0 to 4

If you suspect that you're pregnant, you're probably both excited and anxious to find out if you truly are. The first four weeks are important because the pregnancy is getting established as the implantation process is underway.

During these initial weeks, do the following:

>> **Record your last menstrual period.** Doing so helps your provider better estimate your due date (40 weeks from your last period). Be sure to tell him if your cycles are irregular.

>> **Begin taking a daily prenatal vitamin if you haven't already.** Check to see that the vitamin has at least 400 micrograms of folic acid to make sure your baby is as healthy as possible.

>> **Check for ovulation.** Some women know when they ovulate by a sensation known as *mittelschmerz* (German for "middle pain," due to the mild pain that may be felt when the egg is released from the ovary, typically 14 days after your last period). Others know they've ovulated due to a change in the cervical mucus or a positive reading from an ovulation prediction kit.

Fertilization usually occurs within the fallopian tube. The embryo starts as one cell. During the 1st week, that cell divides many times as it moves down the fallopian tube toward the uterine cavity.

>> **Take your first pregnancy test.** As stated earlier, pregnancy tests check for a hormone called *human chorionic gonadotropin* (hCG), which is produced by the placenta as the embryo implants into the wall of the uterus — usually five to seven days after conception. By the time you miss a period, around ten days after conception, your pregnancy test will most likely be positive.

Don't be too concerned if you have a little spotting around the time when you would expect your period. This is most likely due to the embryo implanting in the womb (implantation bleeding).

At the end of the 4th week, your baby measures 0.2 inches (5 mm) in length.

Weeks 5 to 8

By this time, the pregnancy is well established, and you're feeling the typical signs and symptoms of pregnancy, such as nausea and fatigue. During weeks 5 to 8, most of the baby's organ systems are beginning to form. The first organ to start working is the heart. It's amazing to realize it starts beating at just 5 weeks, although you can't see it beating on ultrasound until 6 weeks. The baby's arms and legs are beginning to develop at this stage. The head is the biggest part of the embryo because the brain is the fastest-growing organ at this time. (Check out Chapter 1 in Book 2 for more on what happens during the first trimester.) The placenta is rapidly growing and is now the way nutrients and oxygen get to your developing baby.

This is an important time to make any necessary lifestyle changes, if you haven't already done so (like stopping smoking or speaking with your doctor about adjusting medications — Book 1, Chapter 2 explains the effects of certain medications, alcohol, and drugs on the developing fetus). Also during this time, begin making these necessary medical appointments:

>> **Call your doctor to make an appointment for your first prenatal visit.** Most doctors want to see their patients before 8 to 10 weeks. Head to Book 1, Chapter 2 for advice on selecting a practitioner and what to expect during your prenatal visits.

>> **Talk to your healthcare provider about scheduling an ultrasound or obtaining a heartbeat by Doppler to confirm a healthy pregnancy.** An ultrasound during this period is very accurate at establishing your due date (it is sometimes called a "dating scan") and can also tell you whether you're having one, two, or even more babies! Your due date is most accurate when it is established by an ultrasound between 8 and 12 weeks.

>> **If you're taking any medications, call or see your doctor earlier than the 8 to 10 weeks mentioned.** You want to make sure that these meds aren't a problem for your developing baby. You should also discuss any over-the-counter or herbal medications you're taking to make sure they aren't a problem, either.

At the end of the 8th week, your baby measures 1.2 inches (3.0 cm) in length. Your uterus is about the size of a medium orange.

Weeks 9 to 12

Although you won't be feeling it this early, this is the time when your baby starts to move around. If you're having an ultrasound at this time, you may actually see these movements on the screen. Before 10 weeks, male and female embryos look the same. After 10 weeks, their external genitalia start to develop differently, although your practitioner may not be able to see this difference on ultrasound until after 16 to 20 weeks, depending on the position of the baby, the amount of abdominal tissue the sound waves have to pass through, the kinds of equipment used, and the experience of the person performing the ultrasound. By the end of the 10th week, all the organ systems have formed. The brain is unique in that it continues to develop throughout pregnancy and even into adulthood.

You want to consider the following counseling and testing at this time:

>> **Schedule an appointment for genetic counseling if you have a family history of genetic problems.** Your doctor may also recommend it, depending on varying circumstances.

>> **Make sure you schedule your first-trimester screen for Down syndrome.** Remember, the best time to screen for Down syndrome is at 11 to 12 weeks (see Book 2, Chapter 1 for detailed information about the first trimester and Down syndrome screening). This screen combines a measurement of the fluid-filled region behind the fetal neck (called a *nuchal translucency*), your age, and blood tests (hCG and PAPP-A) to give you a specific risk for Down syndrome as well as for Trisomy 13 and 18 (other chromosomal disorders).

Talk to your provider to see whether he thinks you're a candidate for a newer type of screening for Down syndrome that extracts fetal genetic material from your blood. This blood sample can be drawn as early as 9 weeks.

>> **If you're considering having a chorionic villus sampling (CVS), weeks 10 to 12 are the best time to do this.** This test can reveal chromosomal conditions as well as other genetic conditions, such as cystic fibrosis. See Book 2, Chapter 1 for more information on this test.

At the end of week 12, your baby is 2.13 inches (5.4 cm) long and weighs less than half an ounce (around 14 g). Your uterus is the size of a large orange.

Weeks 13 to 16

Congratulations! You and your baby made it through the first trimester. You're starting to feel more like yourself — you have more energy and less nausea. After week 14, the majority of the amniotic fluid surrounding your baby is made up of the baby's urine. By week 15, an experienced sonographer can tell by ultrasound whether you're having a boy or a girl. By week 16, your baby starts to grow fine, soft hair (called *lanugo*) and fingernails.

The following considerations apply during this time period:

>> **Between weeks 15 and 18, have your blood drawn to check the alpha-fetoprotein (AFP) level.** This blood test helps to identify fetal abnormalities

such as spina bifida. This is also the time to have the second part of your Down syndrome screening (the quad screen).

» **If you're planning on having an amniocentesis, schedule it between weeks 16 and 18.** See Book 2, Chapter 2 for the reasons to consider an amniocentesis.

» **Consider shopping at a maternity store.** Many women start to show at this time. If you aren't showing, don't worry, because some body types hide pregnancy better than others.

At the end of week 16, your baby is 4.6 inches (11.6 cm) long and weighs about 3.5 ounces (100 g). Your uterus is the size of a large grapefruit.

Weeks 17 to 20

During weeks 17 to 20, your baby begins to put on some fat and looks more like a real baby. The baby's skeleton, which starts out mostly as cartilage, is now transforming into bone. You may notice a little fluttering sensation in your abdomen. This could be gas, but more likely it's early fetal movement. By 20 weeks, the top of the uterus (called the *fundus*) is at the level of your belly button. Twenty weeks is the halfway mark, so you should congratulate yourself. The second half usually flies by faster than the first.

You want to keep the following in mind:

» **Schedule your anatomy ultrasound.** This is the ultrasound where the doctor is able to check the baby's anatomy and make sure he is growing properly and is surrounded by normal amniotic fluid.

» **Pay attention to the baby's movements.** This period is when many women start to feel the baby move, which is called *quickening*. First-time moms, though, don't always feel quickening this early, so don't be alarmed if you haven't.

Your baby now weighs about 10 ounces (300 g) and is about 10 inches (25 cm) long.

Weeks 21 to 24

During this time, your baby's lungs are going through a very important phase of development. The lining of the lungs is beginning to thin out enough to allow for oxygen exchange. You may be experiencing discomfort on either side of your lower abdomen (in the groin area). This discomfort is known as *round ligament pain.* The round ligaments are actual ligaments that attach from the top of the uterus to the labia. Many women feel an uncomfortable pulling sensation, which tends to worsen upon standing and improve upon sitting or lying down. The good news is that after 24 weeks, round ligament pain usually goes away.

At this time, your baby is regularly swallowing large amounts of amniotic fluid and excreting urine back into the amniotic cavity. The baby's fingernails are almost fully formed, and he has started to grow eyelashes and eyebrows. The lanugo is turning from a pale color to a darker hue.

By 24 weeks, your baby is considered *viable.* This means survival on the outside is possible, although the baby would need a great deal of medical attention. The top of your uterus is usually at or above the level of your belly button.

There aren't any actual tasks that you have to schedule with your provider during this time, other than your routine prenatal visits (which should be about every four weeks during this period).

At the end of this period, your baby weighs about 1 pound, 5 ounces (600 g) and measures about 12 inches (30 cm) long.

Weeks 25 to 28

Your baby's bones are continuing to harden, and his fingernails, toes, eyebrows, and eyelashes are fully present. Meanwhile, your baby's skin is still fairly see-through, although it is changing from transparent to a more opaque look. You should still be seeing your provider about every four weeks during this period of pregnancy.

The following considerations are typically addressed during this time:

>> **Get your glucose screen.** This is the blood test to screen for gestational diabetes. You're instructed to drink a 50-gram glucose drink (it tastes like flat soda), and your blood is drawn one hour later. If the glucose level is above a certain value, a definitive test called a GTT (glucose tolerance test) is needed. You're instructed to fast the night before this test so that your fasting glucose level can be determined with the initial blood draw. You then drink a 100-gram glucose drink and have your blood drawn every hour for the next three hours. Two abnormal values are needed for a diagnosis of gestational diabetes. During the glucose screening process, your doctor may draw some additional blood to check for conditions like anemia.

>> **If your blood type is Rh negative (see Book 6, Chapter 2), you need to get a shot of Rh immune globulin.** This shot can prevent any effects of incompatibility between you and your baby.

The top of your uterus is a couple of inches above your belly button. By 28 weeks, your baby weighs about 2 pounds, 4 ounces (1 kg). He is about 14.8 inches (38 cm) long.

Weeks 29 to 32

Your baby's eyes can now open. His permanent teeth have developed, and the lungs and digestive tract are nearly mature. To keep a closer eye on you and your baby, your practitioner will start to schedule your prenatal visits every two weeks.

The following steps are recommended during this time:

>> **If you haven't started childbirth classes, begin them now.** Many alternatives are available, so check with your doctor or the hospital where you'll deliver. Book 1, Chapter 5 discusses several options. If you'll have help taking care of your newborn, remember that it's a good idea for all caregivers (including you and your partner) to take an infant CPR class to be as prepared as possible for your newborn.

>> **Pay closer attention to your baby's movements.** Although fetuses still spend most of their time sleeping, they start to develop clear sleep and wake cycles. A good general rule is that feeling about six movements in an hour is a sign of fetal well-being. You don't have to feel these movements every hour, but if you're ever concerned that you're not feeling your normal fetal movement, lie down and count the movements. If you can feel six movements in an hour, you can rest assured that this is normal.

The nature of the fetal movements may also change. Instead of the big punches and kicks you were feeling earlier, the movements during this time may be gentler, rolling type of movements.

>> **Undergo a follow-up ultrasound if your practitioner orders one.** This ultrasound can confirm that the baby is growing normally and has a good amount of amniotic fluid. Most practitioners also follow growth by measuring your uterine height every time you visit.

The top of your uterus is midway between your navel and your sternum. By 32 weeks, your baby weighs from about 3 pounds, 11 ounces to 4 pounds (1.8 kg) and is 16 to 17 inches (43 cm) long.

Weeks 33 to 36

During this time, you may be feeling lots of rhythmic fetal movements, which are really the baby hiccupping — a normal occurrence. These hiccups can continue even after the baby is born. If you're having twins, you should be well prepared for their arrival now, because on average, twins deliver at about 35 to 36 weeks.

The following considerations come into play now:

>> **Get a culture taken for GBS (group B strep).** Your doctor tests for these common bacteria that can be found in the vagina or rectum. If your GBS culture is positive, your doctor will place you on antibiotics during labor to prevent the baby from contracting the infection. There isn't any point in treating it earlier, because it can just come back again.

>> **Continue to pay attention to the baby's movements.** Even though you're used to feeling kicks and punches, it's normal for the intensity of these movements to decrease during these last weeks of pregnancy. It's the *number* that is important, though, rather than the intensity. See Book 2, Chapter 3 for more about fetal movements in the third trimester.

The top of your uterus is a couple of inches below your sternum. At or just after 36 weeks, your doctor will see you at least once a week until you deliver. Your baby weighs about 5 pounds, 2 ounces (2.3 kg) and is almost 18 inches (46 cm) long.

Weeks 37 to 40

Congratulations — you are now considered *term*. Even though you may not yet be at your due date, any delivery that occurs at or after 37 weeks is considered a full-term delivery. You may notice irregular contractions that come and go in spurts. The big event can happen at any time during this period, so be prepared — day or night.

Do the following to ensure that you're ready for the big day to arrive:

>> **Make sure that your bags are packed and you have the phone numbers of your practitioners handy!** If you have other children at home, make sure you have all the arrangements set for their care, in case you go into labor.

>> **Watch for signs.** Loss of your mucous plug, bloody show, or loose stools may happen during the days before labor to indicate that labor is coming. Unfortunately, they don't determine when labor will happen with any certainty.

The average baby at full-term weighs about 7.5 pounds (close to 3.5 kg), but there is a wide degree of variation in what's considered normal. At this point in pregnancy, your baby will put on about a quarter of a pound per week until delivery. The top of your uterus should be at or just below your sternum or breastbone. Babies at 40 weeks average about 20 to 21 inches (51 to 53 cm) long.

Weeks 40 to 42

Don't worry — the end really is in sight. If you haven't gone into labor on your own, your doctor will likely schedule you for either induction or cesarean section by 41 to 42 weeks. If you're older than 35, and especially if you're older than 40, your doctor may want to deliver you sooner. Because the risks to continuing the pregnancy really increase after 41 to 42 weeks, your baby should be delivered by then. Your doctor makes sure your baby remains healthy during this time:

>> **Your doctor monitors you with non-stress tests to check on fetal well-being.** This is a noninvasive way to make sure the baby is tolerating the in-utero environment. (See Book 2, Chapter 3 for more information.)

>> **Your doctor checks the amount of amniotic fluid present to make sure it's still adequate.** The amniotic fluid volume usually tends to decrease after 36 weeks, so it isn't uncommon for it to be low at this time. Low amniotic fluid volume is a common reason for labor induction during this period.

Although the baby continues to grow after 40 weeks, the rate of growth slows a little, and he may not put on the quarter pound per week that he did in the few weeks before 40 weeks.

Common Tests during Pregnancy

Table 1-1 lists common tests that may be recommended during your pregnancy. Some of these tests may not be recommended for every pregnancy but are included for the sake of those who need them.

TABLE 1-1   ## Common Tests during Pregnancy

Test	Gestational Age (Weeks)	Purpose of Test
Dating ultrasound	7–12	Confirms viability of pregnancy, establishes due date, rules out multiple gestations
Harmony, MaterniT21, Panorama, or Verifi	9–20	Screens for genetic defects in the fetus
Nuchal translucency test (ultrasound)	11–12	Part of the first-trimester screen for Down syndrome
Chorionic villus sampling (CVS)	10–12	Samples the placental tissue for genetic abnormalities; recommended for some women but should be offered to all women
AFP/quad screen	15–18	Screens for defects such as spina bifida and completes the second-trimester screen for Down syndrome
Amniocentesis	16–18	Samples the amniotic fluid for genetic abnormalities; recommended for some women but, again, should be offered to all women
Anatomy ultrasound	18–22	Looks at the baby from head to toe to make sure he is developing normally (to rule out many birth defects)
Glucose screen	24–28	Tests for gestational diabetes
Group B strep (GBS) swab	35–37	Sees if the birth canal is colonized with group B strep bacteria (if so, Mom will be given antibiotics during a vaginal delivery to protect the baby)
Non-stress test (NST)	40–42	Tests the baby's heart rate patterns to determine fetal well-being, despite going past his due date; often done earlier in pregnancy for other complications like high blood pressure and diabetes
Biophysical profile (BPP)	40–42	Determines fetal well-being; often done earlier in pregnancy for other complications; includes an assessment of amniotic fluid volume

Chapter 2

Practitioners, Prenatal Visits, and Maintaining Good Health

Finding the right practitioner to care for you — and your baby — is a decision you shouldn't take lightly. Your healthcare is always important, but your new and sometimes overwhelming condition means you want a practitioner who's in sync with your approach to pregnancy. This person should be someone you trust and feel safe with. If you've had a previous child, you may already have a practitioner. If not, there's no need to feel overwhelmed. This chapter helps you make that important decision and takes you through a typical prenatal visit.

Maintaining good health throughout your pregnancy is a critical step in delivering a healthy baby, so this chapter also includes information on risks and benefits associated with certain medicines and vaccinations, along with the consequences of alcohol and drugs.

Selecting the Right Practitioner for You

Many kinds of professionals can help you through pregnancy and delivery. Be sure to choose a practitioner with whom you feel comfortable. Review this list of the basic five:

>> **Obstetrician/gynecologist:** After completing medical school, this physician receives another four years of special training in pregnancy, delivery, and women's health. She should be *board certified* (or be in the process of becoming board certified) by the American Board of Obstetrics and Gynecology (or an equivalent program if you're from a country other than the United States).

>> **Maternal-fetal medicine specialist:** Also known as a *perinatologist* or *high-risk obstetrician,* this type of doctor has completed a two- to three-year fellowship in the care of high-risk pregnancies, in addition to the standard obstetrics residency, to become board certified in maternal-fetal medicine. Some maternal-fetal medicine specialists act only as consultants; some also deliver babies. You might seek the care of or even a consultation with a high-risk specialist if you've had a history of problem pregnancies (prior preterm delivery, history of preeclampsia, or multiple miscarriages), if you have underlying medical problems (like diabetes or chronic hypertension), or if your fetus has been diagnosed with a disorder.

>> **Family practice physician:** This doctor provides general medical care for families — men, women, and children. She is board certified in family practice medicine. This kind of doctor is likely to refer you to an obstetrician or maternal-fetal medicine specialist if complications arise during your pregnancy.

>> **Certified nurse-midwife:** A certified nurse-midwife is a registered nurse who has completed additional training to obtain a master's degree in nursing and is also licensed to perform deliveries. A certified nurse-midwife typically practices in a setting where there is a physician available and refers patients when complications occur.

>> **Certified registered nurse practitioner:** A certified registered nurse practitioner is a registered nurse who has completed additional training to obtain a master's degree in nursing and is trained to provide routine prenatal care, but she typically doesn't perform deliveries. She usually practices in conjunction with a physician; whether you see the nurse practitioner or the physician for your prenatal visits depends on the individual practice and where you are in your pregnancy. (Whether a certified registered nurse practitioner is allowed by law to deliver differs state to state.)

Before you make a decision, you want to be thorough in your search. Make sure you know what you want out of the experience. When you're deciding on a practitioner, ask yourself the following key questions:

>> **Am I comfortable with and do I have confidence in this person?** You should trust and feel at ease not only with your practitioner but also with the whole constellation of people who work in the practice. Would you feel free to ask questions or express your anxieties to them? Another point to keep in mind is how your general personality fits in with the practice's philosophy. For example, some women prefer a low-key, low-tech approach to prenatal care, while others want to have every possible diagnostic test under the sun. Does this practitioner deliver in a setting where you feel most comfortable having your baby? Your past medical and obstetrical history can also influence the approach you take to your pregnancy and the provider you choose.

>> **How many practitioners are involved in the practice?** You may end up choosing between a practitioner who works with one or more partners and one who is in solo practice. Many group practices rotate you through appointments with each of the doctors, enabling you to get to know them all so you'll feel comfortable having any of them deliver your baby. Some practices utilize nurse practitioners to help render prenatal care. Practically speaking, you're likely to bond more with one or two people in the practice than with others, which is natural, given that practitioners have varied personalities. A provider who practices alone should tell you who handles deliveries when she is ill, off duty, or out of town.

TIP

Ask your practitioner about her policy for after-hours problems or emergencies — including questions you may need to ask by telephone during evening or weekend hours.

>> **Where do I want to deliver?** If your pregnancy is uncomplicated, any good hospital or birthing center will work just fine. Some women may even choose a home birth. If you're at risk for some complications, however, you should consider a hospital delivery and ask whether the hospital you'll be delivering in has a labor and delivery suite and a nursery equipped to handle any problems that may arise if, for example, the baby is born early. You may also want to ask the following questions:

- Is an anesthesiologist on-site 24 hours a day, or can your doctor call in an anesthesiologist quickly in case of an emergency?

- Can the hospital provide you with *epidural* anesthesia (a form of pain control during labor)? If epidural anesthesia isn't readily available or you're not interested in it, find out what other options are available for pain management.

- Are you allowed to *room in* — that is, keep the baby in your room as much as possible — after delivery? Also, are accommodations available for your partner to stay with you during your postpartum hospitalization?

>> **Can this practitioner refer me to a nearby specialist if needed?** Consider whether you may need the services of a maternal-fetal medicine specialist or

a *neonatologist,* a physician who specializes in the care of infants who are born early or who have other medical problems. Ideally, your practitioner can refer you to someone quickly if anything comes up.

>> **Will my insurance plan cover this practitioner?** Now that managed care has become an important part of the health insurance industry, check to see whether your plan covers your practitioner of choice. Some places allow you to select an out-of-network physician if you pay part of the cost yourself.

DETERMINING WHETHER YOU'RE AT HIGH RISK

The question of whether you and your pregnancy are at high risk has no black-and-white answer, especially at the beginning. But it helps to be aware of the kinds of conditions that can put a pregnancy at high risk:

- Diabetes

- High blood pressure

- Lupus

- Blood disorders

- Heart, kidney, or liver disorders

- Twins, triplets, or other multiple fetuses

- A premature delivery in a prior pregnancy

- A previous child with birth defects

- A history of miscarriage

- An abnormally shaped uterus

- Epilepsy

- Some infections

- Bleeding

- Advanced maternal age (35 or older by the due date)

Remember that midwives and most family practice physicians are not equipped to handle high-risk pregnancies. If you have or develop any of these conditions, consult an obstetrician or a maternal-fetal medicine specialist.

Planning Prenatal Visits

Your positive pregnancy test marks a new beginning. The time has come to start thinking about what lies ahead. After you decide who your practitioner will be, give the office a call to find out how to proceed. Some practices want you to come in for a visit with the office nurse to give a medical history and to confirm your good news with either a blood or urine test, whereas others schedule a first visit with the practitioner. How soon your first visit will be scheduled depends in part on your history.

TIP

If you didn't have a preconception visit and you haven't been on prenatal vitamins or other vitamins containing folic acid, let the office know. A prescription for prenatal vitamins can be called in, so you can start taking them even before your first prenatal visit. All over-the-counter adult multivitamins and prenatal vitamins should have the correct dose of folic acid (400 micrograms), so the typical patient doesn't need a prescription for them, but ask the pharmacist if you're not sure. Also, some insurance companies may cover prescription vitamins but not over-the-counter ones, and some women just simply prefer one particular type of vitamin.

Some things are consistent from trimester to trimester — like checking your blood pressure and urine and checking the baby's heartbeat — so these topics are covered in this chapter. In Chapters 1, 2, and 3 in Book 2, you can find specifics on what happens during prenatal visits for each trimester. See Table 2-1 for an overview of a typical schedule for prenatal visits.

TABLE 2-1 **Typical Prenatal Visit Schedule**

Stage of Pregnancy	Frequency of Doctor Visits
First visit to 28 weeks	Every four weeks
28 to 36 weeks	Every two to three weeks
36 weeks to delivery	Weekly

If you develop problems during pregnancy or if your pregnancy is considered high risk (see the risk factors described in Book 6, Chapter 1), your practitioner may suggest that you come in more frequently.

REMEMBER

This schedule of prenatal visits isn't set in stone. If you're planning a vacation or need to miss a prenatal visit, tell your practitioner and reschedule your appointment. If your pregnancy is going smoothly, rescheduling usually isn't a big deal. However, because some prenatal tests have to be performed at specific times during pregnancy (see Book 1, Chapter 1 for details), just make sure that missing an appointment won't affect any of these tests.

Prenatal visits vary a bit according to each woman's personal needs and each practitioner's style. Some women need particular laboratory tests or physical examinations. However, the following procedures are standard during your prenatal visits:

>> **A nurse checks your weight and blood pressure.** For more information on how much weight you should be gaining and when, see Book 1, Chapter 3; for details on healthy ways to manage your weight gain, head to Book 3, Chapter 1.

>> **You give a urine sample (usually an easy job for most pregnant women!).** Your practitioner checks for the presence of protein, which may indicate preeclampsia, or glucose, which may be a sign of diabetes (see Book 6 for information on dealing with special conditions during pregnancy). Some urine tests also enable your doctor to look for any indications of a urinary tract infection.

>> **Starting sometime after 14 to 16 weeks, a nurse or doctor measures your fundal height.** The practitioner uses either a tape measure or her hands to measure your uterus. This gives her a rough idea of how the baby is growing and whether you have an adequate amount of amniotic fluid (see Figure 2-1).

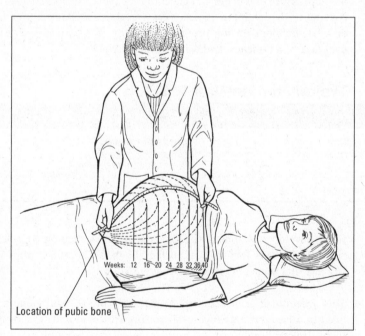

Weeks: 12 16 20 24 28 32 36 40

Location of pubic bone

FIGURE 2-1: Your practitioner may measure your fundal height to ensure that your baby is growing properly.

Illustration by Kathryn Born, MA

The nurse or doctor is measuring the *fundal height,* the distance from the top of the pubic bone to the top of the uterus (the *fundus*). By 20 weeks, the fundus usually reaches the level of the navel. After 20 weeks, the height in centimeters roughly equals the number of weeks pregnant you are. (Being above or below by 2 centimeters is usually within acceptable norms as long as you're consistent from visit to visit.)

Note: The fundal height measurement may not be useful in women who are expecting two or more babies or in women who have large fibroids (in both cases, the uterus is much bigger than normal) or in women who are very obese (because it can be difficult to feel the top of the uterus).

>> **A nurse or doctor listens for and counts the baby's heartbeats.** Typically, the heartbeat ranges between 120 and 160 beats per minute. Most offices use an electronic Doppler device to check the baby's heartbeat. With this method, the baby's heartbeat sounds sort of like horses galloping inside the womb. Sometimes, you can hear the heartbeat as early as 8 or 9 weeks using this method, but often the heartbeat isn't clearly discernible until 10 to 12 weeks. Prior to the availability of Doppler, a special stethoscope called a *fetoscope* was used to hear the baby's heartbeat. Using this method, the doctor can hear the heartbeat around 20 weeks. A third way of checking the baby's heartbeat is by seeing it on ultrasound. The heart beating away can frequently be seen at around 6 weeks.

REMEMBER

In some practices, a medical assistant or nurse performs tasks such as checking your blood pressure; in other practices, a doctor may perform this task. No matter who performs the technical components of the prenatal visit, you should always have the opportunity to ask a practitioner questions before leaving the office.

Keeping Your Medicines and Vaccinations in Check

During your pregnancy, you'll probably experience at least a headache or two and an occasional case of heartburn. The question of whether you can safely take pain relievers, antacids, and other over-the-counter medicines is bound to come up. Many women are afraid to take any medicine at all, for fear of somehow harming their babies. But most nonprescription drugs — and even many prescription drugs — are safe during pregnancy. During your first prenatal visit, go over with your practitioner what medications are okay to take during pregnancy — both over-the-counter medications and medications prescribed to you by another physician. If another physician is treating you for a medical condition, let her know that you're pregnant, in case any adjustments need to be made.

Reviewing your medications

Many medicines — both over-the-counter and prescription — are safe to take during pregnancy. If you're taking medications essential for your health, discuss them with your physician prior to stopping them or changing your dose or regimen. But a few medications can cause problems for the baby's development, so let your doctor know about *all* the medications you take. If one of them is problematic, you can probably switch to something safer. Keep in mind that adjusting dosages and checking for side effects may take time.

Exposure to the drugs and chemicals listed in Table 2-2 is considered to be safe during pregnancy.

TABLE 2-2   ## Medications Generally Considered Safe during Pregnancy

Type of Medication	Example
Pain relievers	Acetaminophen
Antiviral medications	Acyclovir
Antiemetics/antinausea medications	Phenothiazines, trimethobenzamide, and Diclegis, a combination of doxylamine and vitamin B6, which has been approved by the Food and Drug Administration for morning sickness and is in the safest drug classification for pregnancy (category A)
Antihistamines	Doxylamine
Low-dose aspirin	Often used to decrease risk for preeclampsia in patients at risk
Minor tranquilizers and some antidepressants	Meprobamate, chlordiazepoxide, and fluoxetine
Antibiotics	Penicillin, cephalexin, trimethoprim-sulfamethoxazole, and erythromycin
Antiviral agent used in patients with HIV	Zidovudine

Medications to ask your doctor about

The following are some of the common medications that women should ask about before they get pregnant:

>> **Birth control pills:** Women sometimes get pregnant while they're on the Pill (because they missed or were late taking a couple of pills during the month) and then worry that their babies will have birth defects. But oral contraceptives haven't been shown to have any ill effects on a baby. Two to three

percent of *all* babies are born with birth defects, and babies born to women on oral contraceptives are at no higher risk.

>> **Ibuprofen (Motrin, Advil):** Occasional use of these and other *nonsteroidal anti-inflammatory agents* during pregnancy (for pain or inflammation) is okay and hasn't been associated with problems in infants. However, avoid chronic or persistent use of these medications during pregnancy (especially during the last trimester) because they have the potential to affect platelet function and blood vessels in the baby's circulatory system — and because your baby's kidneys process them just like your own kidneys do.

>> **Vitamin A:** This vitamin and some of its derivatives can cause miscarriage or serious birth defects if too much is present in your bloodstream when you get pregnant. The situation is complicated by the fact that vitamin A can remain in your body for several months after you consume it. Discontinuing any drugs that contain vitamin A derivatives — the most common is the anti-acne drug Accutane — at least one month before trying to conceive is important. Scientists don't know whether topical creams containing vitamin A derivatives — anti-aging creams like Retin A and Renova, for example — are as problematic as drugs that you swallow, so consult your physician.

Some women take vitamin A supplements because they're vegetarians and don't get enough from their diet or because they suffer from vitamin A deficiency. The maximum safe dose during pregnancy is 5,000 international units (IU) daily. (You need to take twice that amount to reach the danger zone.) Multiple vitamins, including prenatal vitamins, typically contain 5,000 IU of vitamin A or less. Check the label on your vitamin bottle to be sure.

REMEMBER

If you're worried that your prenatal vitamin plus your diet will put you into that danger zone of 10,000 IU per day, rest assured that it would be extremely difficult to get that much vitamin A in your diet.

>> **Blood thinners:** Women who are prone to developing blood clots or who have artificial heart valves need to take blood-thinning agents every day. One type of blood thinner, Coumadin (warfarin), or its derivatives, if taken during pregnancy, can trigger miscarriage, impair the baby's growth, or cause the baby to develop bleeding problems or structural abnormalities. Women who take this medicine and are thinking of getting pregnant should switch to a different blood thinner. Ask your practitioner for more information. Do not simply stop taking your medications; discuss your options with your provider first.

>> **Drugs for high blood pressure:** Many of these medications are considered safe to take during pregnancy. However, because a few can be problematic, you should discuss any medications to treat high blood pressure with your doctor (see Book 6, Chapter 3).

>> **Antiseizure drugs:** Some of the medicines used to prevent epileptic seizures are safer than others for use during pregnancy. If you're taking any of these

drugs, discuss them with your doctor. Don't simply stop taking any antiseizure medicine, because seizures may be worse for you — and the baby — than the medications themselves (see Book 6, Chapter 3).

» **Tetracycline:** If you take this antibiotic during the last several months of pregnancy, it may, much later on, cause your baby's teeth to be yellow.

» **Antidepressants:** Many antidepressants (like Prozac and Zoloft) have been studied extensively and are considered safe during pregnancy. Recent studies on selective serotonin reuptake inhibitors (SSRIs) showed a small increase in certain birth defects, particularly with paroxetine, while other studies showed no increased risk. Most doctors believe that the absolute risk is very small. Although most data doesn't show an increase in prematurity or low birth weight, some data suggests a possible small increase in the chance of miscarriage in the first trimester. Some reports also show a very small risk (0.6 to 1.2 percent) of a newborn condition called *persistent pulmonary hypertension* with exposure in the latter half of pregnancy.

Some of the newer antidepressants like Cymbalta, Celexa, Lexapro, and Effexor appear to be safe in pregnancy, but because they are new, data is limited. If you need to start an antidepressant during pregnancy, many doctors feel that sertraline (Zoloft) is the best first-line drug. But if you're already taking an antidepressant, ask your doctor whether you'll be able to keep taking the medication while you're pregnant or need to switch to something safer.

» **Bupropion:** Bupropion is an antidepressant, but it's also prescribed to help people stop smoking (for example, Wellbutrin or Zyban). Very little info exists on its use during pregnancy, but the available data doesn't suggest any significant problems with fetal development. Although you shouldn't use it as a first line for depression, its use for smoking cessation may be beneficial.

» **Fluconazole:** Fluconazole is an oral medication used to treat yeast or other fungal infections. A recent study showed that oral fluconazole used during the first trimester was not associated with an increased risk of birth defects overall, but it may be associated, at higher doses, with an increased risk of a specific heart defect known as *Tetralogy of Fallot.*

» **Decongestants:** A mounting body of recent evidence suggests that decongestants like phenylephrine and phenylpropanolamine, when used during the first trimester, may be associated with an increased risk of birth defects. If possible, avoid taking these medications until you've completed your first trimester; however, if you inadvertently took some before you found out that you were pregnant, the likelihood of a resulting birth defect is still very low.

» **Lithium:** Lithium is used occasionally to treat bipolar disorder. It's thought that taking this medication during pregnancy increases your risk of having a child with a specific cardiac abnormality known as *Ebstein's anomaly.* If possible, an alternative medication should be chosen for the first trimester, but if you inadvertently take lithium during the first trimester, the risk is still quite low. Women taking lithium during early pregnancy should have a fetal echocardiogram at around 20 weeks. This is a special type of ultrasound done to diagnose cardiac abnormalities, including Ebstein's anomaly.

REMEMBER

Some drugs are known to have a *teratogenic* effect, which means they have the potential to cause birth defects or problems with growth and development. If you took any teratogenic medications before you knew you were pregnant — or before you knew that the drugs could pose a problem — don't panic. In many cases, the drugs do no harm, depending on when during pregnancy you took them and in what quantities. Some medications can cause problems in the first trimester but are totally safe in the third trimester, and vice versa. In fact, relatively few substances are proven to be teratogenic to humans, and even those that are don't cause birth defects every time. Discuss with your practitioner the medications you've been taking and what tests are available to check on your baby's growth and development.

Continuing medications until you talk to your doctor

Many medications are labeled "Don't take during pregnancy" because they haven't been adequately studied in pregnant women. However, this warning label doesn't necessarily mean that adverse effects have been reported or that you can't use these medications.

Whenever you have a question about a particular medication, ask your practitioner for advice. Don't be surprised if opinions vary among practitioners, especially between nonobstetric providers and obstetricians. Many nonobstetricians are hesitant to prescribe many medications because they're uncertain, whereas your obstetric practitioner may be more secure.

REMEMBER

Certain medical problems, such as high blood pressure, pose more risk to the growing fetus than the medication you'd take to treat it does. Even a common headache, if it's bad enough to cause you to miss a traffic signal when you're behind the wheel, can be more dangerous than a little acetaminophen (Tylenol), which actually isn't dangerous at all when taken in therapeutic doses. Many pregnant women suffer needlessly with common symptoms that could be treated with medications that are safe for the baby.

WARNING

Don't stop taking a prescription medication or change the dosage without talking to your doctor first.

Recognizing the importance of vaccinations and immunity

People are immune to all kinds of infections for one of two reasons:

>> **They've suffered through the disease.** Most people are immune to chickenpox, for example, because they had it when they were kids, causing their immune systems to make antibodies to the chickenpox virus.

>> **They've been vaccinated.** That is, they've been given a shot of something that causes the body to develop antibodies.

Many vaccines are safe, and in fact recommended, while you're pregnant. (See Table 2-3 for information on several vaccines.) Here's some further information on some common vaccinations:

>> **Rubella:** Your practitioner tests to see whether you're immune to rubella (also known as German measles) by drawing a sample of blood and checking to see whether it contains antibodies to the rubella virus. (*Antibodies* are immune system agents that protect you against infections.) If you aren't immune to rubella, your practitioner is likely to recommend that you be vaccinated against rubella at least three months *before* becoming pregnant. Getting pregnant before the three months are over is highly unlikely to be a problem. No cases have been reported of babies born with problems due to the mother having received the rubella vaccine in early pregnancy. If you're already pregnant when you discover that you aren't immune to rubella, your practitioner will recommend that you get the vaccine after you deliver your baby, just before you go home from the hospital.

>> **Flu:** The influenza vaccine is safe and recommended during pregnancy. Pregnant women who get the flu are at an increased risk of complications, including maternal morbidity and mortality. The vaccine poses no harm to your developing baby.

>> **Tetanus, diphtheria, and pertussis:** It's recommended that women get an adult tetanus, diphtheria, and pertussis (Tdap) vaccine during each pregnancy, ideally between weeks 27 and 36 of pregnancy. The pertussis vaccine also protects your baby from whooping cough after birth.

>> **Measles, mumps, and poliomyelitis:** Most people are immune to measles, mumps, and poliomyelitis, and your practitioner is unlikely to check your immunity to all these illnesses. Besides, these illnesses aren't usually associated with significant adverse effects for the baby.

>> **Chickenpox:** There's a small risk that the baby will contract a chickenpox infection from her mother. If you've never had chickenpox, tell your

practitioner so you can discuss possible vaccination before you get pregnant or, if you're already pregnant, after delivery before you go home.

>> **Human papilloma virus:** Vaccines are available for the human papilloma virus (HPV), which is associated with some kinds of abnormal pap smears, genital warts, and cervical cancer. Studies suggest the HPV vaccine is similar to other vaccinations that are safe in pregnancy; however, it's still recommended that pregnant women skip this vaccination. If you inadvertently got vaccinated before realizing that you were pregnant, the risk to your developing baby is very low, but you shouldn't get subsequent doses until after delivery.

TABLE 2-3   **Safe and Unsafe Vaccines before or during Pregnancy**

Disease	Risk of Vaccine to Baby during Pregnancy	Immunization Recommendations	Comments
Cholera	None confirmed	Same as in nonpregnant women	
Hepatitis A (inactivated)	None confirmed	Okay if at high risk for infection or for prevention due to recent exposure	
Hepatitis B	None confirmed	Okay if at high risk for infection	Used with immunoglobulins for acute exposure; newborns need vaccine
Human papilloma virus	None confirmed, but little data	If found to be pregnant after initiating series, give remaining doses postpartum	
Influenza (inactivated)	None confirmed	Recommended	
Measles	None confirmed	No	Vaccinate postpartum
Mumps	None confirmed	No	Vaccinate postpartum
Plague	None confirmed	Selected vaccination if exposed	
Pneumococcus	None confirmed	Okay if high risk	
Poliomyelitis	None confirmed	Only if exposed or if traveling to endemic area	
Rabies	Unknown	Indication same as for nonpregnant women	Consider each case separately
Rubella	None confirmed	No	Vaccinate postpartum

(continued)

TABLE 2-3 *(CONTINUED)*

Disease	Risk of Vaccine to Baby during Pregnancy	Immunization Recommendations	Comments
Smallpox	Possible miscarriage	No, unless emergency situation arises or fetal infection	
Tetanus, diphtheria, and pertussis (Tdap)	None confirmed	Recommended for each pregnancy between 27 and 36 weeks	
Typhoid	None confirmed	Only for close, continued exposure or travel to endemic area	
Varicella (chickenpox)	None confirmed	Immunoglobulins recommended in exposed nonimmune women; should be given to newborn if around time of delivery	If nonimmune, vaccinate postpartum (second dose 4–8 weeks later)
Yellow fever	Unknown	No, unless exposure is unavoidable	

Understanding the Effects of Alcohol and Other Drugs on Your Baby

Alcohol and recreational/illicit drugs can cross the placenta and get into your baby's circulatory system. Some medications can also cross the placenta. Some are completely harmless, whereas others can cause problems. The following sections outline which substances you can safely use and which you should avoid — information that's crucial to your baby's health.

Smoking

Unless you've been living on Mars for the past 30 years, you no doubt are aware that smoking is a health risk for you. When you smoke, you run the risk of developing lung cancer, emphysema, and heart disease, among other illnesses. During pregnancy, however, smoking poses risks to your baby as well.

WARNING

The carbon monoxide in cigarette smoke decreases the amount of oxygen that your growing baby receives, and nicotine cuts back on blood flow to the fetus. Consequently, women who smoke stand an increased chance of delivering babies with low birth weight, which may mean more medical problems for the baby. In fact, babies born to smokers are expected to weigh a half pound less, on average, than those born to nonsmokers. The exact difference in birth weight depends on how much the mother smokes. Secondhand smoke is also a risk.

In addition to low birth weight, smoking during pregnancy is associated with a greater risk of preterm delivery, miscarriage, placenta previa (see Book 6, Chapter 2), placental abruption (also in Book 6, Chapter 2), preterm rupture of the amniotic membranes, and even sudden infant death syndrome (SIDS) after the baby is born.

Quitting smoking can be extremely difficult. But keep in mind that even cutting back on the number of cigarettes you smoke is beneficial to your baby (and yourself).

REMEMBER

If you quit smoking during the first three months you're pregnant, give yourself a pat on the back and be reassured that your baby is likely to be born at a normal weight and have fewer health issues.

WARNING

Some women use nicotine patches, gum, lozenges, or inhalers to help them kick the habit. The nicotine from these products is still absorbed into the bloodstream and can still reach the fetus, but at least the carbon monoxide and other toxins in cigarette smoke are eliminated. The American Congress of Obstetricians and Gynecologists recommends that nicotine replacements such as these may be used when nonpharmacologic treatments have failed. The total amount of nicotine absorbed from the intermittent use of the gum or inhalers may be less than the amount from the patch, which is used continuously. It's very important that you not smoke cigarettes while also using nicotine replacement, and if you relapse, discontinue the nicotine replacement.

The effects on fetal development with the use of bupropion (Zyban or Wellbutrin; see the earlier section "Medications to ask your doctor about") haven't been extensively studied, but one well-designed study showed that pregnant smokers receiving bupropion were much more likely to quit than those not taking the medication.

Drinking alcohol

Clearly, pregnant women who use alcohol put their babies at risk of fetal alcohol syndrome, which encompasses a wide variety of birth defects (including growth problems, heart defects, mental retardation, or abnormalities of the face or limbs). The controversy arises because medical science hasn't defined an absolute safe level of alcohol intake during pregnancy.

Scientific data shows that daily drinking and heavy binge drinking can lead to serious complications, although little information is available about occasional drinking. Two recent studies from Britain, however, demonstrated that light or moderate drinking had little effect on either neurodevelopmental outcomes or balance. In one study, up to two drinks per week was not linked with developmental problems with children. A separate study of 7,000 10-year-olds whose mothers had light (one glass per week) or moderate (three to seven glasses per week) alcohol consumption during pregnancy found that the children had no difference in balance compared to those whose mothers did not drink at all during pregnancy. The authors of the studies still say, however, that abstaining from alcohol during pregnancy is the best choice. Similarly, both the American Congress of Obstetricians and Gynecologists and the Food and Drug Administration (FDA) recommend avoiding any amount of alcohol during pregnancy.

REMEMBER

If you think you may have a drinking problem, don't feel uncomfortable talking to your practitioner about it. Special questionnaires are available to help your doctor identify whether your drinking is excessive enough to pose a risk to you and the fetus. If you think you may have a problem, discussing this questionnaire with your practitioner is crucial to your baby's health — and to yours.

EXPECTANT MOTHERS ASK . . .

Questions about alcohol consumption during pregnancy are very common, so here are the answers to some of the most frequently asked questions:

Q: "On my Caribbean vacation, I enjoyed some piña coladas on the beach. I didn't find out I was pregnant until a few weeks later. Will my baby have birth defects?"

A: No evidence suggests that a single episode of drinking has any increased risk of adverse effects on pregnancy. Now that you know you're pregnant, avoid alcohol.

Q: "Is hard liquor worse for the baby than wine or beer?"

A: They're all considered the same risk. A can of beer, a glass of wine, and a mixed drink with 1 ounce of hard liquor contain roughly the same amounts of alcohol.

Q: "My doctor suggested I have a glass of wine on the evening after my amniocentesis. Is this okay?"

A: While the party line is that avoiding alcohol entirely is best, occasional use is probably okay, especially under these circumstances. Alcohol is a *tocolytic,* which basically means that it relaxes the uterus. After amniocentesis, many women feel a little uterine cramping. The alcohol in a glass of wine minimizes that discomfort without hurting the baby.

Using recreational/illicit drugs

Many studies have evaluated the effects of drug use during pregnancy. But the studies can be confusing because they tend to lump all kinds of drug users together, regardless of which drugs they use and how much they use. The mother's lifestyle also influences the degree of risk to the baby, which complicates the information even more. For example, women who abuse drugs are more likely to be malnourished than other women, they're typically of lower socioeconomic status, and they suffer a higher incidence of sexually transmitted diseases. All these factors, independent of and added to drug use, can cause problems for your pregnancy and for your baby.

Chapter 3

Diet, Exercise, and Expectant Moms

Through the ages, women have received all kinds of advice about what, and how much, to eat while they're expecting. Cultural traditions, religious beliefs, and scientific thinking have all had their influence. Your practitioner's advice is likely to depend on your particular health habits and your size when your pregnancy begins. Also, if you're carrying more than one baby, you're expected to gain more than the average number of pounds.

Of course, health involves more than just eating well. Exercise is as important while you're pregnant as it was before, although what and how much you do to stay fit may change as your pregnancy progresses. This chapter provides you with basic information about proper nourishment and exercise during pregnancy. For more in-depth information, head to Books 3 and 4, which are devoted to nutrition and staying fit and active while pregnant.

Looking at Healthy Weight Gain

Starting pregnancy at a healthy weight and gaining weight at a moderate pace throughout pregnancy can help ensure that your baby grows and develops normally and that you stay healthy as well. So what is *healthy*? This section explains in more depth the weight issues associated with pregnancy.

Determining how much is enough

The best way to figure out your ideal weight — and weight gain — is to look at your *body mass index (BMI)*, a number that takes into account both height and weight.

After you know your body mass index (many BMI calculators are available online), you can figure out your ideal weight gain during pregnancy by consulting Table 3-1. (But don't forget, this number refers to women carrying only one baby!)

TABLE 3-1 **Figuring Out Your Ideal Weight Gain**

Body Mass Index	Recommended Weight Gain
Less than 19.8 (underweight)	28 to 40 pounds (12.5 to 18 kilograms)
19.9 to 26 (normal weight)	25 to 35 pounds (11.5 to 16 kilograms)
26 to 29 (overweight)	15 to 25 pounds (7 to 11.5 kilograms)
29 or more (obese)	15 pounds (7 kilograms) or less

REMEMBER

These numbers refer to total weight gain during the entire pregnancy, so you won't know whether you've hit the target until delivery day. Scientific research hasn't determined the optimal pattern of weight gain throughout pregnancy. Gaining very little weight early on (when you may be in the throes of morning sickness) may have less effect on fetal growth than poor weight gain in the late second or third trimester. Some women gain weight inconsistently, putting on a large number of pounds early and then much less later on. Nothing is necessarily unhealthy about this pattern, either.

Avoiding weight obsession

Use the charts of optimal weight gain as a guide, but don't become fanatical about how much you weigh. Even if the amount you gain is somewhat off course, if your doctor says that the baby is growing normally, you have nothing to worry about. Women who gain more than average can still have healthy babies, and so can women who gain very little.

If your weight gain is way too high or way too low, your doctor can check the baby's growth by measuring the fundal height (refer to Book 1, Chapter 2) or schedule you for a sonogram. If you deviate significantly from the recommended weight gain, your doctor will probably want to evaluate your diet. He may refer you to a nutritionist or dietitian who can give you specific advice about what and how much to eat.

WHERE DOES THE WEIGHT GO?

The good news is that the weight you gain during pregnancy doesn't all go to your thighs. Then again, it doesn't all go to the baby, either. A pregnant woman typically adds a little to her own body fat. It's a myth, however, that you can tell whether she's going to have a boy or a girl based on her pattern of weight gain (more in the hips or more in the belly). Here's a realistic view of your weight gain — assuming it's 27 pounds, which is fairly average:

Baby	7 pounds (3,180 grams)
Placenta	1 pound (455 grams)
Amniotic fluid	2 pounds (910 grams)
Uterus	2 pounds (910 grams)
Breasts	1 pound (455 grams)
Fat stores	7 pounds (3,180 grams)
Body water	4 pounds (1,820 grams)
Extra blood	3 pounds (1,360 grams)

Understanding your baby's weight gain

Your baby's bulking-up pattern is likely to progress slowly at first and then pick up at about 32 weeks, only to slow again in the last weeks before birth. At 14 to 15 weeks, for example, the baby puts on weight at about 0.18 ounce (5 grams) per day. At 32 to 34 weeks, he puts on 1.06 to 1.23 ounces (30 to 35 grams) per day (that's about half a pound or 0.23 kilograms each week). After 36 weeks, the fetal growth rate slows to about a quarter of a pound per week, and by 41 to 42 weeks (you're overdue at this point), minimal or no further fetal growth may occur. In addition to your diet and weight gain, the following factors affect fetal growth:

>> **Cigarette smoking:** Smoking can reduce the birth weight by about half a pound (about 230 grams).

>> **Diabetes:** If the mother is diabetic, the baby can be too big or too small.

>> **Genetic or family history:** In other words, basketball players usually don't have children who grow up to be professional jockeys!

>> **Fetal infection:** Some infections affect growth.

>> **Illicit drug use:** Drug abuse can slow fetal growth.

>> **Mother's medical history:** Some medical problems, like hypertension or lupus, can affect fetal growth.

>> **Multiple pregnancy:** Twins and triplets are often smaller than singles.

>> **Placental function:** Placental blood flow that's below par can slow down the baby's growth.

Your practitioner keeps an eye on your baby's growth rate, most often by measuring fundal height and paying attention to your weight gain. If you put on too little or too much weight, if your fundal height measurements are abnormal, or if something in your history puts you at risk for growth problems, your doctor is likely to send you for an ultrasound exam to more accurately assess the situation.

Taking Stock of What You're Taking In

Sticking to a well-balanced, low-fat, high-fiber diet is important not only for your baby but also for your own health. Consuming adequate protein is also important because protein carries out many of the body's functions. The fiber in your diet helps to prevent or reduce constipation and hemorrhoids. By not consuming too much fat, you help keep your heart healthy and avoid putting on extra pounds that may be difficult to shed.

If your diet is balanced and not too heavy in sugar or fat, you don't need to modify the way you eat dramatically. During pregnancy, you should take in roughly 300 *extra* calories a day, on average. That means that if you're at a healthy weight and you're taking in 2,100 calories per day, while pregnant you should take in an average of 2,400 calories per day (perhaps a little less during your first trimester and a little more during your third trimester).

REMEMBER

You should *not* increase your caloric intake by eating a hot fudge sundae every day. Filling these additional requirements with nutritious foods is key. Your practitioner will likely advise you to take some supplemental vitamins and minerals, too. Keep reading to find out which foods and supplements are best for you, and head to Book 3 for detailed guidance.

Using the USDA MyPlate

No single food can satisfy all your nutritional needs. The USDA MyPlate, shown in Figure 3-1, is a general guideline that illustrates the relative proportions of servings you should eat in each group. To get some specific recommendations tailored for your pre-pregnancy weight and activity level, go to `www.choosemyplate.gov/moms-daily-food-plan` and create a profile to receive a personalized daily food plan.

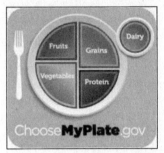

FIGURE 3-1: Use the USDA MyPlate guide to help you eat healthily during pregnancy.

MyPlate includes the following food groups:

» **Grains:** Although many types of grains are healthy to eat, MyPlate refers to fortified dry and cooked cereals. Choose ones that are fortified with folic acid when possible.

» **Vegetables:** Vegetables are divided into five groups, based on their nutrient content. Pregnant women should try to fill half of their plate with fruits or vegetables. The following list orders vegetables from highest nutrient content to lowest and includes examples within each category:

  ● **Dark green vegetables** (spinach, dark green leafy lettuce, romaine lettuce, broccoli, kale, turnip greens, watercress)

  ● **Orange and red vegetables** (carrots, pumpkin, sweet potatoes, certain types of squash, red peppers, and tomatoes)

  ● **Dry beans/peas** (pinto, black, garbanzo, kidney, navy, and white beans; split peas; lentils; soybeans and tofu)

  ● **Starchy vegetables** (potatoes, corn, green peas, green lima beans)

  ● **Other vegetables** (cabbage, cauliflower, iceberg lettuce, green beans, celery, green peppers, mushrooms, onions, asparagus, cucumbers, eggplant)

» **Fruits:** Not only are fruits a good source of vitamins and minerals, but they also provide fiber, which is important during pregnancy to help reduce constipation. You can choose fresh, frozen, canned, or dried fruits. Go easy on the fruit juices, though, because they can contain lots of sugar.

» **Dairy:** Foods that fall in this group include milk, yogurt, and cheese, and all are great sources of calcium. Focus on lowfat or fat-free milk products whenever possible. An average-sized woman needs to consume about 3 cups of milk or milk products per day.

>> **Protein:** Meat, poultry, fish, and nuts fall into this category. Focus on lowfat and lean foods and vary your choices. Baking, broiling, and grilling are the healthiest ways to cook meat, poultry, and fish. During pregnancy, you should eat 5 to 7 ounces of food from this category daily.

What about oils (fats that remain liquid at room temperature) and fats that are solid at room temperature? Healthy fats — unsaturated fats that come from vegetables oils, nuts, seeds, and fish — are good for you, although fewer than 10 percent of your fat intake should come from saturated fats (typically those that remain solid at room temperature). Avoid trans fats (a type of saturated fats that are common in processed foods and have been associated with obesity and heart disease) altogether.

Also, as your pregnancy progresses, your body needs a lot of extra fluid. Early on, some women who don't drink enough liquid feel weak or faint. Later in pregnancy, dehydration can lead to premature contractions. Make a point of drinking plenty of water (or milk) — about six to eight glasses a day, and a bit more if you're carrying more than one baby.

REMEMBER

Experiencing morning sickness during the first trimester is very common (see Book 2, Chapter 1). If you're experiencing this nausea and can't eat a well-balanced diet, you may wonder whether you're getting enough nutrition for you and the baby. You actually can go for several weeks not eating an optimal diet without any ill effects on the baby. You may find that the only foods you can tolerate are foods heavy in starch or carbohydrates. If all you feel like eating are potatoes, bread, and pasta, go right ahead. Keeping something down is better than starving.

IS CAFFEINE SAFE DURING PREGNANCY?

No evidence suggests that caffeine causes birth defects. However, if you consume caffeine in large amounts, it may raise the risk of miscarriage. Most studies suggest that it takes more than 200 milligrams (mg) of caffeine a day to affect the fetus. The average cup of coffee (an 8-ounce cup of regular coffee — not the super-mega size or an espresso or cappuccino!) has between 100 and 150 mg of caffeine. Caffeinated tea has slightly less caffeine — about 50 to 100 mg — and soft drinks have approximately 36 mg per 12-ounce serving. So drinking one 8-ounce cup of coffee (or the equivalent caffeine content in other foods or beverages) per day is usually okay during pregnancy.

Supplementing your diet

If your diet is healthy and balanced, you get most of the vitamins and minerals you need naturally — with the exception of iron, folic acid, and calcium. To make sure you get enough of these nutrients and to guard against inadequate eating habits, your practitioner is likely to recommend prenatal vitamins. In the case of vitamins, more isn't necessarily better; take only the prescribed number of pills each day.

Several different prenatal vitamins are available, and they're generally equivalent. Some are better tolerated than others, so if you find the one you're taking is not agreeable to you, try a different brand. Also, many now contain omega-3 fatty acid supplementation. Some data suggests that omega-3 supplements may decrease the risk of preterm delivery and may have a beneficial effect on the newborn brain, but this hasn't been proven.

REMEMBER

During the early months, if your vitamins make you nauseous, skipping them until you feel better is perfectly safe for the baby. If you're very early in your pregnancy (4 to 7 weeks), you can take just a folic acid supplement, which is sometimes easier to tolerate, until you can handle the complete prenatal vitamin pill. If later on in the pregnancy you get a stomach virus and can't tolerate vitamins for some time, that's not a problem, either. The growing baby is able to get what he needs, even at the expense of the mom (a theme that continues throughout life!).

Iron

You need more iron when you're expecting because both you and the baby are making new red blood cells every day. On average, you need 30 milligrams (mg) of extra iron every day of your pregnancy, which is what most prenatal vitamins contain. Blood counts can easily drop during pregnancy because your body gradually is making more and more blood *plasma* (fluid) and relatively fewer red blood cells (a condition that is called a *dilutional anemia*). If you do develop anemia, you may need to take an extra iron supplement.

TIP

Foods rich in iron include chicken, fish, red meat, green leafy vegetables, and enriched or whole-grain breads and cereals. You can raise the iron content of foods by cooking them in cast-iron pots and skillets.

Calcium and vitamin D

You need about 1,200 milligrams of calcium and 2,000 units of vitamin D every day while you're pregnant. Most women actually get much less. If you're already starting out somewhat deficient in calcium and vitamin D, the calcium requirements of the developing baby will only make matters worse for you. A fetus can extract enough calcium from his mother, even if that means getting it at the expense of the mother's bones. So the extra calcium and vitamin D needed during pregnancy are really aimed at protecting you and your health. The vitamin D helps you store the calcium.

REMEMBER

Prenatal vitamins contain only about 200 to 300 mg of calcium (about one-quarter of the U.S. Recommended Daily Allowance), so you need to get calcium from other sources — your diet or a calcium supplement — as well. Getting enough calcium from your diet alone is possible if you really pay attention. You can get it from three to four servings of calcium-rich foods, such as milk, yogurt, cheese, green leafy vegetables, and canned fish with bones (if your stomach can take it). Supermarkets also stock special lactose-free foods that are high in calcium.

Determining Which Foods Are Safe

Expectant moms often ask about nutrition, and they specifically want to know which foods they should avoid. This section identifies the potentially harmful foods and also debunks some common myths about other foods.

Eyeing potentially harmful foods

If you're healthy, you can probably confidently eat most of the foods you usually eat. Nonetheless, the following list contains some potential dangers that we feel we ought to mention:

>> **Cheeses from unpasteurized or raw milk:** These cheeses may contain certain bacteria, such as *Listeria monocytogenes, Salmonella,* and *E. coli. Listeria,* in particular, has been linked to certain pregnancy complications, such as premature labor or even miscarriage. The FDA mandates that all cheeses sold in the United States be either made from pasteurized milk or aged more than 60 days (which makes the likelihood of listeria extremely low), so most cheeses you buy at your local market are safe. Just check the label to be sure.

>> **Raw or very rare meat:** Steak tartare or very rare beef or pork may contain bacteria, such as *Listeria,* or parasites, such as *Toxoplasma.* Adequate cooking kills both bacteria and parasites, so you want your food to be cooked medium-well to well-done.

>> **Liver:** Liver contains extremely high amounts of vitamin A (more than ten times the amount recommended for a pregnant woman). Consuming more than 10,000 international units (IUs) of vitamin A daily (the recommended

daily allowance for pregnant women is 2,500 IU) was linked to birth defects in one study. Scientists haven't proven this danger unequivocally, but you may want to find a substitute for that liver-and-onions craving in the first trimester.

Debunking popular food myths

Many of the foods that have at one time or another been thought dangerous for pregnant women aren't likely to harm you or your baby. Although you don't have to avoid the following foods, they should be eaten in moderation, especially those that are manufactured (as opposed to natural) products:

>> **Cheeses:** Not only do most people believe that processed and pasteurized cheeses are safe, but these cheeses are also a great source of both protein and calcium. The one caveat? Unpasteurized cheese. Head to the preceding section for details.

>> **Fish:** Fish is a great source of protein and vitamins, and it's also low in fat. In fact, the high levels of protein, omega-3 fatty acids, vitamin D, and other nutrients make fish an excellent food for pregnant mothers and their developing babies.

However, certain fish — shark, mackerel, swordfish, and tilefish — contain high levels of mercury. The FDA currently recommends you avoid fish with high levels of mercury when you're pregnant. The USDA guidelines say you can still enjoy up to 12 ounces (two average meals) per week of fish and shellfish lower in mercury, like salmon, haddock, tilapia, cod, sole, and shrimp, or up to 6 ounces of albacore tuna per week. Avoid tuna steak, due to mercury levels, and raw seafood and oysters due to bacteria (*Vibrio vulnificus* and *Vibrio parahaemolyticus*) that can cause infections.

REMEMBER

Don't let your concern for mercury make you give up fish altogether, because two studies looking at fish consumption in pregnant women showed that women who eat fish may actually have lower rates of preterm delivery, and their children may have higher IQs.

>> **Sushi:** Raw fish (except raw shellfish) actually carries a very small risk of a parasitic infection (about one infection in 2 million servings — less than the risk of getting sick from eating chicken!). Pregnancy doesn't increase the danger, and your fetus is unlikely to suffer any harm from such an infection. Most important is to make sure that the fish comes from a reliable source and that it is stored properly.

>> **Smoked meats or fish:** Many pregnant women worry about eating smoked meats and fish because they've heard that these foods are high in nitrites or nitrates. Although these foods do contain these substances, they won't hurt your baby if eaten in moderation.

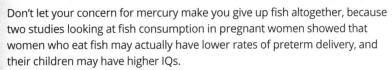

Diet, Exercise, and
Expectant Moms

>> **Sweeteners:** You should limit sweeteners (including sugar) in general, but they should be safe for your baby:

- **Aspartame (Equal or NutraSweet):** Aspartame (a common component of low-calorie foods and beverages) is a type of amino acid, and the body is accustomed to amino acids because they're what all proteins are made of. No medical evidence shows that aspartame causes any problems for the growing baby.

- **Sucralose (Splenda):** Sucralose is a low-calorie sweetener, with less than 2 calories per teaspoon. It's actually a type of sugar, but it's much more potent than regular table sugar, so you only need small amounts to sweeten things up. Because it's a type of sugar, it should have no harmful effects on your developing baby.

- **Stevia leaf extract sweeteners (Truvia or Stevia):** The most recent additions to nonsugar-based sweeteners are derived from the stevia leaf. Although the data is somewhat limited, they appear to be completely safe to use in pregnancy.

Considering Special Dietary Needs

You may find that you need to tailor the rules of healthy nutrition to fit your particular eating habits — for example, if you're a vegetarian. This section addresses some of the issues that arise for women with special nutritional needs.

Eating right, vegetarian-style

If you're a vegetarian, rest assured you can produce a healthy baby without eating steak. But you do have to plan your diet more carefully. Vegetables, whole grains, and legumes (peas and beans) are rich in protein, but most don't have complete proteins. (They don't contain all the essential amino acids that your body can't produce by itself.) To get all the necessary protein, you can combine various proteins — for example, whole grains with legumes or nuts, rice with kidney beans, or even peanut butter with whole-grain bread. The combination doesn't have to occur at the same meal, only on the same day, but a good rule of thumb is to try to get some protein with each meal.

REMEMBER

If you don't eat any animal products, including milk and cheese, your diet may not provide enough of six other important nutrients: vitamin B12, calcium, riboflavin, iron, zinc, and vitamin D. Bring up the topic with your doctor. You may also want to discuss your diet with a nutritionist. In addition, vegetarian and vegan vitamin supplements are available over the counter.

Staying healthy, vegan-style

Vegans, like vegetarians, do not consume meat, fish, or poultry, but they also eliminate all animal products from their diet. So, no milkshakes or eggs-over-easy for vegans! Because many vegans consume fewer calories and may start their pregnancy with a lower BMI, they need to pay extra attention to make sure they're getting enough calories and nutrition for themselves and their growing baby. Here are some helpful hints if you are a pregnant vegan:

» Vitamin B12 deficiency is not unusual for vegans, so make sure you're getting enough vitamin B12, and speak with your doctor about possible supplementation.

» Good sources of protein can be found in soy products, beans, whole grains, lentils, and tofu.

» Pay attention to calcium, because calcium and vitamin D are needed for you and your baby's bones. Good sources of calcium for vegans include calcium-fortified soy milk and juice, calcium-set tofu, soybeans and soy nuts, green leafy vegetables (such as Chinese cabbage, kale, and mustard greens), and okra. Dry cereals are a source of Vitamin D.

» Iron is super important during pregnancy, because your body needs to increase its blood supply for the pregnancy. You can find iron in dried beans, green leafy vegetables, and tofu.

» Folate is another important factor that has been shown to reduce the chance of the baby developing a condition called a *neural tube defect*. It's important to have enough folate onboard before the pregnancy starts and especially through the first trimester. Folate can be found in enriched breads, pasta, cereals, and orange juice.

» DHA (docosahexaenoic acid) is great for the developing fetal brain. Many people think of DHA as occurring only in fish, but a form of DHA can also be found in flaxseed, flaxseed oil, canola oil, walnuts, and soy nuts.

Working Out for Two

During pregnancy, exercise helps your body in many ways: It keeps your heart strong and your muscles in shape, and it relieves the basic discomforts of pregnancy — from morning sickness to constipation to achy legs and backs. The earlier in pregnancy a woman gets regular exercise, the more comfortable she is likely to feel throughout the 40 weeks. Regular exercise may even make for shorter labor.

So if you're in good health and not at risk for obstetrical or medical complications, by all means go ahead and continue with your exercise program — unless your program calls for climbing Mount Fuji, entering a professional boxing match, or some other super-strenuous activity. Go over your exercise program with your practitioner so he knows what you're doing and so you can ask any questions you have.

WARNING

As good as exercise is for most pregnant women, we don't advise it for everyone. If you have any of the following conditions (see Book 6 for details), you may be better off not working out — at least until you discuss the situation with your doctor:

>> Bleeding

>> Incompetent cervix

>> Intrauterine growth restriction

>> Low volume of amniotic fluid

>> Placenta previa (late in pregnancy)

>> Pregnancy-induced hypertension

>> Premature labor or preterm rupture of the membranes

>> Carrying triplets or more

Adapting to your body's changes

Even if you work out in moderation, remember that pregnancy causes your body to undergo real physical changes that can affect your strength, stamina, and performance. The following list details some of those changes:

>> **Cardiovascular changes:** When you're pregnant, the amount of blood that your heart pumps through your body increases. That increase in blood volume usually has no effect on your workout. (Some women feel as though they hear their heartbeat in their ears because of the increased volume.) Also, if you lie flat on your back, especially after about 16 weeks of pregnancy, you may find yourself feeling dizzy or faint — or even nauseous. Known as *supine hypotension syndrome,* this dizziness sometimes happens when the enlarging uterus presses down on major blood vessels that return blood to the heart, thus decreasing the heart's output. It happens even more readily if you're having a multiple pregnancy and your uterus is that much heavier.

TIP

If you're doing any exercises that require you to lie on your back (or if you're accustomed to sleeping on your back), put a small pillow or foam wedge under the right side of your back or your right hip. The pillow tilts you slightly sideways and effectively lifts your uterus off the blood vessels.

- » **Respiratory changes:** Your body is using more oxygen than usual to support the growing baby. At the same time, breathing is more work than it used to be because the enlarging uterus presses upward against the diaphragm. For some women, this difficulty makes performing aerobic exercise a little harder.

- » **Structural changes:** As your body shape changes — bigger abdomen, larger breasts — your center of gravity shifts, which can affect your balance. You notice it especially if you dance, bicycle, ski, surf, ride horses, or do anything else (walk tightropes, maybe?) where balance is important. In addition, pregnancy hormones cause some laxness in your joints, which also can make balance more difficult and may increase your risk of injury.

- » **Metabolic changes:** Pregnant women use carbohydrates faster than non-pregnant women do, which means that they're at a higher risk of developing *hypoglycemia* (low blood sugar). Exercise can be very useful in helping lower and control blood sugar levels, but it also increases the body's need for carbohydrates. So if you exercise, make sure you're eating an adequate amount of starch just before you work out.

- » **Effects on the uterus:** One study of women at *term* (far enough along to deliver) showed that their contractions increased after moderate aerobic exercise. Another study indicated that exercise is associated with a lower risk of early labor. But most studies have shown that exercise has no effect either way, and exercise does not pose a risk of preterm labor in healthy pregnant women.

- » **Effect on birth weight:** Some studies have shown that women who work out strenuously (at high intensity) during pregnancy have lighter-weight babies. The same effect appears to occur in women who perform heavy physical work in a standing position while they're pregnant. But this decrease in birth weight seems to be due mainly to a decrease in the newborn's subcutaneous fat. In other words, more strenuous exercise has no effect on the fetus's normal growth.

Exercising without overdoing it

Your changing body is going to demand a change in exercise routine. Don't beat yourself up if you find that pregnancy makes it harder to continue the workouts you're accustomed to. Modify your program according to what you can reasonably tolerate.

Listen to your body. If weight lifting suddenly hurts your back, lighten up. You may find it easier to perform non-weight-bearing exercises like swimming or stationary bicycling. No matter what your particular exercise regimen may be, keep in mind the basic rules for working out during pregnancy:

>> If you have a moderate exercise routine, keep it up. If you've been pretty sedentary, don't suddenly plunge into a strenuous program; ease in slowly to avoid putting too much strain on your body.

Keeping up a regular schedule of moderate activity is better than engaging in infrequent spurts of intense exercise, which are more likely to cause injury.

>> Avoid overheating, especially during the first six weeks of pregnancy. On very hot or humid days, don't exercise outdoors. Carry a bottle of water to every exercise session and stay well hydrated.

>> Avoid exercising flat on your back for long periods of time; doing so may reduce blood flow to your heart.

>> Avoid anything that puts you at risk of being hurt in the abdomen, like road/mountain biking. Steer clear of high-impact, bouncy exercises that can tax your loosening joints.

>> Throughout the nine months, low- or moderate-impact workouts make more sense than high-impact ones.

>> If you feel fatigued, dizzy, faint, or nauseous, by all means, stop.

>> Eat a well-balanced diet that includes an adequate supply of carbohydrates (see "Taking Stock of What You're Taking In," earlier in this chapter).

>> Talk to your practitioner about what your peak exercise heart rate should be. (Many practitioners suggest 140 beats per minute as the upper limit.) Then regularly measure your heart rate at the peak of your workout to make sure it's at a safe level.

>> Stop exercising and talk to your doctor if you experience any of these symptoms:

- Shortness of breath that is persistent or out of proportion to the exercise you're doing

- Vaginal bleeding

- Rapid heartbeat (that is, more than 140 beats per minute)

- Dizziness or feeling faint

- Any significant pain

Comparing forms of exercise

Now isn't the time to shoot for that Ms. Fitness title, but that certainly doesn't mean you can't exercise. Because your pregnant body demands you take new precautions, choose your style of exercise carefully.

Working your heart: Aerobic exercise

Weight-bearing exercises like running, walking, aerobics, and using a stair-climbing machine or an elliptical trainer are great, as long as you don't do too much. These exercises require you to support all your weight, which is ever-increasing. Because your joints are loosening and your center of gravity is shifting at the same time, you run a slightly higher risk of injuring yourself. Remember to do only what you know you can rather than setting off on a new exercise routine that is too demanding for your current state of fitness, not to mention your pregnancy.

Pilates is a popular mind-body conditioning program focused on strengthening the core postural muscles important in maintaining your balance and supporting your spine. For the most part, continuing Pilates classes while you're pregnant is safe, as long as you avoid lying flat on your back for long periods of time.

REMEMBER

If you choose to take aerobics or Pilates classes, look for those designed specifically for pregnant women. If no classes are available, talk to the instructor to find modifications for exercises that are inappropriate.

You may find it easier, particularly later in pregnancy, to perform non-weight-bearing exercises. Because your weight is supported, you have less chance of injuring yourself, and your joints aren't stressed. If you're new to exercise, a low-intensity workout in the pool or on a stationary bike is ideal.

WARNING

Downhill skiing, waterskiing, and horseback riding put you at risk of falling with significant impact, which could injure you or your baby. Although these activities may be fine early in pregnancy, talk to your doctor before doing them in your second or third trimester. Cross-country skiing is less risky, especially if you're experienced.

Strengthening your muscles

You won't get a great cardiac benefit from weight lifting, yoga, or body sculpting, but you can improve your muscle tone and flexibility, which comes in handy during labor and delivery.

Weight-lifting machines may be preferable to using free weights because you know you won't drop the weights onto your abdomen. Also avoid using very heavy weights, which can cause injury to your joints and ligaments. If you use free weights, do so with caution — and preferably with the help of a trainer or a skilled friend. A trainer can also show you the proper way to exhale and inhale during lifting.

REMEMBER

Breathing well while you lift weights is important because it lessens the chance that you might bear down (otherwise known as the *valsava maneuver*, a method of increasing abdominal pressure), which can reduce blood flow, raise your blood pressure, and stress your heart.

Yoga, which is a great choice for pregnant women, not only is an excellent form of exercise but may also be helpful in mastering breathing and relaxation techniques. Yoga is particularly useful in strengthening lower back and abdominal muscles and increasing stamina and physical endurance — all of which make you better equipped to handle the rigors of pregnancy.

WARNING

Bikram yoga involves performing yoga in a room heated to 105 degrees Fahrenheit with a relative humidity of 60 to 70 percent. Although some doctors feel that this type of yoga is safe for pregnant women during the first trimester, prolonged exposure to high temperatures during the first trimester is inadvisable, given the possible risks of causing a neural tube defect. (See Book 2, Chapter 2 for more on neural tube defects, such as spina bifida.)

PRACTICING SAFE YOGA

Yoga can be a wonderful and relaxing way to work out while you're pregnant but only if you exercise caution. Follow these tips when doing yoga during pregnancy:

- If you're new to yoga, take a beginner class to ease yourself into a new exercise regime.

- Be careful about positions that stretch your muscles too much. Due to elevated levels of progesterone and relaxin (hormones produced during pregnancy), you can easily overstretch your muscles and ligaments.

- When bending forward, try to bend from the hips, not from the back. Also, try to lift your chest high to avoid putting extra pressure on your abdomen.

- After the middle of the second trimester, try to avoid performing poses that require you to lie flat on your back for extensive periods of time, because pressure from a pregnant uterus may decrease blood flow both to your heart and to the baby.

- As a general rule for any exercise, if you feel any pain or discomfort, stop and rest.

Chapter 4

Oh, the Changes You'll See: Physical, Emotional, and Embarrassing Unmentionables

Even though you're pregnant and your body is already undergoing miraculous changes, your day-to-day life goes on. How will you need to change your lifestyle to make your pregnancy go as smoothly as possible? What things in your life don't need to change or need to be modified only slightly? You have a lot to consider: your job, the general level of stress in your life, and what to do about routine things like going to the dentist or hairdresser (among other things!). If you're like most normally healthy women, you'll probably find that for the most part, your life can go on largely as usual.

REMEMBER

In this chapter, you find a general outline for how to plan your life during pregnancy, but all the issues covered are subjects for discussion with your practitioner. If you consider from the beginning how your daily habits and health practices interact with your pregnancy, you're likely to have an easier time getting used to your new state of being.

Bracing for Emotional Changes

When you're pregnant, you know you're probably going to experience mood swings. Watch enough TV comedies featuring pregnant characters, and you'd begin to believe that every pregnant woman must become a raving lunatic at some point in her pregnancy. This section lets you know what you may be in for, without the laugh track. And because one of the most common worries pregnant women have is whether stress is harmful to either the pregnancy or their growing child, this section covers that, too.

Coping with mood swings

You've probably had mood swings before — just not with such intensity. Hormonal shifts affect mood, as most women — especially those who suffer from premenstrual syndrome (PMS) — already know. The hormonal fluctuations that support pregnancy are perhaps the most dramatic a woman experiences in her lifetime, so it's hardly surprising that emotional ups and downs are commonplace. And the fatigue that goes along with pregnancy can easily make these ups and downs more severe. Add to this biochemical mix the normal anxieties that the average expectant mother has about whether the baby will be healthy and whether she'll be a good mother, and you have plenty of fuel to produce good old-fashioned mood swings.

Your moodiness may be especially pronounced during the first trimester because your body is adjusting to its new condition. You may find yourself overreacting to little things: A mushy television commercial may leave you in tears; a careless grocery store clerk who smashes your bread may send you into a teeth-clenching rage. Don't worry — you're just pregnant. Take a few deep breaths, go out for a walk, or just close your eyes and take a short break. These feelings often pass as quickly as they arise.

REMEMBER

If you feel that your mood swings are interfering with your daily life or if you have thoughts of harming yourself or someone else, let your healthcare provider know as soon as possible, or call 911 if you feel that it's an emergency.

HELPING YOUR PARTNER COPE WITH EARLY SYMPTOMS

Early pregnancy brings extreme fatigue, the overwhelming desire to take a nap, food cravings, food aversions, nausea, vomiting, and a constant need to urinate — not to mention hormonal changes that cause pendulum-like mood swings, from crying to euphoria almost before you can ask what's wrong.

Knowing the symptoms ahead of time helps you keep your cool when all around you seems to be falling to pieces. Following are some things you can do to help your partner through these first topsy-turvy months of pregnancy:

- **Accept her limitations.** Maybe you went out to eat several times a week and now the sight of restaurants makes her sick. Hang in there. By the second trimester, she'll be eating everything in sight, and the Szechuan restaurant will still be there.

- **Don't take emotional outbursts seriously.** Not letting her outbursts get to you is hard when they're pointed at you and all your shortcomings, but listen to what she says, accept what may actually be true, and disregard the rest. Don't forget to fix any shortcomings you can, though.

- **Help her.** Shoulder some of her chores, especially the ones that make her nauseated, such as cooking, garbage patrol, dishing out the dog food, and cleaning toilets. Remember that handling cat litter is strictly verboten for pregnant women, so that's your job, too.

- **Let her rest.** Although sitting at home all weekend watching her take two naps a day may not seem like a whole lot of fun, use this time to get projects done around the house or catch up on your parenthood reading.

- **Plan pit stops.** If you're the type of driver who doesn't stop the car unless the road abruptly ends before you reach your destination, realize that pregnant women really do have to pee every five minutes; she's not making up an excuse to go into the gas station shop for a frozen custard. Also, because blood volume increases during pregnancy, blood clots can develop if she doesn't move her legs regularly. Let the woman get out of the car every few hours!

- **Satisfy her cravings.** Not that many pregnant women really want pickles and ice cream, but if your partner does, get some for her. Try not to gag as you watch her eat them; you may have to leave the room yourself.

Experiencing stress

Many women wonder whether stress has any effect on pregnancy. That question is difficult to answer because stress is such an elusive concept. Everyone knows what stress is, but each woman seems to handle it in her own way, and no one can really measure its intensity. Chronic stress — unrelieved day after day — can increase the levels of stress hormones circulating in the bloodstream, and many doctors think that such elevated levels of stress hormones can promote preterm labor or blood pressure problems during pregnancy, but few studies have been able to prove this idea.

Prepping for Physical Changes

When you're pregnant, your body is undergoing a transformation. Pregnancy is a time of joy and excitement, but it can also be a time of some unpleasant and quite possibly embarrassing side effects. You may wonder at times what exactly has taken over inside your body. For example, you can go from feeling so nauseous you can't even stand the smell of food one minute to feeling a burst of energy and a ferocious appetite the next. You may also pass gas, get stopped up, and be so tired you feel like a truck ran over you. But don't worry; this, too, shall pass.

Morning, noon, or nighttime sickness

If you're feeling a bit nauseous, you're not alone! The majority of pregnant women experience nausea and vomiting at some point in their pregnancy, typically beginning in the first month of pregnancy and ending around 14 to 16 weeks (though some women do experience it longer). Nausea and vomiting may be due to low blood sugar and hormone fluctuations that occur in early pregnancy.

Even though pregnancy-induced nausea is called *morning sickness*, it can happen at any time of the day. A completely empty stomach contributes to feelings of nausea, so many women do feel it more in the morning. But nausea can strike at any time, even after you're all ready for bed. To make matters worse, just the sight or smell of food can send a woman running to the bathroom to lose her lunch (or breakfast . . . or dinner). The good news is that nausea and occasional vomiting is not harmful to you or your baby.

REMEMBER

No one likes to feel sick to her stomach. When you're pregnant, you're even more concerned because you're now growing another life inside you. If you're throwing up daily or several times a day, how is that affecting your ability to provide nutrients to your baby? Believe it or not, your baby doesn't suffer from your occasional or even daily vomiting. Your body has reserves of nutrients and energy that the baby can use to grow and develop if food is unavailable in the short term. If you experience vomiting on a regular basis, try to stay hydrated and well-nourished when you're feeling good. Doing so can help build up your fluid and nutrient stores.

WARNING

The main risk of vomiting is dehydration. Mild dehydration can lead to fatigue and headaches, and severe dehydration can cause an imbalance in electrolytes, including sodium and potassium, which can be serious. To prevent either scenario from happening, sip on sports drinks to replenish sodium, potassium, and fluids. If sports drinks don't appeal to you, simply drink water and eat salted crackers or pretzels and fresh, frozen, or dried fruit. And if your nausea is strong enough to interfere with your daily life, talk to your doctor about certain nausea-reducing medications that are safe to use during pregnancy.

Dealing with nausea

TIP

Feeling sick to your stomach is one of the worst feelings. Sometimes you wish you could throw up just to feel better, even if the relief is only temporary. If you're experiencing even mild nausea, try these tips (which are in order of effectiveness) to feel better fast:

» **Go bland early.** Eat something bland (like plain toast or soda crackers) within 15 minutes of getting up in the morning. You may even want to have them on your bedside table to munch on before you get out of bed.

» **Avoid having a completely empty stomach at any time of the day.** When your stomach is empty, the acids in your stomach signal nauseous feelings to your brain. Keep snacks handy so you don't find yourself hungry without something to munch on.

» **Eat small portions.** Just as you don't want an empty stomach, you don't want to get too full either. Limit portions at meals to only small amounts of food and follow those small meals with frequent snacks so you don't get hungry.

» **Eat foods that are low in fat and sugar.** Avoid greasy, creamy, or high-sugar items. Fat takes a long time to digest, and sugar can cause a spike and subsequent drop in energy levels.

» **Stay hydrated.** Nausea can be a side effect of dehydration during pregnancy. To avoid becoming dehydrated, suck on ice chips or sip cold water to count toward your recommended 102 ounces of fluid per day. Why cold water? Not only is it refreshing, but it can also help decrease nauseous feelings and keep you hydrated after you vomit. (For additional tips on staying hydrated, flip to Book 3, Chapter 2.)

- » **Keep cool.** Getting too warm or overheated can make nausea even worse! Keep cool in comfortable, loose-fitting clothing that doesn't press on your stomach (stomach pressure can increase feelings of nausea).

- » **Relax and rest up.** Get plenty of rest at night and nap throughout the day as needed and when possible. Sometimes sleep is the best escape from feeling nauseous because your body is worn down and needs the recovery.

- » **Take your vitamins at night.** Prenatal vitamins have iron, which can aggravate nausea, but if you take yours at night, you may not experience any. Remember to have a small snack with the vitamin so you aren't taking it on an empty stomach.

- » **Suck on lemon drops or sour candy.** Sour foods can stimulate digestion, starting with saliva in the mouth and moving into the stomach.

The preceding tips are some of the standard ways of relieving nausea, but some women swear by less mainstream tactics, such as the following:

- » **Using ginger:** People have used ginger to combat nausea for centuries. Scientists aren't certain how it works, but it has something to do with the unique compounds found in ginger and their effect on the stomach. Look for lowfat gingersnap cookies, ginger tea, or ginger gum.

- » **Smelling lemon scents or eating lemon-flavored foods:** Lemon is a refreshing scent, and many women report feeling less nauseous when eating, drinking, or even smelling lemon. Some companies have special lollipops, lemon drops, and gum just for pregnant women. But plain old lemon drops can do the trick without the premium price tag.

- » **Undergoing hypnosis or acupressure:** These techniques can be beneficial for severe nausea in some women. Hypnosis works by training the unconscious mind to suppress the involuntary feelings of nausea. Acupressure has been used in traditional Chinese medicine to relieve nausea, and acupressure bands for the P6 pressure point on the wrist work for many pregnant women.

TIP

Food smells are often the worst offenders for setting off nausea. Ask someone to help you with food preparation if just smelling food prevents you from eating. Use fans and open windows in the house to get strong smells out as soon as possible. Also, stick with cold foods because they don't have as much aroma as warm foods.

Determining when medical intervention is necessary

For a few women, vomiting becomes so excessive that it can harm them or their babies. This condition is called *hyperemesis gravidarum.* Typically, hyperemesis gravidarum is characterized by severe nausea, vomiting, weight loss of more than 5 percent, and evidence of dehydration. See Table 4-1 to recognize the difference between morning sickness and serious illness.

TABLE 4-1 **Distinguishing between Morning Sickness and Serious Illness**

Morning Sickness	Serious Illness
Your nausea goes away after 14–16 weeks.	Your nausea doesn't go away.
Your nausea leads to occasional vomiting.	Your nausea leads to severe vomiting (several times per day).
Your vomiting doesn't cause dehydration.	Your vomiting causes severe dehydration.
Your vomiting still allows you to keep some food down.	Your vomiting doesn't allow you to keep food down.
Your nausea and vomiting are annoying.	Your nausea and vomiting disrupt your life.
You don't experience any significant weight loss.	You experience weight loss of more than 5% of your body weight.
Nausea and some vomiting are your only symptoms.	Dizziness, weakness, and fatigue accompany your vomiting.

Treatment for severe nausea and vomiting can be as simple as taking antinausea medications prescribed by your doctor, getting enough fluids, and resting. If your symptoms become severe enough, you may have to be treated with intravenous fluids and electrolytes. Some serious cases require hospital stays and bed rest. When in doubt, call your doctor for advice on how to deal with your nausea and vomiting.

WARNING

Even though some vomiting is normal during the first 14 weeks or so of pregnancy, other symptoms that sometimes accompany vomiting are not. Call your doctor or visit your local emergency room for immediate assistance if you

>> Have a fever, diarrhea, and/or severe abdominal pain

>> Experience prolonged vomiting and are also weak, dizzy, or faint

>> Can't keep liquids down for more than 24 hours

Dealing with your newly unruly digestive tract

As you may have already discovered for yourself, pregnant women are known to have problems with their digestive tracts. You can pretty much blame all your digestive tract woes on hormones — specifically progesterone and estrogen.

>> *Progesterone* is one of the most important pregnancy hormones. Some of the side effects of increased levels of progesterone include water retention, sluggish digestion, and nausea. The result of these side effects is feeling bloated, gassy, and constipated.

>> *Estrogen* is to blame for your expanding uterus, which, as the pregnancy goes on, also causes pressure on the digestive tract. This pressure can lead to heartburn and constipation.

Avoiding heartburn with the help of some nutrition tricks

Heartburn, or *gastroesophageal reflux disease* (GERD), is quite common during pregnancy and can happen at any time throughout your 40 weeks, although it often gets worse in the second and third trimesters.

Heartburn has two causes, and both are related to the sphincter muscle that connects the esophagus to your stomach. The progesterone your body produces relaxes that sphincter muscle, and your growing uterus presses on it. The result is that gastric acids, liquids, and food from the stomach travel back up your esophagus, leaving you uncomfortable. Heartburn typically worsens as your belly grows and puts more pressure on your stomach, causing the sphincter muscle to allow acid back into the esophagus (see Figure 4-1).

TIP

You can lessen the symptoms of heartburn by trying the following tips:

>> **Stop eating two to three hours before lying down for bedtime or a nap.** The less you have in your stomach, the less likely you are to experience acid reflux.

>> **Sleep propped up to avoid lying flat.** By elevating your upper body, gravity helps keep your stomach acids down. (If you're past your first trimester, you shouldn't lie flat, anyway, to avoid cutting off circulation to your baby and your legs. Lie on your left side for optimal circulation.)

>> **Practice good posture when sitting.** When you slouch, you put more pressure on your esophagus, which can lead to heartburn.

» **Avoid big meals.** Eat small portions so that you don't overfill the stomach and cause extra food to come back up the esophagus.

» **Sip liquids with meals instead of drinking large amounts.** Because you want to avoid having large amounts in your stomach at one time, drink small amounts at meals and stay hydrated by spreading your liquids out between meals.

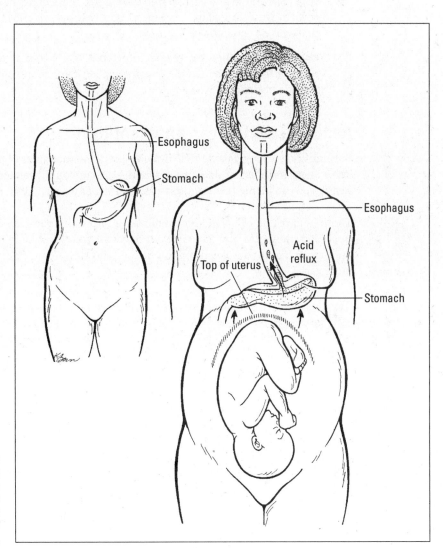

FIGURE 4-1:
Your baby's position in the uterus can lead to increased feelings of heartburn.

Illustration by Kathryn Born, MA

>> **Avoid greasy or fatty foods.** High-fat foods, specifically fried foods, tend to trigger heartburn because they don't stimulate digestion but do take longer to digest (because they just sit in your stomach).

>> **Skip spicy and acidic foods.** Acidic foods, like tomatoes, citrus, and peppers, can be problematic for many women. Onions and garlic are also on some women's problem-foods list.

>> **Avoid caffeinated and carbonated beverages.** These drinks have been known to cause acid reflux. Sorry to say, but chocolate can also irritate the esophagus, so you may want to avoid it, too.

>> **Take an antacid when you're uncomfortable.** Talk to your doctor about which one to choose or about a safe prescription medication if over-the-counter antacids don't work for you.

Reducing gas with an antibloating diet

Burping and passing gas are two of the worst unmentionables of pregnancy. Who knew such an innocent-looking pregnant woman could produce so much gas? Again, you can blame this unpleasant side effect of pregnancy on the hormones.

REMEMBER

Those fun pregnancy hormones combined with certain foods can cause your body to produce more gas, so you may want to adjust your lifestyle to avoid producing even more. Limit your consumption of the following if you find that they cause more gas:

>> Cruciferous vegetables, such as broccoli, cauliflower, cabbage, Brussels sprouts, and bok choy

>> Legumes and beans, such as pinto, kidney, black, cannellini, and garbanzo beans; black-eyed peas; and lentils

>> Onions and garlic

>> Soy and soy-containing foods

>> Sugar-free items that contain sugar alcohols (avoid foods that have maltitol, xylitol, sorbitol, mannitol, and isomalt on the label)

>> Inulin (a type of fiber added to many processed food products)

>> Whole grains, nuts, and seeds

As you can see, most of these common gas-producing foods are good for you, so you still need to be able to enjoy them. To do so while reducing gas production, eat small portions of these (and really all) foods and spread out portions throughout the day. Also, eat slowly so you don't swallow large amounts of air, and chew with your mouth closed.

TIP

One favorite gas-reducing trick is to take Beano, an over-the-counter supplement that contains an enzyme that helps you digest certain parts of carbohydrate-containing foods that cause gas. The trick is to take Beano at the start of the meal, not after you finish. To prevent gas from forming, the enzyme needs to be present in the stomach while you're eating gas-inducing food. Beano is considered to be safe for pregnant women because it's isolated to the digestive tract.

Preventing pregnancy constipation

The digestive tract becomes sluggish during pregnancy, causing the body to eliminate waste at a slower rate, which, in turn, can lead to constipation. If you're anxious about your pregnancy, you don't exercise at all, or you don't eat healthy, high-fiber foods, pregnancy constipation can become a lot worse. Iron supplements or the iron found in prenatal vitamins may also be to blame for some of your constipation.

TIP

About half of women experience constipation during pregnancy, but you can definitely do something about it! Follow these tips to keep things moving in your body:

>> **Drink, drink, and drink more water.** Stool needs water to keep it moving through the digestive tract.

>> **Eat lots of fiber.** Choose whole grains, beans, and plenty of fruits and vegetables.

>> **Move your body to move your bowels.** Exercise, even a low-key activity like yoga, has been shown to stimulate your digestive tract. Stay active throughout all phases of pregnancy. (Flip to Book 4 for some exercises that are safe to do while you're pregnant.)

>> **Spread out your iron supplement throughout the day.** Your prenatal pill has a high iron level, so cut it in half and take half in the morning and half in the evening. Your doctor may also be able to recommend an iron supplement that's easier on the stomach.

>> **Consider taking over-the-counter fiber supplements or a stool softener.** Turn to over-the-counter items only as a last resort, and talk to your doctor about which one is best for you before making a purchase.

>> **Get "good" bacteria from probiotics.** Your digestive tract is full of bacteria, and some of the bacteria (commonly called *probiotics*) help support immune

and digestive health. You can get probiotics by eating yogurt, drinking *kefir* (a type of fermented milk), or taking a probiotic supplement. Unlike stool softeners that you may take only as needed, probiotics are good to have on a daily basis.

WARNING

Don't take a laxative to relieve constipation, because doing so can cause uterine contractions and may also leave you dehydrated. Also, avoid taking mineral oils (which are natural laxatives), because they may inhibit absorption of some important nutrients during pregnancy.

Dealing with hemorrhoids

REMEMBER

Hemorrhoids are essentially dilated, swollen veins in the rectum. The best way to prevent hemorrhoids is to avoid becoming constipated. Read through the recommendations in the preceding section to discover how to avoid constipation. If you find yourself with hard stools that don't pass easily, don't strain yourself trying to get them out. Simply drink lots of fluid and boost the fiber in your diet to 28 grams per day. Go for a walk to get things moving naturally, and avoid sitting for a long time, which puts additional pressure on the rectal area.

Nutritionally speaking, you can also prevent or deal with hemorrhoids by following the dietary guidelines for reducing swollen veins. Basically, these guidelines include the following:

>> Limit the sodium in your diet to less than 2,300 milligrams per day.

>> Avoid processed foods and high-salt condiments, like pickles, salad dressing, and soy sauce.

>> Avoid adding salt to your food.

Hemorrhoids can bleed and be quite painful. If you have hemorrhoids already, take a warm bath with baking soda in the water to help soothe pain, reduce itching, and assist in healing. Witch hazel also helps reduce the swelling.

WARNING

Visit your doctor if hemorrhoids become a concern. If you're losing a lot of blood or if it's too painful to have a bowel movement, you may need medical help.

Steering clear of urinary tract infections

Pregnancy puts you at an increased risk for another pesky problem: urinary tract infections (UTIs). In case you don't remember anatomy and physiology from school, your *urinary tract* includes your kidneys, bladder, and the tubes that connect them.

During pregnancy, your kidneys work overtime to get rid of all your waste products and produce more urine. However, your bladder may not fully empty because your uterus is constantly pressing on it, leaving room for bacteria to multiply and grow until you have a full-blown UTI.

TIP

To reduce your chances of developing a UTI, follow these tips:

» Drink plenty of water to flush out the kidneys.

» Drink cranberry juice, especially if you're prone to kidney infections.

» Eat fruits, vegetables, and whole grains to get plenty of antioxidants to boost your immune system.

» Eat yogurt, drink kefir, and look for other products with added probiotics (or take a probiotic supplement) to increase good bacteria in the urinary tract.

» Avoid caffeinated beverages, which act as a diuretic.

» Wear cotton underwear and avoid tight-fitting pants.

» Wipe front to back when using the bathroom to prevent bacteria from entering the urethra.

» Urinate when you first feel the need to do so instead of trying to hold it.

» Urinate before and after having intercourse.

WARNING

UTIs are easy to treat with antibiotics that are safe during pregnancy, so don't despair if you have any of the symptoms in the following list. Instead, call your doctor:

» Blood or mucus in the urine

» Pain or burning when urinating

» Feelings of urgency to urinate

» Fever or chills

» Urine that looks cloudy or has an unusual odor

» Pain or tenderness in the bladder

WARNING

An untreated UTI is more likely to develop into a kidney infection in pregnant women. So if you have back pain, nausea, vomiting, fever, and chills, don't wait to report these symptoms, all of which can signal a kidney infection.

Fighting fatigue

If you're feeling unusually tired, you're not alone. Most women don't just feel a little bit tired when pregnant; they feel exhausted. It makes sense that in the third trimester, you'd be tired from the extra weight you're carrying, but what could possibly make you feel so tired in the first trimester? Hormones! Between the surge of hormones and the increase in your blood supply, your body is going through a lot of changes. Your breasts and uterus are growing, and your baby is already getting a lot of your energy. The resulting fatigue is also your body's way of telling you to slow down and get plenty of rest.

The good news is that the second trimester is well-known for bursts of energy. Many women find themselves cleaning and organizing in preparation of the baby's arrival, even though their bodies are still working overtime. The third trimester brings some fatigue again, but this time it's mostly because of your larger size. (Chapters 1, 2, and 3 in Book 2 take you on a full-blown road trip through the trimesters.)

TIP

Don't listen to those well-intentioned people who say, "If you think you're tired now, just wait until the baby comes!" Your fatigue right now comes from the physical drain on your body, and you need to take it seriously so that you take care of yourself properly. Follow these tips to beat fatigue:

>> **Take a nap when you need it.** Even resting for 20 minutes without sleeping can make a world of difference.

>> **Ask for help.** Don't be a superwoman and try to do everything yourself. Ask your partner, friends, and family for assistance. Don't be afraid to delegate!

>> **Move your body regularly.** Exercise regularly (unless your doctor has told you not to). Women who exercise tend to have more energy and sleep better at night. See Book 4, Chapters 2 and 3 for recommendations on safe ways to get moving.

>> **Take your prenatal vitamin to ensure that you're getting enough iron.** Fatigue is a major symptom of iron deficiency because iron plays a role in transporting oxygen to the cells.

The most powerful ways to combat fatigue involve eating (specifically, paying attention to how and what you eat) and sleeping (as in getting the amount of sleep your body really needs). The following sections delve into the details of these two fatigue-fighting activities.

Eating for energy

What you eat and, even more important, when you eat it can make a big difference in your energy levels throughout the day. Changing just a few simple things in how you eat can help boost your energy levels.

REMEMBER

>> **Eating small amounts:** Eating small amounts rather than large meals has so many benefits in pregnancy. You can reduce your risk of getting heartburn, prevent excess weight gain, improve sleep, and decrease feelings of nausea, just to name a few. But the biggest benefit may be in the fact that you simply feel more energetic to face your day.

Eating large quantities can make you feel sleepy and lethargic, preventing you from having enough energy for you and your developing baby.

>> **Eating frequently throughout the day:** When you eat smaller meals, you naturally have to eat more often, which really just means you get to enjoy some yummy snacks. Snacks act like a bridge between meals, preventing you from getting too hungry and making poor food choices. When the snacks you choose are also nutritious, you provide you and your baby with more nutrients to properly fuel your activities and your baby's growth.

>> **Eating foods that provide lasting energy:** Certain foods give your body sustained energy throughout the day, but some foods can cause a crash in energy. Avoid foods that are high in simple sugars and refined carbohydrates, like cookies and other sweets, many crackers, and regular soft drinks. Instead, choose foods that contain whole grains. Whole grains have more complex carbohydrates that take your body longer to digest than simple sugars, resulting in more lasting energy.

TIP

For lasting energy in a meal or snack, combine foods rich in complex carbohydrates with protein-rich foods. Aim to include protein, such as a piece of meat, poultry, fish, dairy, eggs, or a vegetarian alternative, at every meal. Protein keeps you feeling full for a longer period of time and prevents blood sugar from rising too quickly, which would lead to the inevitable crash of energy when it drops back down. Look for snacks that have either protein or fiber in them to prevent this type of energy crash at snack time.

Getting the sleep you need

Adults need between seven and nine hours of sleep per night, but you may find that your body needs more sleep while you're pregnant. Plus, poor sleep can affect your labor when you're ready to deliver. Some studies suggest that women who get six hours of sleep or less have longer labors and increased risk of C-section deliveries.

AVOIDING BALLOON-LIKE FEET AND HANDS

Swelling happens because of the increase in fluid in your body. It can also lead to varicose veins and spider veins as your uterus puts pressure on the veins that send blood back up to your heart from your legs, feet, face, and hands. If you're prone to swelling, follow these tips:

- Prop up your feet whenever you can.

- Limit your salt/sodium intake.

- Drink plenty of water and avoid alcohol.

- Avoid standing or sitting for too long. Take breaks if you have a job that requires you to sit or stand a lot.

- Sleep on your side and elevate your legs with pillows.

- Swim laps or join a water aerobics class to take the pressure off your legs. Or just enjoy being weightless while floating in the water.

- Wear medical-grade compression stockings. Get advice from your doctor on the right ones for you.

Remember: Call your doctor if swelling is severe or comes on suddenly. Dramatic or sudden swelling could be a sign of one of the more serious medical conditions.

Many pregnant women face a variety of problems, like frequent urination, heartburn, and restless leg syndrome (RLS), that cause significant disruption to their sleep and therefore increase feelings of fatigue. (RLS causes discomfort in the legs when you're lying down. You relieve the discomfort by moving your legs. To help minimize RLS, exercise regularly and be sure to stretch after exercise. Also, get checked for iron deficiency because it can sometimes contribute to RLS.)

Follow these tips to get a more restful night's sleep:

» **Drink liquids during the day and limit your intake three to four hours before bedtime.** Limiting liquids later in the day may help cut down on the number of trips to the bathroom you need to make in the middle of the night.

» **Develop a good bedtime routine.** Take a warm bath, relax with a book, and dim the lights. Get the TV, computer, and phone out of your bedroom. Use the bedroom for sleep and sex only.

- » **Go to bed at approximately the same time each night.** If possible, don't set an alarm; allow your body to naturally wake up when you feel you've gotten the sleep you need.

- » **Sleep on your left side, especially after the first trimester.** Use a body pillow or just a small pillow in between your knees or under your belly to get more comfortable.

- » **Sleep with your head elevated to keep stomach acids down, and avoid eating two to three hours prior to bedtime.** Doing so helps minimize the possibility of heartburn.

WARNING

Pregnant women, particularly those who are overweight at conception, may develop *sleep apnea*, a disorder in which breathing is repeatedly disrupted during sleep. Untreated sleep apnea is a serious medical condition and increases risk of gestational diabetes, preeclampsia, and having a low-birthweight baby. If your partner notices that you snore much louder or seem to have long pauses between breaths while asleep, alert your doctor.

Living through leg cramps

Leg cramps are a common annoyance of pregnancy, and they're likely to become more frequent as the months go along. They're due to a sudden tightening of the muscles. The muscles may tighten for many reasons, including lack of fluids, muscle strain, or staying in one position for too long. Doctors once thought that leg cramps were due to too little calcium or potassium in the diet, although that hasn't been shown to be true. Some studies suggest that taking an oral magnesium supplement may reduce leg cramps.

To diminish leg cramps, try these suggestions:

- » Apply heat to your calves.

- » Drink plenty of fluids.

- » Avoid staying in one position too long.

- » Stretch and extend your legs and feet.

- » Take a short walk.

- » Ask your partner to give you a foot or leg massage.

Physical, Emotional, and Embarrassing Unmentionables

TIP

Do your stretching nightly before bed. Point your toes up toward the ceiling to really stretch your calves out. Do this about ten times. In the morning, get in the habit of doing this stretching at least a couple of times, before you even open your eyes, if possible. To avoid triggering a spasm, try to avoid extending your feet when you first wake up.

Noticing vaginal discharge

During pregnancy, your vaginal discharge normally increases substantially. Some women find that they need to wear pantyliners every day. The discharge, which tends to be thin, white, and virtually odorless, is technically known as *leucorrhea*. Vaginal douches aren't a good idea because they may alter your natural ability to fight off vaginal infections.

Pregnancy doesn't prevent you from getting a vaginal infection, and the high levels of estrogen in your blood may predispose you to developing a yeast infection. A yeast infection usually produces a thick, white-yellow discharge, and it may cause itchiness or redness. Topical vaginal creams should solve the problem, and they pose no risk to the fetus. Most over-the-counter preparations come in 1-, 3-, and 7-day dosages and are completely safe for the baby. For hard-to-beat yeast infections, talk with your doctor about oral fluconazole, which may be used safely in pregnancy.

WARNING

If your vaginal discharge takes on a brown, yellow, or green color, or if it develops a noxious odor or causes itching, let your practitioner know. (Be sure to use your judgment about how much of an emergency this is — it isn't the sort of problem that requires a 3:00 a.m. phone call to her office.)

Putting up with backaches

Backaches, a common symptom during pregnancy, typically occur in the latter part of pregnancy, although they can occur earlier. The shift in your center of gravity can be one cause. Another can be the change in the curvature of your spine as the baby grows and the uterus enlarges. You may get some relief by getting off your feet when you can, applying mild local heat, and taking acetaminophen (Tylenol).

Some women experience pain extending from their lower back to their buttocks and down one leg or the other. This pain or, less commonly, numbness is known as *sciatica*, which is due to pressure on the sciatic nerve, a major nerve that branches from your back, through your pelvis, to your hips, and down your legs. You can relieve mild cases of sciatica with bed rest, warm baths, or heating pads. If you develop a severe case, you may need prolonged bed rest or special exercises.

WARNING

Occasionally, preterm labor can present itself as low back pain. However, when it's preterm labor, the pain is more cramp-like, and it comes and goes instead of being continuous.

Looking at Lifestyle Changes

Your lifestyle inevitably changes during your pregnancy. You may wonder whether it's still okay to do some of the things you may have done on a regular basis before you were pregnant. This section provides information on activities such as whether you can safely color your hair while you're pregnant, whether you can use saunas and hot tubs, and whether you can travel.

Pampering yourself with beauty treatments

When your friends and relatives hear that you're pregnant, they'll probably tell you how beautiful you look or what a lovely maternal glow you have. And you may feel more beautiful, too, although some women feel the exact opposite. You may find that you're not happy with the physical changes that are happening to your body. Either way, you may wonder whether your customary beauty habits are safe to follow during pregnancy. This list goes over them one by one and shares possible risks:

» **Massages:** Massages are fine, and you'll find that many massage therapists offer special pregnancy massages aimed at accommodating your pregnant belly. Some use special tables with the center cut out so that you can comfortably lie face-down, especially in the latter part of the pregnancy.

» **Manicures and pedicures:** A frequently asked question is "Can I have a manicure/pedicure or have nail tips or acrylic nails placed while I'm pregnant?" The answer is yes. Common sense suggests that you go to a reputable salon where the equipment is properly cleaned and the area is well-ventilated.

» **Hair dyes:** Many different types of chemicals are used in hair dyes, and manufacturers typically change their formulas frequently. Limited data is available on the safety of hair dye, because these chemicals are not usually studied during pregnancy. However, remember that only a fraction of any hair treatment chemicals get absorbed into a woman's body through her skin, and this small amount is probably not enough to cause a problem for the developing baby. In addition, there's absolutely no evidence that suggests that hair dyes cause birth defects or miscarriage. Semi-permanent dyes or highlights are even less controversial. With highlights, foil surrounds the strands of hair coated with the formula, so even less absorption through the skin occurs. Because of the

Physical, Emotional, and Embarrassing Unmentionables

limited hardcore scientific data available, your practitioner may tell you to stick to vegetable hair dyes during pregnancy, while your friend's practitioner may tell her that dyeing her hair is fine.

>> **Permanents:** No scientific evidence suggests that the chemicals in hair permanents are harmful to the developing baby. These preparations usually do contain significant amounts of ammonia, however, so for your own safety, use them in well-ventilated areas.

>> **Standard chemical straightening treatments:** Several standard chemical treatments are available to women who want to have silky-straight locks. Such standard treatments usually include chemicals such as sodium hydroxide (lye), calcium hydroxide and guanidine carbonate (no lye), or thioglycolic acid salts (thio). Although the data is limited, it seems to show that these treatments are generally safe in pregnancy. One study showed no increase of preterm birth or low birth weight but did not look at risks of birth defects. Therefore, it may be best to use after the first trimester.

>> **Brazilian hair treatments:** Brazilian or Brazilian keratin treatments are a popular method for straightening and smoothing the hair. Most of these treatments contain a chemical called *formaldehyde,* which can be absorbed through the skin or by breathing it in. Formaldehyde was used many years ago in hair dyes and was found to be carcinogenic (causing childhood cancers). Therefore, embrace your curls and avoid these products, or stick to blow-drying or flat irons for that super-straight look in pregnancy.

>> **Thermal reconditioning:** Thermal reconditioning, also known as the Japanese straightening technique, is a fairly new method to permanently straighten hair. The process involves applying a variety of chemicals and conditioners to the hair and then using a flat iron to permanently straighten it. No scientific research has studied this technique in pregnancy. Some of the chemicals used are similar to those used for perming hair. The bottom line: Thermal reconditioning is likely okay during pregnancy, but no definitive data is available. If you want to play it as safe as possible, consider avoiding this treatment.

>> **Waxing:** Waxing legs or the bikini line involves applying a heated wax preparation topically and then removing it along with the hair. Nothing in the wax preparations can lead to problems for the baby. So if you like, keep waxing away while you're pregnant to help you remain carefree and hair-free.

>> **Laser hair removal:** The laser used for hair removal works by transmitting heat to the hair follicle and stopping hair regrowth. Often, anesthetic creams are applied to the skin first to reduce pain. This therapy, which is applied locally, should not cause any problem to the baby.

>> **Facials:** You may notice that your complexion has changed over the past few months. Sometimes pregnancy hormones can wreak havoc on your skin.

Facials may or may not help. But go ahead and have one anyway, if only to enjoy the time to sit back and relax!

>> **Chemical peels:** Alpha-hydroxy acids are the main ingredients in chemical peels. The chemicals work topically, but small amounts are absorbed into your system. Chemical peels are probably okay, but first discuss it with your practitioner.

>> **Wrinkle creams:** The two most common antiwrinkle creams used today are Retin-A and Renova. Both of these preparations contain vitamin A derivatives. Substantial data suggests that oral medications containing vitamin A derivatives (for example, Accutane) can cause birth defects, but the information that's available on topical preparations such as Retin-A and Renova doesn't indicate a problem. Due to the significant effects of oral preparations, however, many practitioners discourage the use of any medications containing these compounds, oral or topical, to their patients.

>> **Botox:** The safety of Botox therapy during pregnancy and breastfeeding is controversial, and the data, limited. In one study involving 16 pregnant women injected mostly in the first trimester, there were no reported birth defects. One patient suffered a miscarriage, although she'd had a miscarriage in a prior pregnancy. A few other studies with small numbers showed no untoward effects. To be on the safe side, consider enjoying the beauty from your pregnancy glow while you're pregnant and wait until after you deliver for the Botox. If, however, there is a medical indication for Botox (severe migraines, severe cervical dystonia), it may be a reasonable option. Talk to your practitioner about it.

>> **Injectable fillers:** Injectable skin fillers are used to smooth wrinkles and make lips fuller. Often they're made with collagen or hyaluronic acid. No good data currently exists documenting the safety of fillers during pregnancy, so they're probably best avoided until safety data is available. The good news is that the fluid retention of pregnancy may lessen the wrinkles anyway!

Relaxing in hot tubs, whirlpools, saunas, or steam rooms

A lot of women ask about just taking a nice, relaxing warm bath. In general, soaking in a warm, soothing bath is fine during pregnancy. Just make sure that the water temperature isn't too high.

WARNING

Using hot tubs, whirlpools, saunas, or steam rooms when you're pregnant can be risky because of the high temperatures involved. In laboratory animals, exposure to high levels of heat during pregnancy has been known to cause birth defects or miscarriage. Studies involving humans suggest that pregnant women whose core body temperatures rise significantly during the early weeks of pregnancy may stand an increased risk of miscarriage or having babies with neural tube defects (spina bifida, for example). However, problems typically occur only if the mother's core temperature rises above 102 degrees Fahrenheit (or about 39 degrees Celsius) for more than ten minutes during the first seven weeks of her pregnancy.

Common sense suggests that after the first trimester, occasionally using hot tubs, saunas, and steam rooms for less than ten minutes is probably okay. However, remember to drink plenty of fluids to avoid dehydration.

Traveling

The main potential problem with traveling during pregnancy is that it puts distance between you and your prenatal care provider. If you're close to your due date or if your pregnancy is considered high-risk, you probably shouldn't travel far from home. Your decision to travel, though, depends on what the risk factors actually are. If you have diabetes but it's well controlled, going on a trip is probably okay. But if you're pregnant with triplets, traveling to Timbuktu probably isn't a good idea. If your pregnancy is uncomplicated, traveling during the first, second, and early third trimesters is usually fine.

Traveling by car poses no special risk, aside from requiring that you sit in one place for a long time. On long trips, stop every couple of hours to get out and walk around a bit. Wear your seat belt and shoulder strap; they keep you safe, and they won't hurt the baby, even if you're in an accident. The amniotic fluid surrounding the fetus serves as a cushion against any constriction from the lap belt. Not wearing restraints clearly poses a greater risk; studies show that the leading cause of fetal death in auto accidents is death of the mother.

TIP

Wear your seat belt below your abdomen, not above it, and keep the shoulder strap in its usual position.

Most airlines allow women to fly if they're less than 36 weeks pregnant, but you may want to carry a note from your practitioner indicating that she sees no medical reason why you shouldn't fly. Flying is perfectly safe, especially if you take a couple of precautions:

>> **Get up from your seat occasionally during longer flights and walk around the plane.** Prolonged periods of sitting can cause blood to pool in your legs. Walking around keeps your circulation going.

>> **Carry a water bottle with you and drink water frequently.** Airplane air is always very dry, and you can easily become dehydrated during long flights. In addition to keeping you hydrated, drinking extra water ensures that you get

up frequently to go to the restroom, which keeps the blood from pooling in your legs.

You don't need to worry about airport metal detectors — or any other metal detectors — because they don't use ionizing radiation.

If you're prone to air sickness and have found Dramamine helpful in the past, using it in normal doses while you're pregnant is okay.

WARNING

If you plan to visit tropical countries, where some diseases are particularly prevalent, you may want to be vaccinated before you go. But check with your doctor to see whether any vaccines you're considering are safe to have during pregnancy. (For more information on vaccines, see Book 1, Chapter 2.)

Getting dental care

Pregnancy itself shouldn't affect your dental health. You don't want to avoid the dentist, because neglected cavities can become infected, which is all the more reason to see your dentist when you're pregnant. Some recent studies have shown that pregnant women who suffer from *periodontal disease,* which is infection and inflammation of the gums, are at a higher risk for delivering small or premature babies. This finding is one more reason for making good oral hygiene a priority.

Pregnancy causes an increase in blood flow to the gums. In fact, about half of all pregnant women develop a condition called *pregnancy gingivitis,* which is simply a reddening of the gums caused by this increased blood flow. In this condition, gums have a tendency to bleed easily, so try to be gentle when you brush and floss your teeth.

For those of you who want whiter and brighter teeth, plenty of products are available, including whitening toothpastes and over-the-counter gels, strips, whitening systems, and trays. Although most are frequently used during pregnancy, no large studies document the safety of such treatments. Whitening toothpastes help remove surface stains without using bleach. There's no reason to think they're a problem.

Over-the-counter whitening strips, gels, and whitening systems are peroxide-based and haven't been specifically studied in pregnancy. However, the safety of peroxide can be inferred from other studies. In one such study, pregnant rats were fed up to 10 percent hydrogen peroxide in their diets, and no problems were detected in their offspring. Similarly, when peroxide was tested as a component in hair dyes, it wasn't found to cause birth defects. With in-office bleaching, the technician applies the whitening product to the teeth and uses heat and/or a laser to quicken the process. Many dentists don't perform these procedures on pregnant women because they haven't been well-studied. On the bright side, seeing your dentist for cleaning not only promotes good hygiene but also removes surface stains and leaves you with a brighter smile.

REMEMBER

If you need routine dental work — cavities filled, teeth pulled, crowns placed — don't worry. Local anesthesia and most pain medications are safe to use during pregnancy. Some dentists also recommend antibiotics during dental procedures, most of which are also safe during pregnancy, but you should check with your prenatal care provider to make sure. Even dental X-rays pose no significant problem for the fetus, as long as a lead apron or shield is placed over the abdomen.

Having sex

For most couples, having sex during pregnancy is perfectly safe. In fact, some couples find that sex during pregnancy is even better than before. However, you may have some issues to consider.

In the first half of pregnancy, sex can usually continue as before because your body hasn't changed that noticeably. You may notice that your breasts are particularly sensitive to the touch or even tender. Later, as the uterus grows, some sexual positions become more difficult. You and your partner may find that you have to be a little creative to make things work. If you find that intercourse is too uncomfortable, other forms of sexual gratification may work better for you and your partner.

Many women ask us whether having sex at the end of pregnancy is okay, even if the cervix is a little bit dilated. Having sex then is perfectly fine as long as your membranes haven't ruptured (your water hasn't broken).

WARNING

Avoid intercourse if you're at a high risk for preterm labor (for example, you've been treated for preterm labor or have a cerclage in place), if you have placenta previa (see Book 6, Chapter 2) in the third trimester, or if you've had recent bleeding. Most practitioners suggest refraining from intercourse in these situations because intercourse has the potential to introduce an infection into the uterus, and semen contains substances that are known to make the uterus contract.

Another important aspect to consider is how each of you feels psychologically about having sex during pregnancy. Your libido or sex drive may increase. Often, you may find that you have vivid sexual dreams and that orgasm itself is heightened. On the other hand, you may find that your interest in sex is less than it was before you got pregnant. You may feel less attractive because of the physical changes that have taken place, which is perfectly normal. Your partner may also experience changes in his desire for sex because of the excitement and normal apprehension that go along with being a father and due to (unfounded) fears that intercourse will hurt the baby or that the baby will somehow know what Mom and Dad are up to.

Working during Pregnancy: A Different Type of Labor

Over the last half-century, the number of women who work outside the home has steadily increased. More than 75 percent of pregnant women work during the third trimester, and more than half work until within a few weeks of delivery. Many women find that working until the end of pregnancy keeps them happy and occupied and helps them not to focus on the discomforts. In addition, many women don't have a choice; they may be the main income providers for their families, and their careers are high priority. Although most of the time, working throughout pregnancy doesn't cause any problems for the baby, there can be some exceptions.

TIP

Stress in pregnancy, whether related to work or to home situations, isn't well-studied. Some doctors believe that very high levels of stress may increase the risk of developing preeclampsia or preterm labor, although no study has confirmed this risk (both of these conditions are discussed in Book 6, Chapter 2). Unusual stress may increase your risk of postpartum depression. Too much stress obviously isn't good for anyone. Do whatever you can to decrease the stress in your life, and talk with your practitioner if you find you're becoming persistently blue or anxious.

Considering occupational hazards

Most jobs fall somewhere in between sedentary and demanding, but even then the amount of stress varies according to the individual. If your pregnancy proceeds without complications, you probably can continue to work right up until delivery. However, some complications that may arise during pregnancy may make reducing your workload or stopping work altogether advisable. For example, if you develop preterm labor, your practitioner will most likely advise you to stop working. Other conditions that may warrant a reduction in physical activity are hypertension or problems with the baby's growth.

REMEMBER

If you work at a computer terminal, you may wonder whether you're being exposed to anything harmful. But you have no need to worry — no evidence suggests that the electromagnetic fields that computer terminals emit are a problem.

Occupations that are physically demanding can be problematic. Some studies suggest that women who have jobs associated with physically demanding responsibilities, such as heavy lifting, manual labor, or significant physical exertion, may be at a slightly higher risk of preterm birth, high blood pressure, preeclampsia, or small-for-gestational-age babies. On the other hand, long working hours haven't been found to increase the chances for premature delivery. Other studies have also shown that jobs in which prolonged standing is required (more than eight hours a day) were associated with a greater chance for back and foot pain, circulatory problems, and a slightly increased risk of preterm birth. The good news: The use of support hose, although not particularly attractive, is helpful in decreasing varicose veins.

REMEMBER

Some women believe that if they complain about certain symptoms or take time out from a busy schedule to eat or go to the restroom, they'll garner the disapproval of their superiors at work. Don't let yourself feel guilty about your special needs during this time, and don't let work cause you to ignore any unusual symptoms. If you need time off to deal with complications, take it, and don't feel bad about it. Remember that your health and your baby's health are the highest priority.

Understanding pregnancy and the law

Take the time to understand your rights as they pertain to pregnancy. In the United States, the Pregnancy Discrimination Act, an amendment to Title VII of the Civil Rights Act of 1964, requires pregnant women to be treated in a manner equal to all employees or applicants. According to this act, employers can't refuse to hire a woman because of her pregnancy-related condition, as long as she's capable of performing the job's major functions.

If an employee is temporarily unable to carry out her job due to the pregnancy, the employer must treat her the same as any other temporarily disabled employee, taking such actions as providing alternative tasks, disability leave, or leave without pay. A disability may arise due to the pregnancy itself, such as significant nausea and vomiting. A disability may also occur due to complications of pregnancy, such as bleeding, preterm labor, or high blood pressure, or it may occur due to hazardous job exposures. If your healthcare provider decides that your pregnancy is disabling, you can ask that she send a letter to your employer, verifying your disability.

In the U.S., most maternity leaves are from 6 to 8 weeks. You're entitled to a 12-week leave in a one-year period under the Family and Medical Leave Act, although this may not be a paid leave.

Health insurance should cover expenses for pregnancy-related conditions in a way that's similar to its coverage of other medical conditions, as long as obstetric services are covered. Health insurers are prohibited by law from considering pregnancy a preexisting condition, which means you cannot be denied coverage when you go from one job to another and switch health plans.

Chapter 5

Creating a Birth Plan

Y ou may be wondering how anyone can "plan" birth. Although you obviously can't plan every aspect of what will happen when you give birth, you actually have many options. Creating a birth plan gives you an opportunity to research and consider the many aspects of childbirth that *can* be planned, many of which you may not have known about otherwise. After your plan is put together, you can use it to communicate your wishes to your birth team.

This chapter introduces you to birth plans and their benefits, gives a general overview of birth and postpartum options, explains how you can make informed decisions, and provides tips on avoiding common birth-plan pitfalls.

What's a Birth Plan? And Why Would You Want One?

Put simply, a *birth plan* is a document you create to communicate your wishes and requests to your medical practitioner, the birth team, and your support team (whether that's your partner, a doula, or someone else). You write the plan months before labor begins, when you have time to research and think through your options — preferably before contractions make concentrating difficult! Planning ahead also allows you to switch medical practitioners if your current doctor or midwife isn't on board with your plans.

Despite the name, a birth plan also includes your wishes for the immediate post-partum period, like how you intend to feed your baby and where you want her to sleep if you're giving birth in a hospital. Birth plans also cover the fun options, like who will announce the baby's gender and who cuts the cord. This section explains the reasons you should consider writing a birth plan.

Making informed choices with a clear head

You may wonder why you should bother considering all the many options for dealing with events that may not even happen during your birth. The reason is simple: Thinking straight is much easier when you're not in labor. And unless you bring your laptop into the labor room, researching your choices is difficult when you're in the trenches, so to speak.

Technically, whenever your medical practitioner recommends a birth intervention — like *induction,* or attempting to initiate active labor — he should also tell you the potential risks and benefits. In an ideal world, you'd also be given alternative options to consider. For example, on the subject of induction, your doctor could explain the choices of giving you oxytocin (Pitocin) intravenously, trying something natural first, or taking a "wait and see" approach before augmenting labor. If he thoroughly explains all three options, you can give true *informed consent,* which means agreeing to a procedure only after understanding what's involved.

In practice, informed consent for many procedures is covered extremely quickly, way too fast for you to process the information and make an informed decision. Frequently, procedures are not explained at all, especially if they're routine (which doesn't necessarily mean risk-free), or the procedure is presented as if you have no other options. Even if you have an amazing medical practitioner who really explains your risks and alternatives, you may have difficulty thinking through decisions when you're in the middle of labor.

Creating your birth plan allows you to research your options when you're feeling calm and collected. You still may have to make difficult decisions in the midst of labor — after all, birth isn't completely plan-friendly — but at least for straight-forward issues, you'll be ready.

Visualizing your ideal birth

Everyone's ideal image of birth is different. One mother may consider the perfect birth to be in a well-equipped hospital with an immediate epidural, and another mother may consider her perfect birth to be at home, with no drugs, and in a birthing pool. There's nothing necessarily right or wrong about these different visions (although most people think their ideal birth is the best one!). Every birth choice has its risks and benefits, but many birth choices have more to do with comfort and personal philosophy than statistics.

Don't panic if you're thinking, "But I have no idea what I want. I don't even know what my options are!" Lots of moms and dads have no idea what they want at the beginning of the pregnancy. In fact, their "ideal birth" may change from pregnancy to pregnancy. As you find out more about birth and about birth plans, you'll get a better idea of what you want. For a general overview of your options, skip ahead to the section "Your Birth-Plan Options: An Overview."

Putting what you want on paper for your care providers

A written birth plan helps you communicate your concerns and wishes to your medical practitioner. Discussing your plans for childbirth before you go into labor is essential, and having a written plan in hand can be a huge help.

TIP

Never assume your medical practitioner's idea of the perfect birth is similar to your own. Even if your chosen care provider shares your birth philosophy, you should still write down your wishes to prevent misunderstandings.

If you're giving birth in the hospital, you have very little control over which nurse you get, and you get very little time to discuss your birth plans with her. Most nurses want their patients to have a healthy and positive birth, and a written birth plan makes it easier for them to provide you with what you want.

REMEMBER

Just writing your plan down won't magically make your birth wishes a reality. Not every option is available in every birth location or with every medical practitioner. Even if the option is available, you still need to advocate for yourself beyond handing your nurse, midwife, or doctor a written birth plan.

Your Birth-Plan Options: An Overview

Congratulations on one of the most exciting times of your life: pregnancy and the birth of your baby. Like for any big event, you need to do some planning if you want birth to go smoothly. A birth plan not only helps you to cope during labor and delivery; it also helps you think clearly and logically about the kind of birth you want and what that requires.

Topics your birth plan covers

This chapter mentions birth–plan options a lot, but maybe you're wondering what those options actually are. Here's a list of the basics:

>> **Where do you want to give birth?** You may give birth at home, in a hospital, or at a birth center. You also should consider which hospital or birth center to choose. Finding out whether delivering at home is legal in your state is also important.

>> **What kind of practitioner do you envision?** You may decide on an obstetrician or a midwife. You may or may not want to stick with your current gynecologist or midwife. Refer to Book 1, Chapter 2 for tips on choosing your medical practitioner.

>> **Who will support and advocate for you during labor and delivery?** Your significant other is not the only option for labor support. You may consider hiring a doula to work with your partner or as your sole support. You may also choose a friend or family member for this role.

>> **Whom do you want to invite to the birth?** You can invite friends and family members to the birth, either to wait down the hall or be by your side in the delivery room. You may even consider including your older children at the birth. Or you and your partner can be alone, inviting family after the baby arrives. Rules for how many visitors can be present during the delivery vary from facility to facility and can change based on emergent situations.

>> **Do you want a natural childbirth?** Women choose natural childbirth for a number of reasons, from concerns about epidural risks to wanting a "natural experience." If you decide to use pain medications, you have a number of pain-relief options, from epidurals to walking epidurals to IV narcotics.

>> **What comfort techniques will you try?** Pain drugs are only one way to get relief from labor pains. To name just a few other options, you can use massage, hydrotherapy, or hypnosis. Even if you plan an epidural, you probably won't be able to get one right away, so having an arsenal of comfort techniques is important.

>> **What birthing tools or props do you want to use?** Birthing props and comfort tools are not only fun but also extremely helpful! You may decide to use a birthing pool, a squat bar, a birth ball, or massage tools. Even your music choices can be important for the birth. Checking with each facility to see what's available and what you can bring to the hospital is also a good idea.

>> **How do you expect to stay active during labor?** If you assumed you'd be lying in bed for the entire labor, think again! Many positions and movements can be helpful during labor, and remaining active has lots of benefits.

» **Will you accept an IV for hydration, or do you hope to drink fluids on your own?** IVs are routine in many hospitals but not all, and you have options. You may even be able to eat and drink lightly.

» **What kind of environment do you hope for during delivery?** Perhaps you'd like a meditative environment, with ocean waves playing in the background. Or perhaps you want upbeat music to energize you.

» **What kind of monitoring do you want?** If you're getting an epidural, continuous monitoring is required, but if you're hoping for a natural birth, you may be able to have intermittent monitoring.

» **How do you feel about induction and speeding up labor?** Induction is a controversial topic, especially when done for convenience or when scheduled before your due date. *Labor augmentation* (speeding up labor) is another touchy topic, and your medical practitioner plays a big role in your options.

» **How do you want to push?** Surprise: You don't have to push while lying on your back! In fact, you'll probably have an easier time if you don't. You may even choose to have a water birth.

» **How do you envision the delivery of the baby?** Are you hoping to help guide the baby out (with the help of your practitioner)? Do you hope to watch the delivery in a mirror? If you don't know the sex, do you want your medical practitioner to announce it, or do you want your partner to tell you?

» **Do you prefer to receive an episiotomy (surgical incision) or to tear naturally?** Some (but not all) women prefer to tear rather than be cut, and in an emergency, an episiotomy isn't always an option.

» **What are your feelings about cesarean section (C-section)?** Some women are fearful of C-section, whereas others actually opt for one (sometimes without medical reason). In the past, after you had a cesarean, you always had to have a cesarean with subsequent babies, but now many women can try for a vaginal birth after cesarean (VBAC). If you do need a C-section, you have options — yes, even for a cesarean! — like lowering the drape to watch the delivery or breastfeeding on the surgical table.

» **Who will cut the cord and when? Do you want the baby placed directly on your chest after birth or cleaned up and weighed first?** A number of birth-plan choices are relevant to the moment your baby is born.

» **What do you want to do with the placenta?** You even have options regarding the placenta! For the delivery of the placenta, you may request that the medical practitioner not use controlled traction and allow a natural delivery of the placenta. You also may request that the birth team save the placenta for you so you can make a "placenta print" or bury your placenta in the back yard.

>> **Do you plan to take pictures or video of the birth?** Some parents want pictures only after the baby is delivered, but others want photos of the entire birth experience.

>> **How do you plan to feed your baby?** Will you breastfeed, bottle-feed, or do a little of both? Some bottle-feeding moms face bottle guilt, but breastfeeding isn't always possible or desired. Some hospital routines unintentionally sabotage breastfeeding mothers, but your birth plan can include requests to avoid some potential problems. See Book 5 for more on nourishing your baby.

>> **Where do you want your baby to sleep?** *Full rooming-in* means your baby stays with you around the clock, while *partial rooming-in* means your baby sleeps in the nursery.

>> **What drops, shots, and tests do you want for your baby? If you have a baby boy, do you want the hospital to do a circumcision?** Vaccinations are a hot topic in the United States. Some parents decide to forgo all shots, while others accept them all, choose selectively, or delay them. Circumcision is also a hot topic, and parents who decide to snip may or may not want to do so right after the birth or at the hospital.

Considering alternative birthing methods

More and more women are expressing interest in nontraditional or alternative birthing methods, and more and more options are available. Certainly, the following options aren't for everyone, but knowing what's possible can be helpful.

Delivering without anesthesia

Natural childbirth usually refers to giving birth without any medications or anesthesia. (It's probably not the best terminology, because using pain medication doesn't make the birthing process unnatural.) The theory behind natural birth is that childbirth is an inherently healthy and natural process and that women's bodies are made to handle childbirth without the need for medications.

Natural childbirth allows you to have a great deal of control over the childbirth process and your own body. It emphasizes having you choose which positions are comfortable, how mobile you want to be, and which techniques you want to use to be as comfortable as possible. Natural childbirth can be practiced in a hospital setting, in a birthing center, or even at home. Some practitioners aren't comfortable with every aspect of natural childbirth because they don't want to be limited in doing what they feel is medically necessary and important. Discuss with your practitioner what he feels comfortable with so your delivery can be as great of an experience as possible.

Giving birth at home

For some women, a home birth provides an ideal environment to deliver their baby. Common reasons for choosing a home birth are the desire for a low-intervention birth; a desire for control over the birth process; a desire to give birth in a familiar and comfortable environment, surrounded by family and friends; living in a rural area with lack of access to a hospital; and economic, cultural, or religious issues. Typically, a midwife usually attends a home birth, and an obstetrician is on call in case problems arise. Home births are certainly more appropriate for women who are at very low risk for complications. Although some studies demonstrate that home births are associated with greater risks for both the mother and baby, others show that home births are at least as safe as hospital births for healthy, low-risk women.

Home births are still relatively uncommon in the United States, with fewer than 1 percent of women choosing to deliver at home. Although respecting the right of women to make medically informed decisions about where they want to deliver, the American Congress of Obstetricians and Gynecologists, in agreement with the American Academy of Pediatrics, believes that hospitals and birthing centers are the safest settings for births and has published the minimum criteria for planning a home birth, which include the following:

>> A singleton pregnancy with the fetus's head down

>> No medical or obstetrical conditions

>> No contraindications to vaginal birth

>> A licensed obstetrical caregiver to administer the prenatal, labor, birth, and postpartum care

>> A backup hospital within 15 minutes of the home

In addition, and of prime importance, is that women completely understand that although the absolute risk of home births is low, home birth is still associated with a two- to threefold increase in neonatal death when compared with planned hospital births. Also, home births aren't legal in all states.

Using a doula

A *doula* may be a friend, relative, or trained companion who provides nonmedical, continuous support during labor and delivery. Doulas often meet with prospective moms before delivery so they get to know each other. During labor, they provide both emotional support and physical support — helping to get moms into comfortable positions, massaging their back or legs, getting water or ice chips, and so forth. Some studies have shown that labors attended with doulas may actually be shorter in length, although there is no effect on cesarean delivery rates. Women who used doulas also seemed to have a slightly better overall birth experience and were more likely to rate their labor and delivery as "very good."

Immersing yourself in a water birth

In a *water birth,* much of labor is spent immersed in water, and the baby can even be delivered in the water. Water births usually take place in a birthing center with the help of a midwife, although some hospitals may provide birthing pools or baths. The water temperature is kept about the same as the body temperature, and the woman's temperature should be monitored throughout labor.

A recent review of randomized trials found a somewhat lower rate of anesthesia when water immersion was used in the first stage of labor. Interesting, prolonged immersion for more than two hours may actually slow down labor by decreasing the production of oxytocin. Although some professionals in the medical community feel that a water birth is a safe procedure, others have more serious concerns about its safety for both the patient and newborn. Water immersion during the second stage is not well studied. There have been a few cases reported of water aspiration and snapped umbilical cords, difficulty regulating body temperature, and infections in the newborn. Also, not all facilities are equipped for water births.

Why planning must begin early in pregnancy

Although many options exist, everything isn't available in every birth facility or with every medical practitioner. Birth location policies and your medical practitioner's practices have a big effect on your options and on the chances of getting the birth you want. Planning early for the birth gives you time to do the following:

>> **Interview medical practitioners:** If you start planning early, you'll have more time to consider the right practitioner for you and have time to switch if necessary. Book 1, Chapter 2 discusses choosing a practitioner.

>> **Tour your chosen birth facility:** You can't make a real decision about where to deliver until you've been there. Tour a couple of hospitals or birth centers to evaluate where you'd feel most comfortable. Because where you give birth is often connected to who attends the birth, tour early in your pregnancy in case you need to switch practitioners.

For a home birth, early planning is recommended so you can check your local home-birth laws and find a medical practitioner. Don't make the mistake of thinking all home-birth practitioners share your birth philosophy. You also need to prepare your home, which may include gathering supplies or renting a birthing pool.

Making Smart Choices When You're Not a Doctor

Plenty of mothers-to-be are intimidated at the thought of considering the pros and cons of a medical procedure — especially if they then decide to go against their medical practitioner's protocols or routines. If you feel unqualified to make decisions about childbirth, the good news is you're not the first person to confront all these choices, and you don't have to make them on your own. This section explains how you can educate yourself on your birth options and who you can ask for help when you can't decide what to do.

Getting an education

If you want to make decisions about your birth plan, medical training is not required! You can get the information you need to make informed choices by taking childbirth-education classes and researching birth on your own. Childbirth-education classes aren't only about teaching natural childbirth methods, though most encourage natural labor and spend a great deal of time on comfort techniques. The rest of class time is spent talking about the mechanics of normal childbirth and the pros and cons of various interventions. Your education doesn't have to stop there. Reading about birth in books and doing online research can help you write your birth plan.

Consulting the experienced and the wise

Here's more good news about writing your birth plan: You don't have to do it alone! You can ask for advice from all the following people:

>> **Your medical practitioner:** Although your medical practitioner has his own concerns regarding your birth choices — including malpractice suits and sometimes his own convenience — he is still an excellent resource when you don't understand some issues or want more information.

>> **Your childbirth educator:** Most childbirth instructors are happy to help with birth questions and can even help you write your plan or be willing to read over what you've put together.

>> **Your doula:** Part of a doula's job is to help advocate for your birth choices, and that includes helping you with your birth plan. A doula can also give you inside information on local practitioners and birth locations, which can be a huge help.

>> **Other experienced moms and dads:** Anyone who has gone through childbirth can serve as a resource when you're creating your own plan. Friends and

relatives can tell you what they wish they had done differently and what was just perfect. They may also be able to give feedback on local medical practitioners and birth locations; just be sure to ask *why* they liked a particular place or person. Remember that everyone visualizes the perfect birth differently and that everyone's circumstances are different.

Avoiding Potential Birth-Plan Pitfalls

Birth plans make pretty great advocacy tools, but they aren't always perfect. Here are some common pitfalls and how you can avoid them:

>> **Not making a plan because you feel overwhelmed:** Considering all the options for your birth can be overwhelming. So many choices to make! If you feel exhausted just thinking about it, remember that you don't have to have an opinion on every aspect of birth. Just because you have options doesn't mean you must specifically choose one or the other.

If you don't have strong feelings about an issue, you can go with whatever your medical practitioner suggests or whatever feels right in the moment. Creating your birth plan should be an energizing experience and a chance to really take charge (as much as possible) of your birth experience. The key is to feel empowered, not overwhelmed, by all your choices.

>> **Assuming a birth plan is only for natural births:** Many aspects of the birth and the immediate postpartum period have nothing to do with using drugs or not. Even within the option of using an epidural, you have choices, like when to start it, whether you want a walking epidural, and whether you want it turned down when it's time to push.

>> **Being inflexible:** Critics of birth plans say that they set women up for disappointment. If a couple's birth goes badly, they may feel they failed in some way, like their plan wasn't good enough.

REMEMBER

Creating a birth plan isn't about trying to control birth, and it's not about restricting the possibilities of what's considered a positive birth experience. If you keep in mind that your birth plan isn't a contract but more of a flexible guide, you're less likely to feel disappointed if a few little things go differently than planned.

>> **Not standing up for your decisions:** Writing down your birth wishes is only the first step to getting the birth you want. You also need to speak to your practitioner before labor begins if you want him on your side. During the birth itself, you'll likely need to work with the nurses and advocate for your plan, especially if your wishes run contrary to the hospital's routines.

2

From Twinkle to Term: The Countdown to Labor and Beyond

Contents at a Glance

Chapter 1

The First Trimester

The first trimester of your pregnancy is an exciting time, full of many changes for you and especially for your baby, which — in just 12 short weeks — grows from a single cell to a tiny being with a beating heart and functioning kidneys. With all that change going on in your baby, you can certainly expect many changes in your own body — from fatigue and nausea to newly voluptuous (va-va-voom!) but tender breasts. Through it all, you need to know what's normal and what's worth a call to your practitioner, whom you begin visiting regularly at this point. This chapter gives you a snapshot of what to expect.

REMEMBER

Weeks in this chapter refers to menstrual weeks, which means weeks from the last menstrual period, not weeks from conception. So at eight weeks, the baby is really six weeks from conception. We describe how doctors calculate the timing of pregnancy in Book 1, Chapter 1.

Following the Numbers: How the Embryo Grows

Pregnancy begins when the egg (or *oocyte*) and sperm meet, which happens in the fallopian tube. At this stage, the egg and sperm together form the *zygote* — a single cell. The zygote divides many times into a cluster of multiple cells called a *blastocyst*, which travels down the fallopian tube and into the *uterus* (also called the *womb*). When it reaches the uterus, both you and your baby begin to experience major changes.

On or about the fifth day of development, the blastocyst attaches to the blood-rich lining of the uterus during a process called *implantation*. Part of the blastocyst grows to become the *embryo* (the baby in the first eight weeks of development), and the other part becomes the *placenta* (the organ that implants into the uterus to provide oxygen and nourishment to the fetus and eliminate its waste products).

From the blastocyst, the embryo develops into three tissue layers: the endoderm, mesoderm, and ectoderm. These three layers, which ultimately give rise to all the structures of the body, are initially organized into a flat disk. Around the beginning of the fourth week of embryonic development, the flat disk begins to fold and form a cylinder. At this point, the embryo begins to take on the form of the general body plan, with a mouth region and an anal region. Between weeks four and eight, all the organ systems that you find in an adult will be forming.

After the eighth week of your pregnancy, the developing embryo is referred to as a *fetus.* Amazingly, by this time, almost all the baby's major organs and structures are already formed. The remaining 32 weeks allow the fetus's structures to grow and mature. The brain, although also formed very early, isn't mature at birth; rather, it continues to develop into adulthood.

Your baby grows within the *amniotic sac* in the uterus. The amniotic sac is full of clear fluid, known as *amniotic fluid*. This water balloon–like structure actually comprises two thin layers of membrane called the *chorion* and *amnion* (which together are known as the *membranes*). When people talk about water breaking, they're referring to the rupturing of those membranes that line the uterus's inner walls. The baby "swims" in this fluid and is attached to the placenta by the umbilical cord. Figure 1-1 shows a diagram of an early pregnancy, including a developing fetus and the *cervix,* which is the uterus's opening. The cervix opens up, or *dilates,* when you're in labor.

The placenta begins to form soon after the embryo implants in the uterus. Maternal and fetal blood vessels lie very close to one another inside the placenta, which allows various substances (such as nutrients, oxygen, and waste) to transfer back and forth. The mother's blood and the baby's blood are in close contact, but they don't actually mix.

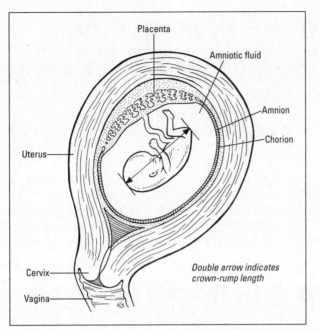

FIGURE 1-1:
An early
pregnancy.

Placenta

Amniotic fluid

Amnion

Chorion

Uterus

Cervix

Vagina

*Double arrow indicates
crown-rump length*

Illustration by Kathryn Born, MA

The placenta grows like a tree, forming branches that in turn divide into smaller and smaller ones. The tiniest buds of the placenta are called the *chorionic villi*, and it's within these villi that small fetal blood vessels form. About three weeks after fertilization, these blood vessels join to form the baby's circulatory system, and the heart begins to beat.

By the end of the eighth week, arms, legs, fingers, and toes begin to form, and the embryo begins to perform small, spontaneous movements. If you have an ultrasound examination performed in the first trimester, you can see these spontaneous movements on the screen. The brain enlarges rapidly, and ears and eyes appear. The external genitalia also emerge and can be differentiated as male or female by the end of the 12th week, although sex differences are not yet detectable by ultrasound.

By the end of the 12th week, the fetus is about 4 inches long and weighs about 1 ounce. The head looks large and round, and the eyelids are fused shut. The intestines, which protruded slightly into the umbilical cord at about week 10, are by this time well inside the abdomen. Fingernails appear, and hair begins to grow on the baby's head. The kidneys start working during the third month. Between 9 and 12 weeks, the fetus begins to produce urine, which you can see within the small fetal bladder on ultrasound.

TAKE TWO: HOW TWINS FORM

Twins can form in two ways: Either two eggs are produced (ovulated) and two sperm fertilize the eggs, or one egg is fertilized by one sperm and the embryo splits into two very early in development (early in the blastocyst stage). If two eggs are fertilized, the genetic information contained in each embryo is different from the other, just like any other siblings. These twins are called *fraternal twins*. If one egg is fertilized and splits, the resulting two embryos are genetically identical, and you have *identical twins*.

Twins (or higher-order multiples) are more common in women who undergo in vitro fertilization (IVF), most often because two (or more) embryos fertilized in a petri dish are placed in the uterus and implanted. It's still possible, however, to have identical twins when a single blastocyst is transferred to the uterus and it splits into two embryos later.

Adapting to Your Body's Changes

Your baby isn't the only one growing and changing during your pregnancy. Your body also has to adjust, and the adjustments it makes aren't always the most pleasant and comfortable for you. Being prepared for what lies ahead can help ease your mind. The following sections let you know what's in store for you during the first trimester.

Breast changes

One of the earliest and most amazing changes in your body happens to your breasts. Even during the first month of pregnancy, most women notice that their breasts grow considerably larger and feel very tender. The nipples and *areolae* (the circular areas around the nipples) also grow bigger and may begin to darken.

Breast changes are caused by the large amounts of estrogen and progesterone your body produces during pregnancy. These hormones cause the glands in your breasts to grow and branch out in preparation for milk production and breast-feeding after the baby is born. Blood supply to the breasts also increases markedly. You may notice large, bluish blood vessels coursing along your breasts.

TIP

Plan to go through several bra sizes while you're pregnant — and don't skimp on buying new bras. Good support helps reduce stretching and sagging later on. Although some women like the way they look with larger breasts, others feel self-conscious. Whichever way you feel, we guarantee other pregnant women feel the same way, so don't be embarrassed about it.

Fatigue

During the first trimester, you're likely to feel overwhelming fatigue. This fatigue may be a side effect of all the physical changes your body is experiencing, including the dramatic rise in hormone levels. Rest assured your exhaustion will probably go away somewhere around the 12th to 14th week of your pregnancy. As your fatigue lessens, you'll probably feel more energetic and almost normal, until about 30 to 34 weeks into your pregnancy, when you may tire out again. In the meantime, remember that fatigue is nature's way of telling you to get more rest. If you can, try to catch a short nap during the day and go to bed earlier than usual at night.

Any-time-of-day sickness

For some women, the nausea that can strike during the first trimester is worse in the mornings, maybe because the stomach is empty at that time of day. But ask anyone who's had morning sickness, also known as *nausea and vomiting of pregnancy* (NVP), and she'll tell you it can hit at any time. It often starts during the fifth or sixth week of pregnancy and goes away, or at least becomes much less severe, by the end of the eleventh or twelfth week. It can last longer, and in fact about 10 percent of women have symptoms up to 16 weeks! If you're carrying twins or more, don't be surprised if the NVP is worse than expected, because the higher hormone levels make the nausea even more extreme.

TIP

Fortunately, there are things you can do to ameliorate your symptoms. If you're less than six weeks pregnant and experiencing NVP, you can take folic acid alone instead of your prenatal vitamin. Folic acid is the main supplement that you need early in your pregnancy, and it's much less likely to upset your stomach than the multivitamin is. Check with your doctor for the correct dose for you, and head to Book 1, Chapter 4, which has other suggestions on ways to keep nausea at bay. Above all, don't compound the problem by worrying about it. The nausea is harmless — to you and the baby. Your optimal weight gain for the first three months is only 2 pounds. Even losing weight probably isn't a big problem.

WARNING

If you're really bothered by the nausea, talk to your doctor about over-the-counter or prescription medications. Occasionally, the nausea and vomiting are so severe that you develop a condition called *hyperemesis gravidarum.* The symptoms include dehydration and weight loss. If you develop hyperemesis gravidarum, you may need to be given fluids and medications intravenously. Again, talk to your doctor.

You may hear some women say that morning sickness is a sign that you're experiencing a "normal" pregnancy, but that claim is a myth — and so is the reverse. If you're not having morning sickness, or if it suddenly disappears, don't worry that your pregnancy isn't normal; just enjoy your good fortune. Similarly, you may hear that the severity of your queasiness indicates whether you're having a girl or a boy. But that's also a myth, so don't buy those pink or blue outfits just yet.

Bloating

Well before the baby is big enough to stretch out your stomach, your belt may begin to feel uncomfortable, and your belly may look bloated and distended. This side effect of the hormone shift starts happening as soon as you conceive. *Progesterone,* one of the two key pregnancy hormones, causes you to retain water. Plus it slows down the bowels, causing them to enlarge and thus increase the size of the abdomen. *Estrogen,* the other key pregnancy hormone, causes your uterus to enlarge, which also makes your abdomen feel bigger. This effect is often more pronounced in second or third pregnancies because the first pregnancy causes your abdominal muscles to relax to a greater degree.

Frequent urination

From early on in your pregnancy, you may feel as if you're spending your whole life in the restroom. During pregnancy, you need to urinate more frequently for a variety of reasons. At the beginning of your pregnancy, your uterus is inside your pelvis. But toward the end of your first trimester (at around 12 weeks), your uterus expands enough to rise up into your abdominal cavity. Your enlarging uterus may compress your bladder, which both decreases its capacity and increases the feeling that you need to urinate. Also, your blood volume rises markedly during pregnancy, and that means the rate at which your kidneys produce urine also increases.

TIP

Drink plenty of fluids during pregnancy to avoid dehydration, but try to drink more during the day and less in the evening so you aren't up all night going to the bathroom. Caffeine is a *diuretic,* which increases the flow of urine, so also try decreasing the amount of caffeine you consume.

WARNING

If you find yourself urinating even more than your pregnancy norm or if you feel any discomfort or burning or notice blood during urination, talk to your practitioner. When you're pregnant, bacteria are more likely than usual to cause a urinary tract infection (UTI; see Book 6, Chapter 3).

Headaches

Many pregnant women notice that they get headaches more often than they used to. These headaches may be the result of nausea, fatigue, hunger, the normal physiologic decrease in blood pressure that starts to occur at this time, tension, or even depression. Simple pain relievers like acetaminophen (for example, Tylenol) or ibuprofen (such as Motrin or Advil) in recommended doses are often the best treatment for headaches, including migraines. Some women find that a little caffeine can also alleviate symptoms of a headache. Food and rest can usually cure headaches that are caused by nausea, fatigue, or hunger, so try eating and getting some extra sleep. If neither of those tactics works, something else is probably causing your headaches.

WARNING

Some women find relief from occasional headaches by taking a combination of acetaminophen and caffeine (such as Excedrin Tension Headache). Although this combination is fine to take once in a while, don't use it on a regular basis. Each tablet contains 65 mg of caffeine, and the package recommends two tablets every six hours — that's a whopping 520 mg of caffeine per day and way beyond the maximum 200 mg recommended for pregnant women. This much caffeine taken on a regular basis could cause problems with your baby's growth or, if consumed early in pregnancy, may increase your risk for miscarriage.

WARNING

Avoid taking regular doses of aspirin unless recommended by your practitioner. Adult doses of aspirin can affect platelet function (important in blood clotting).

If over-the-counter medications don't relieve your headaches, talk with your practitioner about taking a mild tranquilizer or antimigraine medication. Base your decision on whether to use migraine medications on the severity of your problem. If your headaches are chronic or recurrent, you may be better off taking medications, despite their potential effects on your fetus, because feeling bad all the time is likely more harmful to your baby's development than any potential risks from the various medications available. As always, consult with your practitioner before taking these medications.

WARNING

If your headaches are severe and unremitting, you may need a thorough medical evaluation or a referral to a neurologist. Later on in pregnancy, a headache may signal the onset of preeclampsia (covered in Book 6, Chapter 2). In that case, your headache may be accompanied by swelling of your hands and feet and by high blood pressure. If you suffer a severe headache in the late second or third trimester, call your practitioner.

Constipation

About half of all pregnant women complain of constipation. When you're pregnant, you may become constipated because the large amount of progesterone circulating in your bloodstream slows the activity of your digestive tract. The iron in prenatal vitamins may make matters worse.

Eating plenty of high-fiber foods, drinking plenty of water, and exercising regularly can provide relief. Taking stool softeners is another option. A stool softener isn't a laxative; it just keeps the stool soft. Stool softeners are safe during pregnancy, and you may take them two to three times a day. Head to Book 1, Chapter 4 for details on these remedies and to Book 4 for safe exercise options.

WARNING

Avoid laxatives, because they can cause abdominal cramping and, occasionally, uterine contractions. For any person, pregnant or not, chronic laxative use should be avoided. If you're extremely constipated, though, and aren't at risk for preterm labor, you may want to talk to your practitioner about the short-term use of a very mild laxative, like a glycerin suppository or milk of magnesia.

Cramps

You may feel a vague, menstrual-like cramping sensation during the first trimester. This symptom is very common, so don't worry. The cramping is probably related to the uterus growing and enlarging.

WARNING

If you experience cramping along with vaginal bleeding, give your practitioner a call. Although the majority of women who experience bleeding and cramping go on to have perfectly normal pregnancies, sometimes these two symptoms together are associated with miscarriage. Cramping alone, without bleeding, is unlikely to be a problem.

GETTING USED TO STRANGE NEW MATERNAL HABITS

At times, you may look at your partner and wonder who this woman actually is. The sweet-tempered woman you once knew may have been replaced by someone whose head appears to be rotating at times, and the woman who used to party all night long barely makes it into the living room to collapse on the couch after work. You knew having a baby was going to change your life, but you probably didn't expect things to change this much so early in the game.

Take heart: These are temporary changes. After her body adjusts to the new hormone levels, many of the symptoms will decrease, and your original partner will start to emerge again.

In the meantime, some of her new habits may be affecting you in a big way, and you may need to find ways to cope with them. Here are some suggestions to help you deal with a few of your least favorite early pregnancy things.

- **Vomiting:** Although she's the one vomiting, sometimes you may not be far behind, and staying supportive while holding onto your own cookies can be difficult. If the sight, sounds, and smell of vomiting are getting to you, try dabbing something under your nose that smells good to you, like peppermint oil, and stay cool. People are less likely to vomit when cool air is blowing on them.

- **Gaining weight:** When the nausea ends, your partner may start eating like food is going to be taken off the market next week. This can be bad for her waistline, sure, but it can also be not-so-good for yours, because you may find yourself overeating just to keep up with her and matching her weight gain pound for pound. For both of your sakes, try to put a stop to the madness.

  You don't have to remind her how hard this weight is going to be to lose later. Just talk about your own weight gain and how you're afraid you're not going to be able to play Frisbee on the beach with the kid if you keep eating like this. Don't turn into the food police; no one responds well to being told what they should and shouldn't eat.

- **Coping with your cravings:** Sex may be the last thing on your partner's mind in the first trimester. And some types of sex may trigger her gag reflex, which is the last thing you want to associate with a previously enjoyable activity! Although turning into a monk may not be on your list of fun things, you can cope with the words "Not tonight, honey" by being flexible. Be ready to perform when your partner is ready, because the window of opportunity can be slammed shut before you've had a chance to look outside.

  Also experiment with touching: Depending on how open your partner is to experimentation, you can do a lot to pleasure each other that doesn't involve intercourse. You can also practice self-release: Masturbation isn't something most adults like to talk about, but if you have a voracious sexual appetite, and both you and your partner are okay with the idea, there's no shame in taking the matter into your own hands, so to speak.

Going to Your First Prenatal Appointment

After the at-home pregnancy test reveals the news, set up an appointment with a practitioner. Make visits to your practitioner a regular part of your pregnancy, not only to ensure your health but also to ensure your baby's health. Your first prenatal visit may be your first meeting with the practitioner who will guide you through your pregnancy. (If you don't already have a practitioner selected, see Book 1, Chapter 2 for information on the kinds of care available and tips for choosing a healthcare provider.) Or you may have a long-standing relationship with an OB/GYN or family-practice doctor with whom you've already discussed many of the topics that are typically covered at an initial prenatal visit.

TIP

If possible, bring the father-to-be for this initial visit. His family medical history and ethnic roots are important, too. If the father isn't part of the picture, bring your life partner or anyone else who may be helping you through the pregnancy process to the appointment. That person should have a chance to ask questions, address concerns, and find out what to expect in the coming months.

TAKING ON YOUR EMERGING SUPPORT ROLE

Don't think of yourself as your partner's personal assistant or as the pregnancy police. She may become a diva in her pregnancy, but it's not your responsibility to do it all. And try to avoid becoming overprotective of your partner's physical capabilities, especially early in the pregnancy. If everything goes well with the pregnancy, she won't have many restrictions on her activities. But that doesn't mean she's going to be up for taking care of everything she's always managed.

For the first several months — and for the last few — your partner may be too tired/nauseated/hot and so on to make dinner, walk the dog, or perform many of the household chores you used to split. Pick up the slack until she feels good enough to contribute again. When she's back in the swing of things, she can move around and help again. After all, physical activity is beneficial for both mom and baby.

One of your main roles is ensuring that she eats healthfully and exercises if and when possible, but the way to do this is by example, not with a whip and chain in hand and bathroom scales placed in front of the refrigerator. Ask her to take walks with you, and help by preparing meals that settle her stomach and feed baby's growing systems.

Pregnancy doesn't turn your partner into a child, even though she's carrying one around with her. She still gets to make her own choices about what she eats and when (or if) she exercises, and you may have to bite your tongue if she starts exceeding the weight limit for your delicate Queen Anne chairs.

In addition to supporting your partner physically, you need to support her emotionally. She'll likely be weepier and more sensitive than normal. If you're not the kind of guy who likes to talk about feelings, try to become that guy for a month or so.

As hormones surge and wane, roll with the punches. Let the little things go without a struggle, because your partner won't always be able to control her reactions the way she used to. Let her dictate what's for dinner, and if her stomach turns when you plate the exact dinner she asked for, don't take it personally.

Your first prenatal visit usually lasts 30 to 40 minutes or more because your doctor has so much information to provide and so many topics to discuss. Subsequent visits are usually much shorter, sometimes only 5 to 10 minutes long. The frequency of your visits depends on your particular needs and any special risk factors you may have, but in general they're about every four weeks during the first trimester. At these visits, the nurse or practitioner checks your urine, blood pressure, and weight and the baby's heartbeat.

Understanding the consultation

During your first visit, your practitioner discusses your medical and obstetrical history with you. She asks about various aspects of your physical health as well as elements of your lifestyle that may affect your pregnancy.

Lifestyle

Your practitioner asks about your occupation to find out whether your job is sedentary or active, whether you spend your days standing or lifting heavy objects, and whether you work nights or long shifts. She also asks you about your general lifestyle — for example, smoking, heavy alcohol use, dietary restrictions, and exercise patterns.

Date of your last menstrual period

Your practitioner questions you about the start date of your last menstrual period to determine your due date. (For information on calculating your due date, see Book 1, Chapter 1.) If you don't know exactly when your last period began, try to remember the exact date of conception. If you're unsure about either of these dates, your practitioner may want to check on how far along you are by scheduling an ultrasound exam.

Obstetrical and gynecological history

Your provider will ask you about your obstetrical and gynecological history, including any prior pregnancies and any experiences with fibroid tumors, vaginal infections, and other gynecological problems. Your history can help determine how best to manage this pregnancy.

REMEMBER

If you conceived with infertility treatments, inform your practitioner of this during your first prenatal visit because it brings up several points that need to be addressed. Most of the impact of infertility treatment on pregnancy outcomes is related to the higher incidence of multifetal pregnancies — twins and more. In general, children born to couples who have gone through in vitro fertilization (IVF) are as healthy as those who were conceived spontaneously. Recently, some controversy has cropped up in medical literature about an increase in certain birth defects in children born after IVF, as well as an increase in certain chromosomal abnormalities after intracytoplasmic sperm injection (ICSI). Although some studies suggest the incidence may be slightly higher, other studies document no increase at all.

Medical problems

Your practitioner asks you about any medical problems you've had and any surgeries you've undergone, including problems that aren't gynecological in nature. Certain medical conditions may affect pregnancy, and others don't. She also asks you about any allergies to medications you may have. Tell your practitioner so she can know everything about you and your health.

Family medical histories

The family medical histories of both you and the baby's father are important for two reasons. First, your practitioner can identify pregnancy-related conditions that can recur from generation to generation, like having twins or exceptionally large babies. The other reason is to identify serious problems within your family that your baby can inherit. Blood tests can screen for some of these problems, such as cystic fibrosis.

Other available genetic screening tests include the following:

>> **Fragile X:** Fragile X syndrome is the most common inherited form of mental retardation (which can vary from mild to severe disabilities) and is also the most common known cause of autism or autistic-like tendencies. Although many practitioners recommend screening all women for fragile X, the American Congress of Obstetricians and Gynecologists guidelines suggest screening only those women with a family history of fragile X syndrome or undiagnosed mental retardation, developmental delay, autism, or ovarian insufficiency. Certainly, talk with your doctor or healthcare provider if you're interested in fragile X screening.

>> **Spinal Muscular Atrophy (SMA):** Spinal Muscular Atrophy (SMA) is an autosomal recessive neurodegenerative disorder that occurs due to degeneration of nerve cells in the spinal cord. The disease is caused by mutations in a gene known as SMN1 (survival motor neuron gene 1). SMA is not very common (1 in 10,000 live births), although it is thought to be the most common genetic cause of infant death. Currently, couples with a family history of SMA are being offered carrier screening, although many obstetricians offer routine screening. In fact, the American College of Medical Genetics has recently recommended offering carrier testing to all couples, regardless of race or ethnicity.

» **Expanded Carrier Screening for other genetic diseases:** Several companies have come out with tests to screen for over 100 different genetic disorders (including the ones that are mentioned in the following section for certain ethnic groups). Almost all are autosomal recessive, meaning that you and your partner would have to be carriers for there to be a 1 in 4 chance of the fetus inheriting the disease. You may want to discuss the option of screening with your healthcare provider, as the test has to be ordered by a healthcare professional.

» **Cystic fibrosis (CF):** Cystic fibrosis is one of the most common genetic diseases in the United States, with an incidence of about 1 in 3,500. CF is also a recessive condition, and it's more common among the non-Hispanic white population compared with other racial and ethnic groups. Obstetricians and geneticists recommend that CF screening, through a blood test, be offered to all pregnant couples. Speak to your doctor about CF screening during your first prenatal visit.

Ethnic roots

Even if you and your partner have family histories that are free of any known genetic disorders, your ethnic backgrounds are important because some genetic disorders occur more frequently in one ethnic group than others:

» **Tay-Sachs:** Jewish people of Eastern European descent are ten times more likely than others to carry the rare gene for *Tay-Sachs,* a disease of the nervous system that is usually fatal in early childhood. French Canadians and Cajuns (from Louisiana) also have a higher-than-normal risk of carrying this gene. Most of the time, a simple blood test can determine whether you're a carrier of this disease.

REMEMBER

Although Tay-Sachs and some other conditions are found more frequently among the Jewish population, individuals from other ethnic groups can still be carriers (but that's much less common). For this reason, even if only one member of a couple is Jewish, both should still be tested, if possible.

» **Sickle-cell anemia:** This blood disorder is especially prevalent among people with African or Hispanic ancestors. This condition, too, is recessive, so both members of a couple must be carriers for the baby to be at risk of inheriting the disease.

» **Beta-thalassemia (also known as Mediterranean anemia or Cooley's anemia) and alpha-thalassemia:** People whose ancestors come from Italy, Greece, and other Mediterranean countries are at an elevated risk of having — and passing to their children — genes for beta-thalassemia, a blood disorder. Among Asians, the analogous blood problem is alpha-thalassemia. Both of these disorders produce abnormalities in hemoglobin (the protein in red blood cells that holds onto oxygen) and therefore result in varying degrees of anemia. Both parents have to carry the gene in order for their baby to be at risk of having the disease.

The risks of inheritable diseases overlap from one ethnic or geographic group to another. Genes get passed around among the various populations whenever the parents are from different ethnic groups. But you can roughly gauge whether your ancestry puts you at an elevated risk of carrying genes for certain diseases.

REMEMBER

Some people don't know very much about their ethnic background or family medical history, perhaps because they were adopted or haven't had much contact with their biological families. If this is your situation, don't worry. Keep in mind that the chances of both you and your partner carrying a gene for a particular disorder are extremely low.

OTHER TESTS FOR THOSE OF JEWISH DESCENT

Here's a list of genetic disorders for which screening is available to couples of Jewish descent (although at this time, the American Congress of Obstetricians and Gynecologists recommends only Tay-Sachs, cystic fibrosis, Canavan disease, and familial dysautonomia testing):

- Tay-Sachs
- Cystic fibrosis
- Canavan
- Familial dysautonomia
- Gaucher
- Neimann-Pick
- Mucolipidosis IV
- Fanconi anemia

- Bloom syndrome
- Familial hyperinsulinemia
- Lipoamide dehydrogenase deficiency
- Maple syrup urine disease
- Glycogen storage disease 1a
- Nemaline myopathy
- Usher syndrome

Although recommended for the Ashkenazi Jewish population, these tests are available to everyone.

Considering the physical exam

At your first prenatal visit, your practitioner examines your head, neck, breasts, heart, lungs, abdomen, and extremities. She also performs an internal exam. During this exam, your practitioner evaluates your uterus, cervix, and ovaries and performs, if due, a Pap test (cervix cancer and pre-cancer screening). Also, in many (if not all) states, screening for sexually transmitted infections (STIs) is mandated by law. If your state isn't one in which this screening is required, be sure to let your physician know if you feel you also should be tested for the possibility of sexually transmitted diseases.

After the exam, you and your practitioner will discuss the overall plan for your pregnancy and talk about any possible problems. You can also discuss what medications you can take while you're pregnant, when you should call for help, and what tests you can expect to undergo throughout your pregnancy.

Eyeing the standard tests

Brace yourself: You're probably going to be stuck with a needle and have to pee in a cup during your first prenatal visit. Here's a look at the standard procedures, including blood and urine tests.

Get ready for the prick: Blood tests

On your first prenatal visit, your practitioner will draw your blood for a bunch of standard tests to check your general health as well as to make sure you're immune to certain infections. The following tests are routine:

>> **A standard test for blood type, Rh factor, and antibody status:** The blood type refers to whether your blood is type A, B, AB, or O and whether you're Rh-positive or Rh-negative. The antibody test is designed to tell whether special blood-group antibodies to certain antigens (like the Rh antigen) are present. (See Book 6, Chapter 2 for more about the Rh factor and the implications of blood incompatibilities.)

>> **Complete blood count (CBC):** This test checks for *anemia,* which refers to a low red blood cell count. It also checks your *platelet count* (a component of blood important in clotting).

>> **VDRL or RPR:** These tests check for syphilis. They're very accurate, but sometimes they produce a false positive result if the patient has other conditions, such as lupus or antiphospholipid antibody syndrome (see Book 6, Chapter 3). However, these kinds of false positive results are usually weakly positive. These tests are nonspecific, so in order to confirm the diagnosis of

syphilis, another, more specific blood test should be performed. Because it's essential that syphilis be adequately treated, make sure you receive a test. In fact, most states require it. Unfortunately, the incidence of syphilis is on the rise in the United States.

>> **Hepatitis B:** This test checks for evidence of the hepatitis viruses. These viruses come in several different types, and the hepatitis B virus can be present without producing actual symptoms. In fact, some women are diagnosed only during a blood test, such as the one performed during pregnancy.

>> **Rubella:** Your practitioner also checks for immunity to rubella (also called German measles). Most women have been vaccinated against rubella or, because they've had the illness in the past, their blood carries rubella antibodies, which is why contracting German measles during pregnancy is so rare. Most practitioners test to see that the mother is immune to rubella during the very first prenatal visit. Any woman who isn't immune is counseled to be careful to avoid contact with anyone who has the illness. A practitioner also advises these women to get vaccinated against rubella soon after they deliver so that they aren't susceptible in subsequent pregnancies.

>> **HIV:** Some states require that healthcare providers routinely ask whether you want to be checked for HIV, the virus that causes AIDS. Because medication is available to reduce the risk of transmission to the baby as well as to slow disease progression in the mother, being aware of your HIV status is very important. A doctor can usually perform this test at the same time as the other prenatal blood tests.

Doctors sometimes need to perform other tests during your first prenatal visit. These additional tests include the following (head to Book 6, Chapter 3 for information on many of the conditions and illnesses identified in this list):

>> **Glucose screen:** You usually get this test around 24 to 28 weeks, but your doctor may administer it in the first trimester if you're at a high risk of developing gestational diabetes.

>> **Varicella (chickenpox):** Your doctor may conduct this test to check for immunity to varicella. If you're unsure whether or not you've had chickenpox or you know that you haven't had it, let your practitioner know so you can be tested for immunity.

>> **Toxoplasmosis:** Sometimes a doctor administers a test in order to check for immunity to *toxoplasmosis,* a type of parasitic infection. In the United States, testing for toxoplasmosis isn't considered routine unless you're at a higher risk for contracting it. For example, if you have an outdoor cat and you're the one who changes the litter box, your practitioner is likely to send off a test to check for past or recent exposure. If you're in France, where the incidence of

toxoplasmosis is much higher, your practitioner will probably recommend that you be tested.

» **Cytomegalovirus (CMV):** Testing for CMV, a common childhood infection, isn't routine during pregnancy. However, if you have a lot of contact with school-age children who may have the infection, your practitioner may suggest you have this test. As with toxoplasmosis, the blood test looks for evidence of past or recent infection.

» **Vitamin D:** Vitamin D deficiency is more common in pregnancy than previously thought. In fact, it's quite common in certain high-risk groups, including vegetarians, women who have limited sun exposure, and ethnic minorities. Babies born to vitamin D-deficient moms are also at risk of vitamin D deficiency. When severe, this can lead to problems in the development of the bones in the newborns. A simple blood test for 25-OH-D can indicate vitamin D status. If you do find that you're vitamin D-deficient, your provider may recommend a supplement (in addition to your prenatal multivitamin).

» **Lead screening:** Prenatal lead exposure has been linked to a variety of adverse outcomes for mom and baby. Recently, the Centers for Disease Control and Prevention (CDC) and the American Congress of Obstetricians and Gynecologists (ACOG) have addressed the issue of screening for elevated lead levels in maternal blood. Although they don't recommend routine screening, they do suggest evaluating pregnant women for risk factors and testing those women at high risk. Some risk factors for lead exposure include the following:

- Recent emigration from a place where lead contamination is high

- Living near a high source of lead, such as land mines or battery recycling plants

- Being in close contact with someone who works with lead

- Eating nonfood substances such as soil or paint containing lead or glazed ceramic pottery (*pica* is a disorder where individuals eat nonnutritive substances)

- Using home remedies or certain therapeutic herbs traditionally used by East Indian, Indian, Middle Eastern, West Asian, and Hispanic cultures that may be contaminated with lead

- Having a history of previous lead exposure or living with someone identified as having an elevated lead level

If testing shows you have a high lead level, you need to speak with your doctor about treatment. A diet containing adequate amounts of calcium, iron, zinc, and vitamins C, D, and E is also known to help decrease lead absorption.

Take a quick trip to the bathroom: Urine tests

Each time you visit your practitioner during your pregnancy, including the first prenatal visit, you're asked to give a sample of urine. Your practitioner uses the urine sample to check for the presence of glucose (for a possible sign of diabetes) and protein (for evidence of preeclampsia) and to screen for a UTI.

Sneak the first look at your baby: Ultrasound

An ultrasound uses sound waves to create a picture of the uterus and the baby inside it. Ultrasound examinations don't involve radiation, and the procedure is safe for both you and your baby. Your practitioner may suggest that you undergo a first-trimester ultrasound exam. Often, this ultrasound is performed transvaginally, which means that a special ultrasound probe is inserted into the vagina. The advantage to this technique is that the probe, or transducer, is closer to the fetus, so a much clearer view is attained than with a standard transabdominal ultrasound examination.

REMEMBER

Some women worry that a probe inserted into the vagina could harm the baby. Although understandable, you don't need to worry. The probe is completely safe.

The following are evaluated during a first-trimester ultrasound exam:

>> **The accuracy of your due date:** An ultrasound can show whether the fetus is any larger or smaller than the date of your last menstrual period would suggest. An ultrasound in the first trimester is actually more accurate than a later ultrasound in confirming or establishing your due date.

>> **Fetal viability:** By five to six weeks into your pregnancy, an ultrasound can detect a fetal heartbeat. After a fetal heartbeat has been identified, the risk of miscarriage drops significantly (to about 3 percent). Prior to five weeks, the fetus itself may not be visible; instead, the ultrasound may show only the gestational sac.

>> **Fetal abnormalities:** Although a complete ultrasound examination to detect structural abnormalities in the fetus usually isn't performed until about 20 weeks, some problems may already be visible by 11 to 12 weeks. Much of the brain, spine, limbs, abdomen, and urinary tract structures can be seen with a transvaginal ultrasound. In addition, the presence of a thickening behind the neck of the fetus (known as *increased nuchal translucency*) may indicate an added risk for certain genetic or chromosomal conditions (see Book 2, Chapter 2).

>> **Fetal number:** An ultrasound shows whether you're carrying more than one fetus. In addition, the appearance of the membrane separating the babies, as well as the placental locations, helps indicate whether the babies share one

placenta or have separate placentas. Book 6, Chapter 1 goes into greater detail about this topic.

>> **The condition of your ovaries:** An ultrasound can reveal abnormalities or cysts in your ovaries. Sometimes an ultrasound shows a small cyst, called a *corpus luteal cyst,* which forms at the site where the egg was released. Over the course of three or four months, it gradually goes away. Two other types of cysts, called *dermoid cysts* and *simple cysts,* are unrelated to the pregnancy and may be found incidentally during an ultrasound exam. Whether removal of these types of cysts is necessary and when they should be removed depends on the size of the cyst and any symptoms you may be having.

>> **The presence of fibroid tumors:** Also called *fibroids,* these are benign overgrowths of the muscle of the uterus. Book 6, Chapter 3 goes into more details about these.

>> **Location of the pregnancy:** Occasionally, the pregnancy may be located outside the uterus, which is called an *ectopic pregnancy* (see the "Ectopic pregnancy" section later in this chapter for more information).

Detecting Genetic Abnormalities in the First Trimester: Your Options

With the explosion of genetic technology, there's a whole menu of options for detecting genetic abnormalities in your baby, and many of them can be done in the first trimester. The options fall mainly into two categories: screening tests and diagnostic tests:

>> **Screening:** A screening test collects bits of information about the developing fetus that can be used to estimate the probability that your baby has certain genetic abnormalities; the odds are usually expressed as a ratio (1/100, 1/1,000, 1/10,000, and so on). The bits of information can be substances produced by the placenta that can be measured in the mother's blood, measurements on an ultrasound, or fragments of fetal DNA that circulate in Mom's bloodstream.

>> **Diagnostic:** A diagnostic test uses tiny pieces of placental tissue (chorionic villus sampling, or CVS), fetal skin cells that have flaked off the surface of the baby (amniocentesis), or fetal lymphocytes (fetal blood sampling) to directly look at the tissue to see whether the genetic makeup is normal or abnormal. CVS is the only diagnostic test performed in the first trimester.

The diagnostic tests involve checking the developing baby's chromosomes. Chromosomes carry the genetic information (DNA) that determines what a person is like. People normally have 46 chromosomes — 23 inherited from their mother and 23 from their father. The 23 from each side are paired inside the nucleus of each human cell. Twenty-two of these pairs are *autosomes*, which are the chromosomes that aren't sex-related. The 23rd pair of chromosomes are the sex chromosomes, which can be either XX (girl) or XY (boy).

Certain abnormalities in chromosome number or structure can lead to problems in the baby. For example, *Down syndrome*, one of the more common chromosomal abnormalities associated with severe mental retardation, may occur if the fetus has an extra copy of chromosome 21. (The condition is also known as *trisomy 21*, because the fetus has three copies of the chromosome.)

Amniocentesis, CVS, and other tests detect abnormalities in chromosome number and structure by yielding a *karyotype*, which is an enlarged picture of the individual chromosomes. In addition, if you and the baby's father have a known risk for carrying a genetic disease that runs in your family or ethnic group (Tay-Sachs or cystic fibrosis, for example), your practitioner can use the material obtained during these procedures to test for such diseases. However, unless you're specifically at risk for one of these rare genetic disorders, your practitioner won't routinely administer this testing; the chromosomes are checked only for number and structure.

LOOKING AT MATERNAL AGE

In the past, women who were going to be age 35 or older at their due date were offered the chance to undergo prenatal diagnosis to check the fetal chromosomes. Age 35 was chosen as the target age because a woman's risk of having a baby with a chromosomal abnormality increases significantly after she reaches that age. The cutoff age of 35 is somewhat arbitrary, however, and not followed in all countries. In Great Britain, for example, women are offered prenatal chromosomal testing at age 37 or after.

When nuchal translucency testing became available, the American Congress of Obstetricians and Gynecologists recommended that doctors stop using age to determine who should have a diagnostic test. The current practice is to offer every woman the same thing and allow her to choose which test or tests she wants to undergo.

Even among women at risk for a chromosomal problem, some choose not to be tested, either because they don't want to run any risk of miscarriage associated with the test or because of their personal beliefs about terminating a pregnancy. Even if pregnancy termination isn't something you would consider, prior knowledge of a fetus's abnormalities can give you time to make preparations for a child who may have special needs.

Chorionic villus sampling (CVS)

Chorionic villi are tiny, budlike pieces of tissue that make up the placenta. Because they develop from cells arising out of the fertilized egg, they have the same genetic makeup as the developing fetus. By checking a sample of chorionic villi, the laboratory can see whether the chromosomes are normal in number and structure, determine the fetal sex, and test for some specific diseases (if the fetus may be at risk for these diseases).

Your doctor performs a chorionic villus sampling (CVS) by withdrawing placental tissue (containing chorionic villi) either through a hollow needle inserted through the abdomen (*transabdominal CVS*) or through a flexible catheter inserted through the cervix (*transcervical CVS,* seen in Figure 1-2), depending on where the placenta is located within the uterus and the uterus's general shape and position. Your doctor uses ultrasound equipment as a guide as she performs the procedure. She then examines the tissue under a microscope, and the cells are cultured in a laboratory.

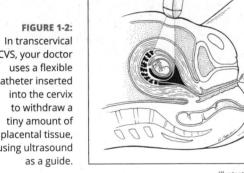

FIGURE 1-2: In transcervical CVS, your doctor uses a flexible catheter inserted into the cervix to withdraw a tiny amount of placental tissue, using ultrasound as a guide.

Illustration by Kathryn Born, MA

Like amniocentesis, CVS raises the risk of miscarriage slightly — about 1/1,000. Neither CVS method is riskier than the other. The person performing the test should have plenty of experience doing the procedure, and experience reduces the risk.

CVS results are typically available in seven to ten days. The main advantage that CVS has over amniocentesis is that it can provide information earlier in the pregnancy. This time factor may be important to women who feel that termination is an option if severe abnormalities are present.

REMEMBER

If you undergo CVS and are Rh-negative, you should receive an injection of Rh-immune globulin (such as Rhophylac or Rhogam) following the procedure to prevent you from developing Rh disease (see Chapter 2 in Book 6).

Noninvasive screening in the first trimester

CVS and early amniocentesis (which is no longer recommended due to concerns about causing birth defects) are the only tests that can give definitive information about fetal chromosomes during the first trimester. There are two screening tests now available in the first trimester.

First Trimester Screen

The First Trimester Screen uses a combination of a special ultrasound measurement, called *nuchal translucency*, and two substances found in Mom's blood. Eighty to 90 percent of fetuses with Down syndrome may be detected through this type of screening.

These first-trimester screening tests are usually performed between the approximate gestational ages of 10 weeks, 4 days and 13 weeks, 6 days. Here's how they work:

>> **Nuchal translucency (NT):** This test uses ultrasound to measure a special area behind the fetal neck. Only physicians specially trained in the procedure should conduct a nuchal translucency test. Combining measurements of nuchal translucency with blood screening tests probably increases the accuracy of these tests.

>> **Serum screening:** Tests that check the levels of PAPP-A, a substance produced by the placenta, and hCG, a hormone in the mother's blood, may help screen for Down syndrome in the first trimester. Usually, this blood test is done around the same time as the ultrasound to measure the nuchal translucency.

The equation to calculate the risk for Down syndrome takes into account the nuchal translucency, the two blood components mentioned previously, a measurement of the length of the embryo called the *crown to rump length* (CRL), and your age at your expected due date. The results come as a risk ratio — like 1/310.

>> If the screening shows your chances of having a baby with Down syndrome are high, your doctor will recommend that you have a diagnostic test. CVS (see the preceding section) can be done in the first trimester, but for amniocentesis, you have to wait until the second trimester.

>> If your results are good (for example, if they show that you have a low risk for Down syndrome), you may want to wait until the second trimester and have a Quad Test (see Book 2, Chapter 2). The results of this test will be integrated with the First Trimester Screen to even further refine your risk for Down syndrome. Doing the tests this way will detect almost 96 to 98 percent of fetuses with Down syndrome.

NIPS (noninvasive prenatal screening)

The newest way of screening for Down syndrome is called NIPS, or *noninvasive prenatal screening.* For this procedure, a sample of blood is drawn from Mom and sent to the lab, where tiny fragments of the baby's DNA (which are normally present in small quantities in Mom's blood) are isolated and analyzed. This method can detect about 98 to 99 percent of babies with Down syndrome.

The sample of blood can be drawn and sent anytime during pregnancy, but it's best to do it in the first trimester so you can get the results back in time to make reproductive choices that are right for you. You can also predict the gender with this test. NIPS also detects many cases of trisomy 13 and 18 (which are disorders similar to Down syndrome, but different chromosomes are involved) but not at the same detection rate as for Down syndrome.

The original studies on NIPS were done on high-risk women (women over the age of 35, with a family history of chromosomal abnormalities, or with high-risk First Trimester Screen results), so that's whom the test was recommended for. Recently, however, data suggests that NIPS may be useful in low-risk women too.

Recognizing Causes for Concern

In each trimester, a few things may go less than smoothly. This section describes some of the things that can happen during the first trimester of your pregnancy and what they may mean to you.

Bleeding

Early in pregnancy, around the time of your missed period, experiencing a little bleeding from the vagina isn't uncommon. The amount of bleeding is usually less than what you'd expect with a period and lasts for only one or two days. This is called *implantation bleeding,* and it happens when the fertilized egg attaches to the uterus's lining. Bleeding due to implantation isn't a cause for concern, but many women may be confused by it and mistake it for their period.

Bleeding also may occur later in the first trimester, but it doesn't necessarily indicate a miscarriage. About one-third of women experience bleeding during the first trimester, and the majority of them go on to have perfectly healthy babies. Bleeding is especially common in women carrying more than one fetus — and again, most go on to have normal pregnancies. Bright red bleeding usually indicates active bleeding, while dark staining usually indicates old blood that is making its way out from the cervix and vagina. Most of the time, an ultrasound exam doesn't show any evidence of the source of the bleeding. However, sometimes a collection of blood, known as a *subchorionic* or *retroplacental hemorrhage* or *collection*, is visible and indicates an area of bleeding from behind the placenta. It usually takes several weeks for this blood to be reabsorbed. During this time, some dark blood continues to pass out through the cervix and vagina.

WARNING

In some cases, bleeding can be the first sign of an impending miscarriage (see the next section for more information). In this case, the bleeding often accompanies abdominal cramping. However, keep in mind that the vast majority of women who experience bleeding go on to have a completely normal pregnancy.

WARNING

If you notice some bleeding, let your practitioner know. If the bleeding is a small amount and not associated with a lot of abdominal cramping, it isn't an emergency. However, if you're bleeding heavily (much more than a period), call your practitioner as soon as you can. She may want to do an ultrasound and perform a pelvic exam to investigate the cause of the bleeding and see whether the pregnancy is still viable and located inside the uterus. Most of the time, your practitioner can do very little about the bleeding. Some doctors may suggest that you rest at home for a few days and avoid exercise and sex. No scientific data supports these instructions, but given that no really good alternatives exist, they certainly don't hurt.

Miscarriage

The great majority of pregnancies proceed normally. But about one in five ends in early miscarriage, often before a woman even knows she's pregnant. If a miscarriage occurs early in a pregnancy, you may mistake it for a regular menstrual period. About half the time, chromosomal abnormalities in the embryo cause the miscarriage. In another 20 percent of cases, the embryo may have structural defects that are too small to be detectable by ultrasound or pathological examination. *Note:* Having one miscarriage doesn't mean that you have an increased chance of its happening again. Also, no routine everyday activities can cause a miscarriage.

WARNING

Miscarriage may lead to cramping and bleeding. You may feel abdominal pains that are stronger than menstrual cramps, and you may pass fetal and placental tissue. In cases where all the tissue is passed, your practitioner doesn't need to do anything else. Often, though, some tissue remains in your uterus, and you may need medication to encourage its passing or have a D&C *(dilation and curettage)* procedure, designed to empty the uterus. Your doctor dilates, or gently opens, the cervix with surgical instruments and then empties the remaining contents of the uterus with a suction device and/or a scraping of the uterus. A D&C can be performed either in the doctor's office or in an operating suite, depending on the doctor, the gestational age, and any other important medical problems.

Sometimes, you may have no overt signs of miscarriage. Your practitioner may discover during a routine prenatal visit that the fetus is no longer alive, which is known as a *missed abortion.* If you have a missed abortion very early in your pregnancy, a D&C may not be necessary. But if it happens later in the first trimester, you may need to have a D&C to reduce the risk of heavy bleeding or incomplete passage of tissue. Depending on your obstetrical history and your desire to try to determine the cause of the miscarriage, you may decide to have the tissue sent for genetic analysis (to find out whether the chromosomes were normal or abnormal). Because half of all miscarriages are due to chromosomal abnormalities, it may be useful to find out whether this was the cause.

REMEMBER

Unfortunately, most miscarriages can't be prevented. Many, if not most, of them may simply be nature's way of handling an abnormal pregnancy. However, having a miscarriage doesn't mean that you can't have a perfectly normal pregnancy in the future. In fact, even in women who have had two consecutive miscarriages, the chances are very good (about 70 percent) that the next pregnancy will be successful without any special treatment.

TECHNICAL STUFF

Any woman who experiences two or three consecutive miscarriages *may* have some underlying condition that can be identified and possibly treated. She should have a complete physical examination and undergo special tests to look for causes. Some women who have even one miscarriage may want to be examined. If you miscarry, discuss with your practitioner the possibility of undergoing certain tests or sending fetal or placental tissue to a laboratory for chromosomal analysis.

Ectopic pregnancy

An *ectopic pregnancy* occurs when the fertilized egg implants outside the uterus — in one of the fallopian tubes, the ovary, the abdomen, or the cervix. An ectopic pregnancy is a serious threat to the mother's health. Fortunately, ultrasound has advanced to the point that it can detect ectopic pregnancies very early.

WARNING

Signs of an ectopic pregnancy include vaginal bleeding, abdominal pain, pelvic pain, dizziness, and feeling faint. You may not have any symptoms, in which case your doctor identifies the condition during an ultrasound. Your doctor can treat the problem in one of several ways, depending on the location of the embryo or fetus, how far along the pregnancy is, and the symptoms you're experiencing. Unfortunately, a doctor can't move the embryo or fetus to the uterus so that the pregnancy can continue as normal.

Chapter 2

The Second Trimester

The second trimester, which encompasses the three months between weeks 13 and 26, is often the most enjoyable part of pregnancy. The feelings of nausea and fatigue so common during the first trimester are usually gone, and you feel more energetic and comfortable. The second trimester is a very exciting time because you can feel the baby moving within you and you're finally starting to show. During the second trimester, blood tests, prenatal tests, and ultrasound (sonogram) can confirm that the baby is healthy and growing normally. And many women find they can finally grasp the concept that they'll soon be having a baby. The second trimester is often the time you start sharing the exciting news with family, friends, and coworkers.

Following Your Baby's Development

Your baby grows rapidly during the second trimester, as you can see in Figure 2-1. The fetus measures about 3 inches (8 centimeters) long at 13 weeks. By 26 weeks, she's about 14 inches (35 centimeters) and weighs about 2¼ pounds (1,022 grams). Somewhere between weeks 14 and 16, the limbs begin to elongate and start to look like arms and legs. Coordinated arm and leg movements are observable on

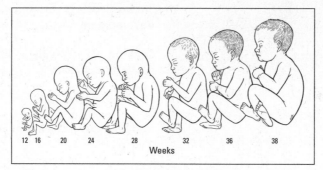

FIGURE 2-1: During the second trimester (13 to 26 weeks), your baby grows and develops at an astounding rate.

12 16 20 24 28 32 36 38
Weeks

Illustration by Kathryn Born, MA

ultrasound, too. Between 18 and 22 weeks, you may begin to feel fetal movements, although they don't necessarily occur regularly throughout the day.

The baby's head, which was large in relation to the body during the first trimester, becomes more proportional as the body catches up. The bones solidify and are recognizable on ultrasound. Early in the second trimester, the fetus looks something like an alien (think E.T.), but by 26 weeks, she looks much more like a human baby.

The fetus also performs many recognizable activities. She not only moves but also undergoes regular periods of sleeping and wakefulness and can hear and swallow. Lung development increases markedly between 20 and 25 weeks. By 24 weeks, lung cells begin to secrete *surfactant,* a chemical substance that enables the lungs to stay expanded. Between 26 and 28 weeks, the eyes — which had been fused shut — open, and hair (called *lanugo*) appears on the head and body. Fat deposits form under the skin, and the central nervous system matures dramatically.

At 23 to 24 weeks, the fetus is considered *viable,* which means that if she were born at this time, she would have a chance of surviving in a center with a neonatal unit experienced in caring for very premature babies. A premature baby born at 28 weeks (nearly three months early) and cared for in an intensive care unit has an excellent chance of survival.

Most mothers begin to feel their babies move at about this time. Knowing for sure when you first feel your baby moving inside you is difficult. Many women sense fluttering movements (called *quickening*) at about 16 to 20 weeks. Not every woman can tell that sensation is actually the baby moving. Some think it's just gas (and maybe you *did* eat too much chili), but most likely, it's the baby. Around 20 to 22 weeks, the fetal movements are much easier to identify, but they still aren't consistent. Over the course of the next four weeks, they fall into a more regular pattern.

Different babies have different movement patterns. You may notice your baby tends to move more at night — perhaps to prepare you for all the sleepless nights you'll have after she's born! Or you may simply be more aware of the baby's movements at night because you're more sedentary at that time. If this is your second (or third or fourth. . .) child, you may start to feel movements a couple of weeks earlier.

REMEMBER

Just because you haven't felt your baby move at all by 22 weeks doesn't mean you need to worry. A common explanation for not feeling the baby's movements is that the placenta is implanted on the anterior (front) wall of the uterus between the baby and your skin. The placenta acts as a cushion and delays the time when you first feel movements. Just let your practitioner know. He may recommend an ultrasound, especially if you haven't had one already, to check the baby.

WARNING

After 26 to 28 weeks, if you stop feeling the baby move as much as usual, call your practitioner. By 28 weeks, you should feel movement at least six times an hour after you eat dinner. If you aren't sure whether the baby is moving normally, lie down on your left side and count the movements. If the baby moves — any movement counts — at least six times in an hour, be reassured that the baby is okay. On the other hand, if you feel that the baby's movements are still less than they should be, call your practitioner.

CLOTHING YOURSELF IN MATERNITY GARB

Thank goodness the fashion industry has recognized that women continue to care about looking chic and professional when they're pregnant — which doesn't necessarily mean wearing those choir-boy blouses with big bows at the neck. Many women look forward to shopping for maternity clothes, while others aim to stay in their usual clothes for as long as possible. Keep in mind that you're going to need maternity clothes only for a few months, and they're not cheap. So don't be shy about accepting hand-me-downs (your friends are probably happy to see their clothes get more use) and check out consignment shops, secondhand stores, and garage sales, where you can often buy inexpensive, gently used maternity clothes. Or forgo maternity clothes altogether: You can often go a long way through your pregnancy in regular leggings and big shirts or sweaters.

Perhaps the most important items to buy are comfortable shoes and roomier bras. Both shoe size and bra size can increase during pregnancy. (And you don't have to wear special maternity underwear — unless you find it especially comfortable. Many kinds of regular underwear, especially the bikini kind, fit well under a bulging belly.)

Understanding Your Changing Body

By 12 weeks, your uterus begins to rise out of your pelvis. Your practitioner can feel the top of the uterus through your abdominal wall. By 20 weeks, the top of your uterus reaches the level of your navel. Then each week, your uterus grows by about 1 centimeter (½ inch). Your doctor may run a tape measure from your pubic bone to the top of your uterus to measure the *fundal height* (see Book 1, Chapter 2) to see that your uterus and the baby are growing appropriately. Many women begin to show at 16 weeks, although looking pregnant varies a great deal. Some women look pregnant at 12 weeks; others aren't obvious until 28 weeks.

FOR PARTNERS: WATCHING MOM GROW

"Honey, do you think I'm fat and ugly now?" You may start to hear this question during the second trimester when the mother's body really begins to change. Tread lightly when making comments about your partner's belly size. Maybe you're just being observant, but it's a great way to get the cold shoulder without intending it! Here's a tip: It's not a multiple-choice question. You have only one answer, and you may as well commit it to memory so that you can answer without hesitation: "Absolutely not, honey. You're the most beautiful woman I've ever laid eyes on."

Enjoy the second trimester. Often, it's the most fun part of pregnancy for both parents. Morning sickness fades away, fatigue subsides, and your partner begins to feel the baby move around inside her. Often, you, too, can feel the baby move by placing your hand on the mom's abdomen.

During this trimester, many mothers get an ultrasound exam to check the baby's anatomy. Try to go along to see the ultrasound exam; it's one of the most enjoyable prenatal tests. You get to see the baby's hands, feet, and face, and you get to watch the baby move around. For the first time, you see the living, moving, growing little human inside, and suddenly the whole enterprise seems so much more real!

By the end of the second trimester, you may begin prenatal classes. Don't make excuses! Go with your partner. The classes are designed for both the partner and mother. During this time, you can find out how to be useful during labor and delivery. And you can also ask questions about what to anticipate — to relieve some of your own anxiety.

Many of the changes you experience have little to do with your belly's size. Rather, they involve your baby's development and your body's continuing adaptation to pregnancy. You may experience some, none, or all of the symptoms in this section.

Forgetfulness and clumsiness

You may have heard that misplacing keys, bumping into furniture, and dropping things are side effects of pregnancy. Although there seems to be no medical explanation for these effects, some women do feel they're more scatterbrained and clumsy. If it happens to you, don't worry. You're not losing your mind. Look at it this way: Now you have an excuse for having forgotten your best friend's birthday. And rest assured you'll go back to being your brilliant, coordinated self after your baby is born.

Gas

You may find that you develop the annoying and embarrassing tendency to burp and pass gas at inopportune times during this trimester. If it's any consolation, you're not the first pregnant woman to run into this problem. Unfortunately, though, you can do very little about it — besides getting a dog to blame it on. Try to avoid becoming constipated (see Book 2, Chapter 1) because that can make things worse. Also avoid eating large meals that may leave you feeling bloated and uncomfortable or foods that you know make the problem even worse.

Hair and nail growth

While you're pregnant, your fingernails and toenails may become stronger than they've ever been before and grow at an unprecedented rate. Manicures are safe when done in a reputable, clean salon, and they often relieve stress, so sit back and enjoy your beautiful nails!

Pregnancy also speeds up hair growth. Unfortunately, some women find hair also begins growing in unusual places — on their face or stomach, for example. Waxing, plucking, or shaving the unwanted hair is safe, but hair removal creams (depilatories) contain chemicals that haven't been extensively studied. Because safer alternatives are readily available, avoid these creams. Take comfort in the likelihood that the unwanted hair will disappear after your baby is born.

Heartburn

Heartburn — the burning sensation you feel when stomach acids rise into your esophagus — is common during pregnancy. Heartburn has two basic causes (neither of which validates the myth that heartburn means your baby will have a lot of hair):

>> The high level of progesterone your body is producing can slow digestion and relax the sphincter muscle between the esophagus and the stomach, which normally prevents the upward movement of stomach acids.

>> As the uterus grows, it presses upward on the stomach, which can push stomach acids into the esophagus.

For tips on how to avoid or manage heartburn, refer to Book 1, Chapter 4. And if it becomes intolerable, talk to your doctor about taking a prescription treatment. Many effective heartburn treatments are considered safe for use during pregnancy. The use of famotidine (Pepcid), ranitidine (Zantac), and omeprazole (Prilosec/Nexium) in the first trimester has been studied, and researchers found no increased risk for birth defects, preterm labor, or problems with fetal growth. (The first trimester is the period of greatest risk, so medications proven safe for use in the first trimester are presumably safe in the second trimester, too.)

Lower abdominal/groin pain

REMEMBER

Between 18 and 24 weeks, you may feel a sharp pain or a dull ache near your groin on either or both sides. When you move quickly or stand, you may notice it worsen, and it may fade if you lie down. This pain is called *round ligament pain.* The round ligaments are bands of fibrous tissue on each side of the uterus that attach the top of the uterus to the labia. The pain occurs because as the uterus grows, the ligaments stretch. The pain can be quite uncomfortable and sometimes can stop you in your tracks, but it's normal. The good news is that it usually goes away — or at least lessens considerably — after 24 weeks.

Sometime in the middle of the second trimester (the exact time varies), you may start to feel mild, short-lived contractions or cramps. These are referred to as *Braxton-Hicks contractions* and are nothing to worry about. They often are more noticeable when you're walking or physically active and then go away when you get off your feet. If they become uncomfortable and regular (more than six in an hour), call your practitioner.

Nasal congestion

The increased blood flow that occurs during pregnancy can cause stuffiness and some swelling of the mucous membranes inside your nose. This, in turn, can lead to postnasal drip and, ultimately, a chronic cough. Nasal saline drops may provide some relief and are perfectly safe to use during pregnancy. Keeping the air in your home or office well humidified also helps. Nasal sprays and decongestants work, too, but avoid using these medications for more than a few days at a time.

You (or your partner, especially) may notice that suddenly you're snoring like never before! This common symptom again relates to the increase in nasal congestion. To treat this? Lovingly suggest that your partner buy a good set of earplugs!

Nosebleeds and bleeding gums

Because of the higher volume of blood coursing through your body to support your pregnancy, you may experience some bleeding from small blood vessels in your nose and gums. This bleeding usually stops by itself, but you can help by applying slight pressure to the point of bleeding. If bleeding becomes particularly heavy or frequent, call your doctor.

TIP

Using a softer toothbrush may help minimize bleeding when you brush your teeth.

Skin changes

The hormones coursing through your body at soaring levels may make strange things happen to your skin. These changes, illustrated in Figure 2-2, don't occur in all women, and if they do happen to you, rest assured they usually fade away after the baby is born.

>> You may notice a dark line, called the *linea nigra,* on your lower abdomen running from your pubic bone up to your navel. This line may be more noticeable in women with relatively dark skin. Fair-skinned women often don't develop this line at all.

>> The skin on your face may darken in a masklike distribution around your cheeks, nose, and eyes. This darkening is called *chloasma* or the *mask of pregnancy.* Sun exposure makes it even darker. Use a facial cream with sunblock to minimize the effects of the sun on chloasma.

>> Red spots, called *spider angiomas,* may suddenly appear anywhere on your body. Press on them, and they probably turn white. These spots are concentrations of blood vessels caused by the high level of estrogen in your body. They'll probably disappear after delivery.

>> Some women notice a reddish coloring on the palms of their hands known as *palmar erythema.* This coloring is another estrogen effect, and it, too, will go away.

>> *Skin tags* (small, benign skin growths) are a common occurrence, although it isn't totally clear why they develop. Fortunately, they, too, fade away or disappear after pregnancy. Because they're likely to resolve in time, you don't need to rush to the dermatologist to have them removed, unless they're really bothersome.

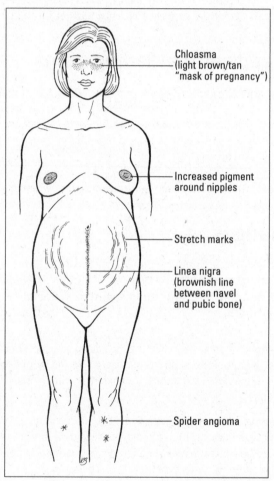

Chloasma (light brown/tan "mask of pregnancy")

Increased pigment around nipples

Stretch marks

Linea nigra (brownish line between navel and pubic bone)

Spider angioma

FIGURE 2-2: Some common skin changes associated with pregnancy.

Illustration by Kathryn Born, MA

Checking In: Prenatal Visits

In the second trimester, you're likely to see your practitioner about once every four weeks. At each visit, he checks your weight, your blood pressure, your urine, and the fetal heart rate. You may want to bring up any questions you have about fetal movement, childbirth classes, your weight gain, and any unusual symptoms or discomfort you have.

As your baby grows and changes, so does the range and scope of possible prenatal tests. In the second trimester, you'll likely undergo a blood test or two and an ultrasound for a general scan of your baby's anatomy, growth, and well-being. At this point, you can find out the sex of your baby. Amniocentesis may also be performed in the second trimester. This section outlines the tests you may undergo.

Second-trimester blood tests

The blood tests covered in this section usually yield normal results, but if yours are at all unusual, you may need further testing — an ultrasound examination, perhaps. But keep in mind that further testing doesn't necessarily mean that anything is wrong — only that your practitioner is being careful to ensure that everything is okay.

Alpha-fetoprotein screen

MSAFP stands for *maternal serum alpha-fetoprotein*, a protein made by the fetus that also circulates in the mother's bloodstream. Doctors use a simple blood test to check the level of MSAFP, usually sometime between 15 and 18 weeks. The test result is affected by weight, race, and preexisting diabetes, so it has to be adjusted for those factors. An elevated MSAFP is expressed as more than 2.0 or 2.5 *multiples of the median*, or MOMs, for women carrying only one baby and more than 4.0 or 4.5 MOMs for mothers of twins. (In triplets and quadruplets, the measurement hasn't been well studied.)

Abnormal MSAFP can usually indicate whether a pregnancy is at risk for certain complications and *may* indicate

>> Underestimation of the fetus's age (how far along you are)

>> The presence of twins or more

>> Bleeding that may have occurred earlier in the pregnancy

>> Neural tube defects (spina bifida, anencephaly, and others)

>> Abdominal wall defects (protrusion of the fetus's abdominal contents through a defect in the abdominal wall)

>> Rh disease (see Book 6, Chapter 2) or other conditions associated with *fetal edema* (abnormal fluid collection in the fetus)

>> Increased risk for low birth weight, preeclampsia, or other complications (see Book 6, Chapter 2)

>> A rare fetal kidney condition known as *congenital nephrosis*

>> Fetal death

>> Other fetal abnormalities

REMEMBER

Remember that the MSAFP test is only a screening test. Most women with an elevated MSAFP have a normal fetus and continue to have a completely normal pregnancy. Only about 5 percent of women with a positive maternal serum screen actually have a fetus with a neural tube defect. On the other hand, the test isn't perfect, and therefore it can't identify all abnormal fetuses. To reduce the risk of getting a false positive result (that is, an abnormal test result but a normal fetus), a positive test should be repeated (especially if it's only mildly elevated or under 3.0 MOMs), and an ultrasound should be performed to confirm the fetus's age. If a test comes back elevated a second time or if it's greater than 3.0 MOMs on the first screen, a detailed ultrasound exam should be done to look for abnormalities.

UNDERSTANDING NEURAL TUBE DEFECTS

The baby's central nervous system begins as a flat sheet of cells that rolls up into a tube as it matures. The front of the tube, which closes at about day 23 of life, becomes the brain. The other end of the tube, which closes at about day 28 of life, becomes the lower end of the spinal cord. If either end fails to close for some reason (nobody knows why it sometimes doesn't), a *neural tube defect* occurs. The most common neural tube defects are *spina bifida* (an opening in the spine), *anencephaly* (absence of the skull), and *encephalocele* (an opening in the skull). These defects cause abnormalities in the nervous system such as paralysis, extra fluid in the brain, or mental retardation. Fetuses with anencephaly usually don't survive more than a few days after birth.

This all sounds pretty scary, but fortunately, these defects are rare. In the United States, a neural tube defect occurs about once in every 1,000 babies born. The incidence in the United Kingdom is higher: 4 to 8 cases in every 1,000 babies. In Japan, the incidence is quite low, at about 1 case per 2,000 babies. No one knows exactly why the incidence varies among countries, but it has something to do with the interaction between the environment and one's genetic makeup. If you or your baby's father has a family history of neural tube defects, let your practitioner know at your first visit, because that slightly raises your risk of having a baby with a neural tube defect, and you can discuss your options for prenatal diagnosis (ultrasound or amniocentesis).

You can reduce the likelihood of having a baby with a neural tube defect by taking folic acid before you conceive and by getting your blood sugar under control if you have diabetes. If you had a previous pregnancy in which a neural tube defect was diagnosed or if you have a family history of this condition, increase the amount of folic acid you take at the beginning of pregnancy to 4 mg per day. The earlier in pregnancy you start taking it, the better it is at preventing neural tube defects.

If you have two elevated MSAFP tests, a very high single test, or a questionable ultrasound for spine and head defects, you may want to have an amniocentesis to check the level of AFP in the amniotic fluid (see the section "Testing with amniocentesis" later in this chapter). Your practitioner can also check the amniotic fluid for a substance called *acetylcholinesterase,* which is present if the fetus has an open neural tube defect (see the nearby sidebar "Understanding neural tube defects").

In most cases, the amniotic fluid AFP is negative and the pregnancy continues normally. Some studies suggest, however, that women who have an abnormal MSAFP and then a normal amniotic fluid AFP *may* be at risk for preterm delivery, low birth-weight babies, or hypertension. If you fit the pattern, your doctor may suggest that you and your baby be closely observed, either with ultrasound or with other tests of fetal well-being, such as nonstress tests (see Book 2, Chapter 3). Specific protocols for fetal monitoring vary from doctor to doctor.

The quadruple test for Down syndrome

Another test that can be performed with the same sample of blood that's used for the MSAFP during the second trimester is a screening test for Down syndrome — the most common chromosomal abnormality in babies. This test can also help identify women at risk of having babies with other chromosomal abnormalities, like trisomy 18 or trisomy 13 (an extra copy of the number 18 or 13 chromosome). These particular chromosomal abnormalities are associated with severe birth defects and are often incompatible with life.

Your practitioner performs this test by measuring four substances in the blood: MSAFP, hCG (human chorionic gonadotropin), estriol (a form of estrogen), and inhibin A (a substance secreted by the placenta).

Your practitioner uses the results of these tests to calculate risk for Down syndrome. In women under the age of 35, the test detects Down syndrome in about 80 percent of the cases where it's present. (In other words, if 100 women carrying fetuses with Down syndrome had the test, the condition would be diagnosed in about 80 of them.) This test is only a screening, so even if the result is abnormal, the fetus is normal in the majority of cases. If your test is abnormal, your practitioner will discuss with you the possibility of having an amniocentesis to check the baby's chromosomes. The quad test is often combined with the first-trimester tests described in Book 2, Chapter 1 to improve the detection of Down syndrome.

TIP

Unlike the screen for neural tube defects, which yields a high MSAFP and is often repeated when abnormal, the screens for Down syndrome should *not* be repeated, because doing so will only provide a less accurate result.

Cell-free fetal DNA

If abnormalities are suspected on your baby's ultrasound, your doctor may recommend sending off a sample of your blood to check the baby's chromosomes. This test examines the cell-free fetal DNA that circulates in your blood and is the same test that is discussed in Book 2, Chapter 1.

Glucose screen

The *glucose screen* is a test to identify women who may have gestational diabetes. Your practitioner conducts the test by first having you drink a super-sweet glucose mixture (it tastes like flat soda) and then, exactly one hour later, drawing a sample of blood. He checks this sample for the level of glucose (sugar). High levels indicate that you're at risk for gestational diabetes. To understand why treating gestational diabetes is important, go to Book 6, Chapter 3.

The one-hour screening test is usually performed between 24 and 28 weeks, though some doctors do it twice — once early in the pregnancy and again at 24 to 28 weeks. About 25 percent of obstetricians test only those women who are at risk for gestational diabetes. The risk factors, which follow, are broad, and about 50 percent of all pregnant women have one of them:

>> Maternal age greater than 25 years

>> Previous birth of a large infant

>> Previous unexplained fetal death

>> Previous pregnancy with gestational diabetes

>> Strong family history of diabetes

>> Obesity

If your initial glucose screening test is abnormal, you don't necessarily have gestational diabetes. (Remember, it's only a screening test.) Only about 5 percent of pregnant women actually develop gestational diabetes (although 15 percent may screen positive). Your practitioner will recommend another test that tells whether gestational diabetes is really present. This three-hour test involves drawing blood after you fast overnight, having you drink a different glucose mixture, and then drawing blood three more times, at one, two, and three hours later. Some practitioners recommend eating an extra helping of pasta or rice for the three days before the test (called *carbohydrate loading*) in order to get your body ready for the test.

A test is considered *positive* — or abnormal — if two (or more) of the four blood levels are in the abnormal range. If you test positive for gestational diabetes, your doctor will put you on a special diet and check your glucose levels throughout the remainder of your pregnancy. If you have elevated glucose levels despite adhering to this special diet, you may need to be on insulin or an oral medication to keep your sugars well controlled. (See Book 6, Chapter 3 for more on this topic.)

Complete blood count (CBC)

Many obstetricians check a complete blood count at the same time that they do your glucose test in order to see whether you've developed significant *anemia* (iron deficiency) or a variety of other (less-common) problems. Anemia is common during pregnancy, and some women need to take extra iron. A CBC also gives your physician a platelet count (platelets help with clotting).

Looking at sound waves: Ultrasound

An *ultrasound* (also referred to as a *sonogram*) exam is an incredibly useful tool that allows you and your doctor to see the baby inside your uterus. A device called a *transducer* emits sound waves. The sound waves are reflected off the fetus and converted into an image that appears on a monitor. You can see almost all the structures in the fetus's body, and you can see the fetus moving around and performing all her normal activities — kicking, waving, and so on. The best time to view the baby's anatomy is around 18 to 22 weeks.

An ultrasound exam doesn't hurt. Your practitioner spreads gel or lotion over your abdomen and then moves the transducer around through the gel (see Figure 2-3). A full bladder isn't necessary, because the amniotic fluid surrounding the fetus provides the liquid needed to transmit the sound waves to create a clear or detailed picture. Picture quality varies, depending on maternal fat, scar tissue, and the fetus's position.

A doctor (an obstetrician, a perinatologist, or a radiologist) or an ultrasound technologist may perform the ultrasound. Sometimes a technologist does a preliminary exam, and the doctor comes in later to check on images or review the printed pictures.

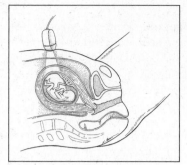

Illustration by Kathryn Born, MA

What an ultrasound can reveal

Ultrasound is like a checkup for the fetus. It can provide information about the following:

>> Number of babies

>> Gestational age

>> Rate of fetal growth

>> Fetal position, movement, and breathing exercises (the fetus moves her chest and abdomen as if she were breathing air)

>> Fetal heart rate

>> Amount of amniotic fluid

>> Location of placenta

>> General fetal anatomy, including the identification of some birth defects

>> The baby's sex (after 15 to 16 weeks), although depending on the position of the fetus, the sex may be difficult to discern

Typically, the examiner measures the fetus first and then studies her anatomy. The extent and degree of detail of the exam varies from woman to woman and doctor to doctor. A detailed ultrasound can examine these structures:

>> Arms and legs

>> Bladder

>> Brain and skull

>> Face

>> Genitalia

>> Heart, chest cavity, and diaphragm

>> Kidneys

>> Spine

>> Stomach, abdominal cavity, and abdominal wall

REMEMBER

The technology used in ultrasounds has been in widespread use for more than 40 years, and overwhelmingly most studies show no harmful consequences for the baby or mom. In addition, the information provided by an ultrasound examination has been shown to have many health benefits. For example, certain conditions (such as bladder outlet obstruction) may be treated during the pregnancy, and the diagnosis of others (such as a congenital heart defect) allow for careful planning for delivery. Detection of problems with fetal growth or amniotic fluid volume lets your doctor know that close surveillance of the pregnancy may be indicated.

Reasons for having an ultrasound

Whether and how often you need an ultrasound depends on your particular risk factors, your doctor's preferences, and your insurance coverage. Some doctors recommend that all women have an ultrasound exam at about 20 weeks; others feel that it's unnecessary if your risks are low. Multiple ultrasound examinations may be needed if any of the following conditions arise:

>> You're carrying twins or more.

>> Your doctor suspects that the baby is too small or too large for her age.

>> Your doctor suspects that you have too little or too much amniotic fluid.

>> You're at risk for preterm labor or incompetent cervix (find out more later in this chapter and Book 6, Chapter 2).

>> You have diabetes, hypertension, or other underlying medical conditions (see Book 6, Chapter 2).

>> You're bleeding.

>> Your doctor wants to do a *biophysical profile,* which is an assessment of fetal well-being that looks at movement, breathing exercises, amniotic fluid volume, and fetal tone (ability to flex the muscles).

Recently, doctors have also used ultrasound to get an accurate measurement of the *cervix* (the uterus's opening) in women at risk for preterm delivery or incompetent cervix. Your practitioner places a transducer in the vagina to measure the cervix's length and check the appearance of the lower part of the uterus.

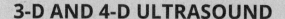

3-D AND 4-D ULTRASOUND

Most perinatal ultrasound centers now have special machines with the capability of showing three-dimensional images of the fetus, known as *3-D ultrasound*. *4-D ultrasound* is similar, but instead of seeing a still (static) 3-D picture, you can see the fetus move. These high-tech ultrasound machines aren't available everywhere, and no medical data has shown that a 3-D or 4-D ultrasound is better at detecting problems than the usual 2-D image. However, you may see certain features in the fetus better, such as the face, hands, and feet. Also, many women experience a real bonding with the fetus, seeing it three-dimensionally. If a 3-D or 4-D ultrasound is available, you may enjoy and benefit from the experience. If not, don't feel bad; you'll have the baby — all four dimensions of it — in real life soon enough.

Testing with amniocentesis

Amniocentesis is a test performed by inserting a thin, hollow needle into the amniotic fluid and then withdrawing some of the fluid through the needle into a syringe (see Figure 2-4). The amniotic fluid can then be tested in a variety of ways. If your practitioner performs a *genetic amniocentesis* — a check of fetal chromosomes — he usually conducts it at 15 to 20 weeks. Your practitioner may perform amniocentesis for other reasons, like checking for lung maturity in the baby, at any time later in the pregnancy.

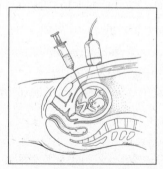

FIGURE 2-4:
An amniocentesis procedure.

Illustration by Kathryn Born, MA

During the amniocentesis procedure, you lie flat on your back on top of a table. Your doctor cleans your abdomen with an iodine solution. Using ultrasound to locate an area of amniotic fluid that is away from the baby, your doctor inserts a thin needle through your abdomen and uterus into the amniotic sac. After withdrawing enough amniotic fluid (usually about 15 to 20 cc, or 1 to 2 tablespoons), he removes the needle.

A common misconception is that the needle is inserted through the navel. The exact point of insertion depends on where the fetus, the placenta, and the amniotic sac are located within the uterus. You may have heard that the amniocentesis needle is exceptionally long, and you may be afraid of long needles. But the needle's length, which enables it to reach the amniotic sac, doesn't make it painful. A needle's thickness determines how uncomfortable it is, and an amniocentesis needle is very thin.

The procedure, which typically lasts no longer than one to two minutes, is mildly uncomfortable but not terribly painful. Many women feel a slight, brief cramping sensation as the needle goes into the uterus and then a weird pulling sensation as the fluid is withdrawn through the needle. Some women worry about moving too much during an amniocentesis. This usually isn't a problem. If you really are flinching or moving too much, your doctor will let you know. Also, it's a common misconception that the risk of an amniocentesis is that the needle may hurt the baby. Your doctor will place the needle in a place well away from the baby. Sometimes a fetus moves toward the needle, but this doesn't cause any harm. Your doctor will simply reposition the needle to a safe place and wait for the baby to stop moving.

Afterward, your doctor may advise you to rest and avoid strenuous activity and sex for one to two days. Most women cramp a bit the day of the procedure, which is expected and normal.

A genetic amniocentesis primarily tests to see that 23 chromosome pairs are present and that their structure is normal. It doesn't routinely test for all possible genetic diseases or birth defects. The amniotic fluid cells must be incubated before your doctor can read the results of a genetic amniocentesis. Results are usually available in one to two weeks.

If prenatal blood studies show that you're Rh-negative, your doctor will give you an injection of Rh-D immune globulin (such as Rhogam or Rhophylac), which helps prevent Rh sensitization.

Risks and side effects of amniocentesis

Following are some side effects that may occur, although not all patients have these symptoms or problems after an amniocentesis:

>> **Cramping:** Some women experience cramping for several hours after the procedure. The best treatment for this cramping is rest. Some practitioners recommend a single glass of wine to help ease the discomfort.

>> **Spotting:** This may last one to two days.

>> **Amniotic fluid leak:** A leakage of 1 to 2 teaspoons of fluid through the vagina occurs in 1 to 2 percent of patients. In the great majority of these cases, the membrane seals over within 48 hours. Leakage stops and the pregnancy continues normally. If you experience a large amount of leakage or persistent leakage, call your doctor.

>> **Fetal injury:** Injury to the fetus is extremely rare, given the use of ultrasound guidance.

>> **Miscarriage:** Although amniocentesis is considered very safe, it's still invasive and is associated with a small risk of pregnancy loss. Recent studies have shown that the risk of pregnancy loss after amniocentesis is much less than the 0.5 percent risk previously quoted and is probably closer to about 1 in 1,000.

An amniocentesis performed later in the pregnancy — later than 20 weeks — doesn't carry the same increased risk of miscarriage. It carries only a very small risk of infection, rupture of membranes (breaking the water), or onset of labor.

REMEMBER

Your decision to undergo the procedure must weigh both risks and benefits, which vary according to the individual. For example, a 40-year-old woman with a history of infertility may not want to undergo any test that carries an increased risk of miscarriage, even though she stands a higher risk of carrying a fetus with a chromosomal abnormality. On the other hand, a 32-year-old maternal–fetal medicine specialist who sees patients with a multitude of problems every day may opt to undergo an amniocentesis even though her risk of having a fetus with a chromosomal abnormality is relatively low — lower, in fact, than her risk of miscarriage because of the test. The peace of mind may be worth the small increased risk of miscarriage.

Reasons for having an amniocentesis

Your practitioner may recommend a genetic amniocentesis for the following conditions or situations:

>> Your age is 35 or more at your due date. This age recommendation also depends on the number of babies you're carrying. For example, if you're carrying twins, your practitioner may offer an amniocentesis at age 33.

>> You had an elevated MSAFP (see the "Alpha-fetoprotein screen" section earlier in this chapter).

>> You had abnormal results from Down syndrome screening (during either your first or second trimester).

>> Your ultrasound exam was abnormal, indicating, for example, poor fetal growth or suspected structural abnormalities.

>> You had a previous child or previous pregnancy with a chromosomal abnormality.

>> You're at risk of having a baby with a certain genetic disease.

>> You and your partner have concerns and want to confirm that the chromosomes are normal.

Your practitioner may perform amniocentesis for other reasons:

>> **Infections leading to preterm labor:** An infection within the amniotic fluid may be a cause of preterm labor. Your practitioner can send the fluid to a lab for tests to look for any such infection. If an infection is present, your doctor may want to deliver your baby right away to minimize harm to you and the baby.

>> **Other infections:** Some patients may find that they're at risk of developing infections such as toxoplasmosis, CMV (cytomegalovirus), or parvovirus (see Book 6, Chapter 3). The amniotic fluid can be tested for evidence of such problems in patients at risk.

>> **Rh sensitization:** Patients with Rh sensitization are sometimes monitored with a test known as *delta OD-450,* in which the amniotic fluid is examined for evidence of broken-down fetal red blood cells. However, most doctors instead perform a special type of Doppler ultrasound called an *MCA (middle cerebral artery) Doppler* (see the section "Doppler studies" later in this chapter). Go to Book 6, Chapter 2 for info on Rh sensitization.

>> **Lung maturity studies:** Sometimes your doctor needs to find out whether the fetus's lungs are mature enough for the baby to be delivered. Certain tests on the amniotic fluid can determine the maturity of the lungs.

Other prenatal tests and procedures

Not all the tests or procedures in this section are performed in all pregnancies — only when a specific problem is present. In fact, most of these tests are rarely done and are usually done in centers that specialize in fetal medicine. If needed, they're usually performed in the second or third trimester.

Fetal blood sampling

For fetal blood sampling — also known as *PUBS (percutaneous umbilical blood sampling)* or *cordocentesis* — a doctor withdraws fetal blood from the umbilical cord. This test lets your doctor obtain blood for rapid chromosomal diagnosis when time is critical, although testing cell-free fetal DNA in the mother's blood can also be used in this situation (see the earlier section "Cell-free fetal DNA").

Your doctor may do fetal blood sampling in order to diagnose fetal infections, detect evidence of fetal anemia, or diagnose and treat a condition called *non-immune hydrops,* in which fluid accumulates abnormally in the fetus. A maternal–fetal medicine specialist performs the procedure under ultrasound guidance. The procedure is similar to an amniocentesis, except that the doctor directs the needle into the umbilical cord rather than into the amniotic fluid. Risks are low but include infection, rupture of the membranes, or fetal loss. (The risk of fetal loss is about 1 percent.)

Some fetuses develop anemia, which can be treated *in utero* (within the womb) with a blood transfusion directly into the umbilical cord. Conditions that may lead to anemia include certain infections (like parvovirus), genetic diseases, or certain blood group incompatibilities (see Book 6, Chapter 2).

Fetal echocardiogram

A *fetal echocardiogram* is basically a sonogram focused on the fetal heart. A maternal–fetal medicine specialist, a pediatric cardiologist, or a radiologist usually performs this procedure. You may need a fetal echo if you have a history of diabetes or a family history of congenital heart disease, or if an ultrasound shows any signs of a heart abnormality. Sometimes your practitioner recommends a fetal echo if he sees *any* structural problem on ultrasound, because heart abnormalities are often associated with other birth defects.

Doppler studies

Ultrasound can be used to perform Doppler studies of fetal and umbilical blood flow. These studies are a way of assessing blood flow to various organ systems and also within the placenta. A Doppler study is sometimes used as a test of well-being in fetuses with IUGR (intrauterine growth restriction) — see Book 6, Chapter 2 for more on IUGR. MCA Dopplers measure the blood flow through a major blood vessel in the fetal brain and can detect fetuses who may be anemic from an infection or a blood group incompatibility.

Recognizing Causes for Concern

This section covers certain problems that can develop during the second trimester and symptoms that you should discuss with your practitioner.

The following is a list of second-trimester symptoms that require some attention. If you experience any of them, call your practitioner:

>> Bleeding

>> An unusual sense of pressure or heaviness

>> Regular contractions or strong cramping

>> A lack of normal fetal movement

>> High fever

>> Severe abdominal pain

Bleeding

Some women experience bleeding in the second trimester. Possible causes include a low-lying placenta (*placenta previa*), premature labor, cervical incompetence, or placental abruption (all covered in Book 6, Chapter 2). Sometimes the doctor can't find a cause. If you do experience bleeding, it doesn't necessarily mean you'll have a miscarriage, but you should call your doctor. He'll probably recommend you have an ultrasound exam and be monitored to make sure that you're not contracting. Bleeding may increase the risk for premature delivery, so your doctor may recommend that your pregnancy come under extra-close surveillance.

Fetal abnormality

Although the vast majority of pregnancies proceed normally, about 2 to 3 percent of infants are born with some abnormality. Most of these abnormalities are minor, although some do lead to significant problems for the newborn. Some are due to chromosomal problems, and others stem from abnormal development of organs and structures. Many of these problems, though not all of them, can be diagnosed on a prenatal ultrasound exam (see the earlier section "Looking at sound waves: Ultrasound"). When confronted with any such problem, the most important first step is to gather all the available information about it so you know what to expect and what the treatment options are. Keep in mind that even specialists may not be able to tell you everything to expect until your baby is born and they can further evaluate the situation.

Cervical insufficiency/incompetent cervix

During the second trimester, usually between 16 and 24 weeks, some women develop a problem known as *cervical insufficiency* or *incompetent cervix*. The cervix opens up and dilates, even though the woman feels no contractions. This condition may lead to miscarriage. A woman who develops this condition ordinarily doesn't notice any symptoms, although sometimes she may report feeling pelvic heaviness or pressure that's out of the ordinary, or she may notice some spotting. Most women who experience cervical insufficiency do so for no identifiable reason. Others may have one of the following risk factors:

» **Cervical trauma:** Some evidence suggests that multiple *D&Cs* (dilation and curettage; see Book 2, Chapter 1) or procedures called *cervical cone biopsy* or *LEEP* (in which a cone-shaped portion of the cervix is removed in the diagnosis or treatment of cervical abnormalities) can increase the risk of cervical insufficiency. A significant tear of the cervix during a prior delivery may also increase the risk for this disorder.

» **Multiple gestations:** Some obstetricians believe that carrying multiple babies, especially triplets or more, may increase the risk for cervical insufficiency and advocate that all patients with triplets or more have a *cerclage* (a stitch in the cervix) put in. Some patients who have undergone a procedure called *multifetal pregnancy reduction* (see Book 6, Chapter 1) may also be at increased risk for incompetent cervix, although routine cerclage placement isn't recommended for them at this time.

» **Prior history of cervical insufficiency:** After you've had a cervical insufficiency, your risk of having it again in a subsequent pregnancy is increased.

In cases in which a cervical insufficiency is diagnosed before the pregnancy is lost, attempts can be made to hold the cervix shut with a stitch, called a *cerclage*, around the cervix. The cerclage is usually placed at 12 to 14 weeks, although it's occasionally performed as an emergency procedure later in the pregnancy. Doctors most commonly perform the procedure in the hospital under spinal or epidural anesthesia, but the woman is usually discharged later the same day.

Some women with a cerclage notice they have a heavy discharge throughout pregnancy. If you need to have a cerclage, talk to your doctor about how active you can be — whether you can have sex and how much exercise is advisable. Complications associated with emergency cerclage include infection, contractions, rupture of membranes, bleeding, and miscarriage. The same complications can occur with elective cerclage, but they're unusual.

Many doctors are now using a *pessary*, a plastic/rubber device that is inserted into the vagina to take some of the pressure off of the cervix. The device is easily inserted and removable, so it doesn't carry the same risks as a cerclage because no needles are involved.

FOR PARTNERS: HAVING SEX IN THE SECOND TRIMESTER

For many women, the libido is back on the ascent during the second trimester, which is a big sigh of relief for any guy who has patiently waited through her nausea, exhaustion, discomfort, and lack of sexual energy for some long-awaited sex. In fact, some women become very sexual during this time because they're flush with hormones and feeling in touch with their bodies. So forget what you may have heard — sex during pregnancy is safe as long as your partner is having a normal pregnancy. Your baby is protected by an amniotic sac and the cervix, which is sealed tightly by a thick mucus plug, which keeps out foreign and unwanted intruders. (So, no, your penis isn't long enough to hit or poke the baby during sex. The baby can't see your penis when you're having sex and isn't afraid of your penis during sex. Your semen won't get all over the baby upon completion of sex.)

Don't be surprised if your partner needs to take it slowly in the beginning. Stop at any signs of discomfort. As the baby bump continues to expand, you'll likely find yourselves exploring new positions that offer support for your partner's stomach. Many women are most comfortable on their sides or even up on their knees and can use pillows for stomach support. Spotting and cramping that can last up to 24 hours can occur after sex. If you or your partner has any questions or concerns about either, call her medical practitioner.

One warning: If your partner desires oral sex, it's absolutely safe. Just make sure not to blow air into the vagina because this can cause an embolism, which can be fatal for the baby and the mother-to-be.

In a few instances, sex during pregnancy isn't recommended. Talk with your partner's doctor or midwife prior to having sex if your partner has dealt with any of the following issues:

- **Bleeding:** Sometimes vaginal bleeding ranging from normal to potentially life-threatening can occur during the early months of pregnancy, and sex can cause the cervix to bleed.

- **Leaking amniotic fluid:** Any time amniotic fluid is leaking, the sterile barrier between the baby and the outside world is broken, and infection can enter into the uterus and infect the baby. No sex after her water breaks!

- **Miscarriage:** If your partner has ever had a miscarriage, or if a medical professional has said that she's at risk for having one, check before having sex.

- **Multiple pregnancy:** Because multiples often deliver early, you need to avoid anything that can upset the delicate balance between no children and two (or more)

(continued)

(continued)

children — sex included. Semen contains substances that may bring on labor if the tendency for preterm delivery exists. Besides, your partner probably has enough going on in there already.

- **Placenta previa:** With the placenta close to or overlying the cervix in placenta previa, having sex can cause life-threatening bleeding.

- **Preterm labor:** If your partner gave birth to a previous child prematurely, get clearance to make sure having sex is safe.

- **Weakened cervix:** Sometimes called an *incompetent cervix,* this condition can lead to the cervix dilating before the baby is full term, which can lead to miscarriage. A stitch is often placed into the cervix to keep it closed. Sex can cause uterine contractions that disrupt the stitch.

A female orgasm during low-risk pregnancy won't cause your partner to go into labor prematurely. Contractions of the uterus associated with sex aren't the same as those experienced during labor (and your partner is *very* thankful for this!). However, orgasm achieved by any method can start contractions that can lead to preterm labor in high-risk pregnancy, so put the vibrator away for the duration as well.

Some medical practitioners recommend avoiding sex during the final weeks of pregnancy because of the *prostaglandins* in semen, which are hormones that can stimulate contractions. On the flip side, if your partner is overdue, you may get a "prescription" for sex to jump-start the contractions.

Chapter 3

The Third Trimester

You're finally ready for the third act — your pregnancy's final trimester. By now, you're probably accustomed to having a protruding belly, your morning sickness is long gone, and you've come to expect and enjoy the feeling of your baby moving around and kicking inside you. In this trimester, your baby continues to grow, and your practitioner continues to monitor you and your baby's health. You also begin making preparations for the new arrival, which may mean anything from getting ready to take a leave of absence from your job to taking childbirth classes (or otherwise finding out what to expect during labor and delivery).

Your Baby Gets Ready for Birth

At 28 weeks, your baby measures about 14 inches (about 35 cm) and weighs about 2½ pounds (about 1,135 grams). But by the end of the third trimester — at 40 weeks, your due date — she measures about 20 inches (50 cm) and weighs 6 to 8 pounds (about 2,700 to 3,600 grams), sometimes a bit more, sometimes a bit less. The fetus spends most of the third trimester growing, adding fat, and continuing to develop various organs, especially the central nervous system. The arms and legs get chubbier, and the skin becomes thicker and smooth.

During the third trimester, your baby is less susceptible to infections and to the adverse effects of medications, but some of these agents may still affect her growth. The last two months are usually spent getting ready for the transition to life in the world outside the uterus. The changes are less dramatic than they were early on, but the maturation and growth that happen now are very important.

By 28 to 34 weeks, the fetus generally assumes a head-down position (called a *vertex presentation*), like in Figure 3-1. This way, the buttocks and legs (the bulkiest parts of its body) occupy the roomiest part of the uterus — the top part. In about 4 percent of singleton pregnancies, the baby may be positioned buttocks-down (breech) or lie across the uterus (transverse). (See the "Breech presentation" section later in this chapter for details.)

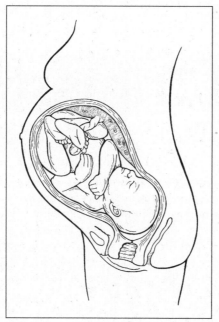

FIGURE 3-1: How your baby may look inside your uterus during the third trimester.

Illustration by Kathryn Born, MA

By 36 weeks, growth slows, and amniotic fluid volume is at its maximum level. After this point, the amount of amniotic fluid may start to decline because blood flow to the baby's kidneys decreases as the placenta ages, and the baby produces less urine (and therefore less amniotic fluid). In fact, most practitioners routinely check the amniotic fluid volume on ultrasound or by feeling your abdomen during the last few weeks to make sure that a normal amount remains.

Movin' and shakin': Fetal movements

Look down at your belly during times of fetal activity during the third trimester, and it may appear that an alien from outer space is doing an aerobic dance inside you. Although fetal movements don't actually diminish as your due date approaches, the timing and quality of the movements change. Toward the end of pregnancy, fetal movements may feel less like jabs and more like tumbles or rolls, and you notice longer periods of quiet between movements. The fetus is adapting to a more newborn-like pattern, taking longer naps and having longer active cycles.

WARNING

If you don't sense a normal amount of activity, let your practitioner know. A good general rule is that you should feel about six movements in one hour after dinner, while resting. Any movement, no matter how subtle, counts. Some women find that they go for periods of feeling less fetal movement, but then the movements pick up again and are normal. This is very common and isn't a reason to be concerned. However, if you notice a pattern of diminishing fetal movements or you feel absolutely no fetal movements over several hours (despite resting or eating), give your practitioner a call right away.

If you have certain risk factors or if you need specific guidelines to track the adequacy of fetal movements, your practitioner may suggest that you keep a diary to chart fetal movement, starting at 28 weeks. You can track fetal movements in a couple of ways:

>> Lie down on your left side after dinner to count fetal movements, and write down how long it takes to count ten movements.

>> Count fetal movements while lying down for an hour each day (it doesn't have to be the same hour every day) and plot the number of movements on a chart given to you by your practitioner. This method shows the pattern of the baby's movements throughout the day.

Flexing the breathing muscles

Fetuses undergo what are called *rhythmic breathing movements* from 10 weeks onward, although these movements are much more frequent in the third trimester. The fetus doesn't actually breathe, but her chest, abdominal wall, and diaphragm move in a pattern that is characteristic of breathing. You don't notice these movements, but a doctor can observe them with ultrasound. These movements are signs that the baby is faring well. During the third trimester, the amount of time a fetus spends performing the breathing movements increases, especially after meals.

Hiccupping in utero

At times, you may feel a quick, rhythmic pattern of fetal movements, occurring every few seconds. These movements are most likely hiccups. Some women feel fetal hiccups several times throughout the day; others sense them only rarely. Occasionally you may actually see the baby hiccupping during an ultrasound exam. These hiccups are completely normal.

Keeping Up with Your Changing Body

As the baby grows, so does your belly! Big is beautiful, but it can become uncomfortable. You may notice that your uterus pushes up on your ribs, and sometimes you notice kicking in one spot in particular — that is probably where the baby's extremities are, either feet or arms. If you're pregnant with twins or more, the discomforts are even more pronounced. Women with twins may feel one baby move more than the other, which is usually related to the babies' positions — one baby may be oriented with the arms and legs facing out and the other with them facing in. Whether you are carrying one, two, or more babies, you notice that moving around like you used to becomes more and more difficult as you get bigger.

TIP

If you find rising after lying on your back is difficult and no one is around to help, try turning on your side first and then pushing yourself up to a sitting position (see Figure 3-2).

Accidents and falls

REMEMBER

Being pregnant may make you more cautious about taking obvious risks, but it doesn't prevent you from stumbling or otherwise having an occasional mishap. If you do fall, don't worry. Chances are good that the baby remains well protected in your uterus and within its sac of amniotic fluid, which is an excellent natural cushion. But just to be careful, let your practitioner know of any falls. She may want you to come in to check that the baby is fine.

WARNING

If, after your fall, you suffer severe abdominal pain, contractions, bleeding, or leakage of amniotic fluid, or if you notice a decrease in fetal movements, call your practitioner immediately or go to the hospital where you receive care. If the fall or injury involves a direct blow to your uterus (for example, the steering wheel hits your belly in a car accident), your practitioner will probably want to monitor your baby for a while.

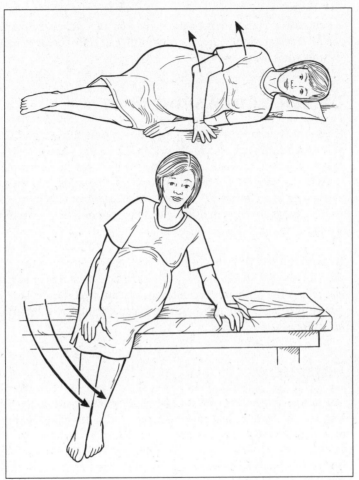

FIGURE 3-2:
To give your back a break when you get up after lying down, roll over to your side and then push yourself up as you swing your legs down.

Braxton-Hicks contractions

In the late second trimester or beginning of the third trimester, your uterus may, from time to time, become momentarily hard or feel as though it's balling up. Most likely, you're experiencing *Braxton-Hicks contractions.* They're not the kind of contractions you have in labor; they're more like practice ones.

Braxton-Hicks contractions are usually painless, but at times they may be uncomfortable, and they may occur with more frequency when you're active and subside when you rest. Women who have already had children tend to notice more Braxton-Hicks contractions. You may have a hard time distinguishing Braxton-Hicks contractions from fetal movements, especially if this is your first pregnancy. Other times, Braxton-Hicks contractions can become uncomfortable and progress to false labor.

WARNING

If you're less than 36 weeks along and you experience contractions that are persistent, regular, and increasingly painful, call your doctor to make sure you're not in premature labor.

Carpal tunnel syndrome

If you feel numbness, tingling, or pain in your fingers and wrist, you're probably experiencing *carpal tunnel syndrome.* It occurs when swelling in the wrist puts pressure on the median nerve, which runs through the carpal tunnel from the wrist to the hand. It can happen in one or both hands, and the pain may be worse at night or upon awakening. Carpal tunnel syndrome is more common in women who are pregnant than in those who aren't because of the swelling that goes along with pregnancy.

If carpal tunnel syndrome becomes persistent or bothersome, discuss it with your practitioner. Wrist splints, available at some drugstores or surgical supply stores, can relieve the problem. Try not to be discouraged if it doesn't seem to get better during pregnancy, though, because it usually improves (often dramatically fast) after delivery.

Fatigue

The fatigue you felt early in your pregnancy may return in the third trimester. You may feel as if you're just slowing down. You're tired all the time, you're carrying around more weight, you're not very comfortable much of the time, and you may feel that you can't accomplish everything you need to. Women may find their second or third pregnancies more tiring than the first because they have to care for one or more older children.

TIP

Try to be realistic about what you can do, and don't feel guilty about what you can't get done. Take time for yourself and get as much rest as you can. Delegate tasks. Whenever possible, let other people help with household chores and other responsibilities. Do whatever you can to take advantage of the quiet times. Rest as much as you can now, because after delivery, the work really picks up!

Feeling the baby "drop"

During the month before delivery, you may notice that your belly feels lower and that breathing is suddenly easier. If you've experienced regular heartburn, you may notice that that has improved as well. At the same time, however, you may feel more pressure in your vaginal area — many women feel heaviness there.

Some women report feeling strange, sharp twinges as the baby's head moves and exerts pressure on the bladder and pelvic floor. These feeling are because the baby has *dropped,* or descended lower into the pelvis, and no longer presses up against your diaphragm or stomach. This movement is also called *lightening.* It typically happens two to three weeks before delivery in women who are having their first child. Those who've had children before may not drop until they're in labor. Having the baby drop doesn't predict when labor will happen.

You may not notice that you've dropped. During your prenatal visit, your doctor may be able to tell by an external or internal exam how low the baby's head is and whether it's engaged. The fetal head is *engaged* when it has reached the level of the *ischial spines,* which are bony landmarks in your pelvis that can be felt during an internal exam (see Figure 3-3).

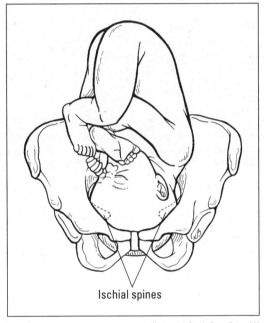

Ischial spines

FIGURE 3-3: The baby's head reaches the bony ischial spines in your pelvis and is engaged.

Illustration by Kathryn Born, MA

If the baby's head is engaged prior to labor, you're more likely to deliver vaginally, although obviously there are no guarantees. Similarly, although a floating (unengaged) head isn't every obstetrician's dream, it doesn't mean that you won't have a completely normal delivery.

If you're having your second child or more, the baby's head may not engage until well into labor.

Hemorrhoids

No one wants to talk about them, but *hemorrhoids* — dilated, swollen veins around the rectum — are a common problem for pregnant women. The enlarging uterus causes hemorrhoids by pressing on major blood vessels, which leads to pooling of blood and ultimately makes the veins enlarge and swell. Progesterone relaxes the veins, allowing the swelling to increase. Constipation makes hemorrhoids worse. Straining and pushing hard during bowel movements puts added pressure on the blood vessels, causing them to enlarge and possibly protrude from the rectum.

WARNING

Hemorrhoids sometimes bleed. This bleeding doesn't harm the pregnancy, but if it becomes frequent, talk to your doctor and possibly see a colorectal specialist or general surgeon. If hemorrhoids become very painful, you may want to discuss whether treatment is necessary. Meanwhile, you can try the suggestions in Book 1, Chapter 4 to avoid or relieve the discomfort of hemorrhoids.

Pushing during the second stage of labor can make hemorrhoids worse or make them appear where they weren't before. But most of the time, hemorrhoids go away after delivery.

Insomnia

During the last few months of pregnancy, many women find sleeping difficult. Finding a comfortable position when you're eight months along isn't easy. You feel a little like a beached whale. Getting up five times a night to go to the bathroom doesn't make things any easier. However, you may find relief in the following:

>> **Drink warm milk with honey before bedtime.** If you have gestational diabetes, see Book 6, Chapter 3.

>> **Exercise during the day.** Activity helps to tire you out, which means you'll fall asleep sooner.

>> **Go to bed a little later than usual.** You'll spend less time *trying* to fall asleep.

>> **Limit your liquid intake after 6 p.m.** Don't limit it to the point that you become dehydrated, however.

>> **Invest in a body pillow.** You can tuck it around your body in various places, making it easier to find a comfortable position.

>> **Take a warm, relaxing bath before going to bed.** Many women say a bath makes them feel sleepy.

FOR PARTNERS: DEALING WITH TEARS, PANIC, AND DOUBTS

Doing anything for the first time can be stressful, overwhelming, and scary. Facing labor, delivery, and motherhood for the first time certainly qualifies. Yes, you're also facing fatherhood for the first time — dealing with the prospect of labor, seeing your partner in pain, and managing a host of doubts and fears — but her concerns are fueled by hormones and the knowledge that some form of delivery, be it labor or surgery, is the only way to emerge with a baby after nine months of pregnancy. The inevitability of the end of pregnancy can be overwhelming at times.

Your partner won't be the first woman to ever express the feeling that she can't do this, that having a baby was a mistake, or that she's changed her mind about the whole thing and wants to call it off. These feelings will intensify when she's in labor, so if you deal with them rationally now, you'll be better prepared for them then.

Allow your partner to vent and express doubts and concerns, but never fail to reassure her that you know she'll be a great mom, that she was born to do this, and that you'll be helping her every step of the way. Feel free to express your own fears and doubts about being a really good parent, but never in a "Can you top this?" way.

Many women at the end of pregnancy have vivid dreams about the baby or develop fears that something may be wrong with him. You can't do much about these fears except let her talk them out and reassure her that no matter what happens, you're there for her and the baby. However, if your partner becomes fixated on thoughts that she may harm the baby or that something is wrong with the baby, she may be experiencing a severe depressive disorder. Make sure she sees her medical practitioner promptly.

Rashes and itches

Pregnant women are subject to the same rashes that nonpregnant women get. One rash is unique to pregnancy, however: *pruritic urticarial papules of pregnancy,* or PUPP. It sounds scary, but it's really more of a nuisance than anything else because it can cause some intense itching. It occurs more often during a first pregnancy and in women having twins or more (the more fetuses, the greater the likelihood).

PUPP tends to occur late in pregnancy and is characterized by hives or red patches that first appear in the stretch marks on your abdomen. These patches can spread to other areas on the abdomen and to the legs, arms, chest, and back. They almost never spread to the face (thank heaven for small favors). The good news is that the condition poses no risk to the baby. But if you develop this rash, your doctor may recommend that you have some blood tests to make sure you don't have other conditions that can be associated with itching.

TIP

The only surefire way to make PUPP go away is to deliver. If delivery is still weeks away, it sometimes helps to bathe in a solution of colloidal oatmeal (Aveeno makes a good one). Skin lotions containing Benadryl can also help, but these products sometimes dry the skin, which only makes the itching worse. In very severe cases (which are rare), the doctor may prescribe a short-term course of steroids or other medications.

Even if you don't have a rash, you may notice that you itch a lot, especially where stretch marks develop. This itching is very common and usually is caused by the stretching of your skin as the baby gets bigger.

Up to 2 percent of pregnant women develop *cholestasis of pregnancy,* which is a condition where an increase of bile acids in the blood causes the itching. If the itching is mild, you can treat it with skin moisturizers, topical anti-itching medications, or oral antihistamines such as Benadryl (but remember to talk to your doctor first before taking them). If the itching is severe, your doctor may recommend oral medications that help to clear the bile acids from the bloodstream. Some studies have suggested that the baby should be monitored with nonstress tests (see the later section "Nonstress test [NST]") when the mother has this condition, because it's associated with an increased risk of complications. The itching goes away shortly after delivery, but the condition may recur in future pregnancies.

PREPARING FOR BREASTFEEDING

If you plan on breastfeeding, you may want to take steps now to prepare yourself. Head to Book 5, where you can find the information you need.

Many women notice from early on in pregnancy that their breasts occasionally secrete a yellowish discharge. This discharge is *colostrum,* and it's what the newborn baby sucks out and swallows in the first few days of life before actual milk comes in. Colostrum has a higher protein and lower fat content than milk; most importantly, it contains antibodies from your immune system that help protect your baby against certain infections until her own immune system matures and can take over.

Don't worry if you don't produce any visible colostrum during pregnancy; not producing colostrum in no way means that you won't produce adequate milk if you're planning to breastfeed your baby. Each woman is different; some leak from the breasts during pregnancy, and some don't. Even if it isn't obvious, your baby will still get colostrum the first few times she breastfeeds.

Sciatica

Some women experience pain extending from their lower back to their buttocks and down one leg or the other. This pain or, less commonly, numbness, is known as *sciatica*, because it's due to pressure on the sciatic nerve, a major nerve that branches from your back, through your pelvis, to your hips, and down your legs. You can relieve mild cases of sciatica with bed rest (shift from side to side to find the most comfortable position), warm baths, or heating pads applied to the painful areas. If you develop a severe case, you may need prolonged bed rest or special exercises. Ask your doctor.

Shortness of breath

You may find that as pregnancy proceeds, you become increasingly short of breath. The hormone progesterone affects your central breathing center and may cause these feelings of breathlessness. Furthermore, as your enlarging uterus presses upward on your diaphragm, your lungs have less room to expand normally.

In most cases, shortness of breath is perfectly normal. But if it comes on very suddenly or if it comes with chest pain, call your doctor.

WARNING

Stretch marks

As your skin stretches to accommodate the enlarging uterus and weight gain, stretch marks form. Some women probably also have some genetic predisposition for stretch marks. The marks typically appear as pinkish-red streaks along the abdomen and breasts, but they fade to silvery gray or white several months after delivery. Their exact color depends on your skin tone — they appear browner on dark-skinned women, for example.

No cream or ointment is completely effective in preventing stretch marks, although products continue to enter the market. Many people think that rubbing vitamin E oil on the belly helps prevent stretch marks or helps them fade faster, but the effectiveness of vitamin E has never been proven scientifically. Your best bet is to avoid excessive weight gain and to exercise regularly to maintain muscle tone, which eases the pressure of the uterus on the overlying skin.

Recently, some dermatologists have started offering a special laser procedure that may help reduce stretch marks after delivery. Also, some advise using a cream containing retinoic acid to treat stretch marks after delivery. However, don't use these creams during pregnancy; also, you shouldn't use some of them when you're breastfeeding. If your stretch marks are particularly noticeable, consult a dermatologist a few months after your pregnancy is over.

TIP

The Third Trimester

Swelling

Swelling (also called *edema*) of the hands and legs is very common in the third trimester. It most often occurs after you've been on your feet for a while, but it can happen throughout the day. Swelling tends to be even more common in warm weather. Contrary to popular wisdom, no evidence indicates that lowering your salt intake or drinking a lot of water prevents swelling or makes it go away. Here's what you can do to relieve ordinary swelling:

>> Keep your legs elevated whenever possible.

>> Stay in a cool environment.

>> Wear supportive pantyhose or stockings that aren't tight around your knees.

>> When in bed, don't lie flat on your back; try to lie on your side.

WARNING

Although swelling is a normal symptom of pregnancy, it can be a sign of pre-eclampsia (see Book 6, Chapter 2). If you notice a sudden increase in the amount of swelling or a sudden, large weight gain — 5 pounds or more in a week — or if the swelling is associated with significant headache or right-sided abdominal pain, call your practitioner immediately.

Urinary stress incontinence

Leaking a little urine when you cough, laugh, or sneeze isn't unusual when you're pregnant. This kind of *urinary stress incontinence* occurs because your growing uterus is putting pressure on your bladder. Relaxation of the pelvic floor muscles increases the problem during the late second and third trimesters. And sometimes the baby may give the bladder a swift kick and cause it to leak urine. *Kegel exercises* — in which you repeatedly contract the pelvic floor muscles as if you're trying very hard not to urinate — can prevent or markedly reduce the problem. Some women continue to experience a little stress incontinence even after delivery, but it usually goes away after about 6 to 12 months.

If you have a particularly difficult labor, where you push for a long time, or have a very large baby, the stress incontinence may not completely go away. Give it at least six months to see whether it stops. After that, talk to your doctor about how to proceed.

Varicose veins

You may notice that a small road map has suddenly appeared on your lower legs (and sometimes the vulvar area). These marks are dilated veins, referred to as *varicose veins.* They're caused by the pressure of the uterus on major blood vessels — the *inferior vena cava* (the vein that returns blood to the heart) and the pelvic veins, in particular. Pregnancy also causes the muscle tissue inside your veins to relax and your blood volume to increase, and these conditions add to the problem. Women with light skin or with a family history of varicose veins are particularly susceptible. Very often, the bluish-purple highways fade after delivery, but sometimes they don't disappear completely. They're most often painless, but they may be associated with discomfort, achiness, or pain.

In rare instances, a blood clot develops in the superficial veins of the legs. This condition, called *superficial thrombophlebitis,* isn't a serious problem; it's often successfully treated with rest, leg elevation, warm compresses, and special stockings. A clot that forms in the deep veins of the leg is more serious (see Book 6, Chapter 3 for a discussion of deep vein thrombosis).

BRACING FOR YOUR PARTNER'S EMOTIONAL CHANGES

Hormone levels are very high in the last few months of pregnancy, and, for many women, with hormones come mood swings. Be prepared for the following emotional changes in the last trimester:

- **Irritability:** When you don't feel your best physically, everything irritates you. Try not to be one of the "everythings" that drives your partner crazy.

- **Self-image issues:** Expect to hear your partner make negative comments, and don't respond to them in kind. The answer to "Do I look fat?" is never "Yes."

- **Weepiness:** During the last few months of pregnancy, women cry because they're happy, or sad, or frustrated, or angry. They cry for reasons they can't even express to you, which can, of course, be frustrating to you, but you'll get over it.

Some degree of moodiness, sadness, or depression is normal in late pregnancy. These mood changes should be fleeting, but as many as 10 percent of women become clinically depressed during pregnancy and need medical intervention. Additionally, up to 20 percent develop some depressive symptoms that may also need medical treatment.

Symptoms of clinical depression include sadness that doesn't lift, feelings of hopelessness or guilt, difficulty sleeping, constant fatigue, or behavior not typical for your partner. Don't ignore depression that seems extreme or that doesn't lift after a few days. Head to Book 2, Chapter 7 for information about depression and pregnancy.

TIP

You can't prevent varicose veins — you can't fight heredity — but you can reduce their number and severity by avoiding standing for prolonged periods of time or wearing clothes that are very tight around one part of your leg. If you must be relatively stationary, move your legs around from time to time to stimulate circulation, and keep your legs elevated whenever you can. You can also wear support stockings or talk to your doctor about a prescription for special elastic stockings.

Hitting the Home Stretch: Prenatal Visits in the Third Trimester

Between 28 and 36 weeks, your practitioner probably wants to see you every two to three weeks, and then weekly as you close in on delivery. She takes the usual measurements: blood pressure, weight, fetal heart rate, fundal height, and urine tests. These visits are a good time to discuss issues related to labor and delivery with your practitioner.

If you don't deliver by your due date, your practitioner may want to start performing nonstress tests (see the later section "Nonstress test [NST]" for details). These tests assess fetal well-being. After 40 to 41 weeks, placental function and amniotic fluid may decline, and ensuring that both remain adequate to support the pregnancy is important. By 42 weeks, many practitioners recommend inducing labor (see Book 2, Chapter 4) because the risk of problems for the baby rises significantly after that time.

As your pregnancy winds down, your practitioner may perform certain tests to make sure that your baby is as healthy as possible. Some tests, like Group B strep cultures, are done so you can take measures to avoid certain problems. Other tests, like a nonstress test or a biophysical profile, are performed to ensure fetal well-being.

Taking Group B strep cultures

The only routine test that may be performed during one of your final prenatal visits is a culture for *Group B strep*, bacteria commonly found in the vagina and rectum. The Centers for Disease Control and Prevention (CDC) and the American Congress of Obstetricians and Gynecologists now recommend that all women be routinely screened for Group B strep at around 36 weeks gestation. About 15 to 20 percent of women harbor this organism. If the culture is positive at 36 weeks, your doctor will recommend that you receive antibiotics during labor to reduce the risk of transmitting the bacteria to the baby. Treating the bacteria any earlier doesn't help, because it can come back by the time you're in labor. Currently, no tests that yield immediate results are available, so you can't test for Group B strep at the time of labor; it must be done in advance.

Assessing your baby's current health

At certain times, your practitioner may suggest that you undergo tests for the baby. These tests, also referred to as *antepartum fetal surveillance,* check the baby's well-being. Your practitioner can perform these tests at any time after about 24 to 26 weeks if cause for concern exists or after 41 weeks if you haven't delivered. Several different tests can be used, as described in the following sections.

Nonstress test (NST)

Nonstress testing consists of measuring the fetal heart rate, fetal movement, and uterine activity using a special monitoring machine. Your practitioner hooks you up to this device, which picks up uterine contractions and the baby's heart rate and generates a tracing of both. The NST is similar to the device used during labor to monitor the fetal heart rate and contractions. You also receive a button to press each time you perceive fetal movement. The monitoring goes on for about 20 to 40 minutes. The doctor then looks at the tracing for signs of *accelerations,* or increases, in the fetal heart rate. If accelerations are present and occur often enough, the test is considered *reactive,* and the fetus is thought to be healthy and should continue to be so for three to seven days. (The fetus is healthy in more than 99 percent of cases.) If the accelerations aren't adequate (that is, the test is *nonreactive*), you still have no cause for alarm. In 80 percent of cases, the fetus is fine and probably just in sleep cycle, but further evaluation is needed.

GAUGING LUNG MATURITY (FOR REPEAT CESAREAN DELIVERIES)

If you're planning a repeat cesarean delivery (meaning that you had one in an earlier pregnancy) or an elective induction at less than 39 weeks, some practitioners may recommend that you have an amniocentesis to establish that the fetus's lungs are mature and ready to function. Over the past few years, there has been a movement across the country to stop performing elective deliveries before 39 weeks because newer studies have shown that these place newborns at increased risks for problems in the newborn period, so the need for fetal lung maturity amniocenteses is declining. The American Congress of Obstetricians and Gynecologists and the March of Dimes both strongly discourage such deliveries.

Your practitioner may perform this test (which is usually repeated once or twice a week) for a variety of reasons, including the following:

>> You're past your due date.

>> The baby isn't growing properly.

>> You have a decreased volume of amniotic fluid.

>> Your blood pressure is high.

>> You have diabetes.

>> You notice decreased fetal movement.

Your doctor may perform a vibracoustic stimulation test during a nonstress test. During the test, the fetus's response to stimulation by sound or vibrations is observed. The practitioner "buzzes" the mother's belly with a vibrating device, which causes a transmission of sound or vibrations to the fetus. Normally, the fetal heart rate accelerates when the fetus is stimulated in this way. Vibracoustic stimulation can often cut down the time necessary to perform a nonstress test, because you see accelerations in the heart rate more quickly. It is often performed if the NST is still not reactive after 20 to 30 minutes.

Contraction stress test (CST)

The contraction stress test is similar to a nonstress test except that the fetal heart is timed in relation to uterine contractions. The contractions sometimes occur by themselves, but more often are brought on with low doses of oxytocin (Pitocin) or by nipple stimulation.

WARNING

Don't stimulate your nipples at home to bring on contractions. Perform nipple stimulation only under your doctor's supervision, because you doctor wants to monitor you and make sure that the uterus doesn't contract too much.

Three good contractions in a ten-minute period need to be present in order for the test to be interpreted. If the fetal heart rate doesn't drop after the contractions, the test is considered *negative,* and the baby is thought to be fine for at least one more week. If the test is *positive* (the fetal heart rate does drop after the contractions) or suspicious, your practitioner investigates the situation further. Proper management depends on your particular situation. A CST is performed if the results of the nonstress test are inconclusive or if your doctor wants additional testing of fetal well-being.

A CST shouldn't be performed under certain circumstances, such as if you have placenta previa (see Book 6, Chapter 2) or if you're at risk of preterm delivery.

Biophysical profile (BPP)

A biophysical profile, which combines ultrasound with a nonstress test (NST), may be performed instead of the NST alone or in addition to the NST if further testing is warranted. Which test is performed (NST or BPP) is often just a matter of physician preference.

The BPP evaluates the following, all by ultrasound: fetal movements, fetal body tone, fetal breathing, and quantity of amniotic fluid.

A perfect score is 10 (2 points for each parameter that's normal and 2 points for a normal nonstress test). Babies who score 8 out of 10 or better are considered okay. A score of 6 out of 10 is probably fine but usually calls for follow-up testing. A score of less than 6 out of 10 needs further evaluation.

Doppler velocimetry

A doctor performs a Doppler velocimetry test only in certain situations — for example, if certain fetal problems exist (like intrauterine growth restriction; see Book 6, Chapter 2) or if you have high blood pressure. Basically, with this test, your doctor performs a special type of ultrasound exam that assesses the blood flow through the umbilical cord.

Preparing for Labor

Toward the end of your third trimester, you're likely to think more about delivery and anticipate what that's going to be like. Many patients want to know when their labor may start and whether they can do anything to influence the timing or to bring it on sooner. This section helps you plan your labor, provides some insight on some classes you can take to get ready for labor, discusses what you can tell your doctor if you want a cesarean section, and gives you some pointers on how to prepare yourself as labor nears.

Making a birth plan

A *birth plan* is a statement of your preferences for how you want to manage your labor and delivery. It's about educating yourself about your options and feelings rather than making hard-and-fast, "I absolutely will/won't" decisions. It involves sorting through things like where you want to deliver, whom you want to have with you during the process, and how you want to manage any pain you may experience. It can be something you simply sort out in your mind and convey verbally, or it can be something you put in writing.

SYMPATHIZING WITH HER DESIRE TO HAVE THIS OVER, ALREADY

Around the seventh month, many women start expressing a strong desire to have this pregnancy over and done with. Before you jump in with long-winded explanations of how the baby isn't fully developed yet, it's too early, or other pompous statements about why being pregnant for just two more months is a good idea, realize that your partner doesn't really want to have the baby early (well, maybe she does, a little); she's just tired and frustrated with being pregnant.

The last few months of pregnancy are no picnic, and unfortunately, you can't truly understand what she's going through. When she starts talking about getting this baby out by hook or crook the minute she hits 37 weeks, take it with a grain of salt. She's every bit as concerned about the welfare of this baby as you are, and she's not going to do anything rash.

Let her vent without giving her a lecture, and in five minutes, she'll probably be telling her mom how pregnancy has been the best time of her life. That's how hormones go sometimes.

No matter how you develop your plan, make sure you discuss your wishes with your provider well in advance of the big day because obstetric practices vary widely by provider and hospital. The most important part of a birth plan — be it written or verbal — is to provide a platform that fosters an open discussion between you and your provider about your preferences wherever there is a choice. For information on creating a birth plan, refer to Book 1, Chapter 5.

Going back to school: Classes to take

To prepare yourself for labor, you may want to consider taking some birthing classes to find out about breathing, relaxation, and massage techniques that help alleviate the fear, anxiety, and pain associated with labor. Today, a great majority of first-time expectant parents attend childbirth classes.

REMEMBER

As you look toward your labor, you need to have a basic understanding of the different types of birthing methods in order to determine which classes may be right for you. The following is a primer on birthing methods:

>> **Lamaze:** Developed in the 1940s by Dr. Fernand Lamaze, a French obstetrician, this birthing method is probably the best known. Lamaze focuses on

deep breathing techniques and other exercises aimed at distracting you from the pain associated with childbirth. For more info, go to www.lamaze.org.

>> **Bradley:** Developed in the 1940s by an American obstetrician named Dr. Robert Bradley, this method focuses on a "natural" (drug-free) childbirth. This method involves training in deep breathing and other techniques to control the pain of labor and uses a coach. Check out www.bradleybirth.com.

>> **Leboyer:** The cornerstone of this method is to minimize the shock for the baby of transitioning from inside the uterus to outside. It involves being born in a dimly lit room and immediate bonding with Mom. Although there's no specific website devoted to this method, you can read the original text of Dr. Leboyer's book at http://ebookbrowsee.net/birth-without-violence-leboyer-pdf-d123360765.

>> **Alexander:** This method focuses on intensive conditioning of your body to promote balance, flexibility, and coordination, thereby enhancing comfort during labor. Find out more at www.alexandertechnique.com/articles2/pregnancy.

>> **HypnoBirthing:** The origins of this technique were originally described in 1944 by Dr. Grantly Dick-Read, an English obstetrician, in a book called *Childbirth without Fear*. The focus of this method is to use hypnosis to break the fear-tension-pain cycle, thereby making labor easier. For more information, go to http://hypnobirthing.com.

TIP

If you decide to take a class, make sure the one you choose provides reliable and accurate information. Ask your healthcare provider for recommendations, or ask friends who have already attended classes.

Most contemporary childbirth education classes teach a combination of some of these techniques. The greatest benefit of childbirth classes is probably the opportunity they provide to find out what to anticipate during labor, because a little information goes a long way in reducing anxiety and fear about the big event. Other benefits to the classes include

>> **Bringing your partner into the process of pregnancy:** If attending your prenatal visits isn't always possible for your partner, a class may be the best time for your partner to find out about what's ahead and to ask questions.

>> **Meeting other parents-to-be:** You may make friends and ultimately find playmates for your child.

>> **Touring the hospital or childbirth center where you plan to deliver:** Seeing where it's all going to happen is often very helpful. (If your class doesn't include a tour, ask your practitioner to arrange one.)

BEING PREPARED: INFANT CPR

No one wants to think about finding their newborn unresponsive or having difficulty breathing, but the truth is that being prepared helps pull babies through these scary situations. Hence, infant and child CPR are recommended to all parents and childcare providers.

Infant CPR is a technique that all parents should be familiar with. Many people think it requires intensive training to master, but the American Heart Association has simplified the training so that almost anyone can do it with a minimum of effort. In fact, check out www.americanheart.org. Do a search for "Infant CPR Anytime" for information about a valuable 20-minute training session for parents and family members.

REMEMBER

You don't have to believe everything you hear at a childbirth class. If you plan to use medication or anesthesia to reduce the pain of labor and the instructor warns you that all such medications are to be avoided, don't be bullied into accepting her point of view. In class, just find out whatever you can that may be helpful and take the rest in stride. Ultimately, it's your labor, and you need to do what makes you feel comfortable.

Childbirth education isn't for everyone. Some women feel that becoming fully informed about what's ahead only adds to their nervousness — and that's a valid concern. Every woman should make her own decision about whether to attend childbirth classes. Also, if for some reason you deliver before you finish your classes, don't be overly concerned. Most nurses in labor and delivery are trained to show you the techniques you need to know during labor.

Asking for a c-section on demand

Cesarean section on demand (also known as a *cesarean delivery on maternal request*) is having a cesarean delivery just because the mom asks for it, even though no medical or obstetrical reasons for a cesarean exist. If you want to have a c-section on demand, make sure you discuss your wishes with your doctor well in advance of your delivery. She'll talk to you in depth about the risks and benefits of doing this to help you make an informed decision. If you plan on having lots of children, having a c-section on demand probably isn't a good idea because the risks for some problems increase with each subsequent cesarean delivery.

Over the past ten years or so, having a c-section on demand has become increasingly popular. In fact, statistics show that about 2.5 percent of all deliveries in the United States each year are by c-section on demand.

The potential benefits of this mode of delivery are a lower risk of postpartum bleeding or hemorrhage (see Book 2, Chapter 7) and a lower risk of urinary incontinence. The latter has been shown to be true in the first year after delivery, but after that time, the risk of this problem is equal between moms who deliver vaginally and those who have c-section on demand.

The downsides to c-section on demand are a longer stay in the hospital, transient breathing problems for the baby, and higher risks in your subsequent pregnancies for problems like uterine rupture (see the information in Book 6, Chapter 1 on TOLAC and VBAC) and an adherent placenta (also known as *placenta accrete*). Also, not all physicians will agree to c-section on demand.

Timing labor

"When am I going to have this baby?" a lot of soon-to-deliver moms want to know. Unfortunately, there's no foolproof way of knowing, and not even a crystal ball works. Some uncertain signs that something may happen include loss of the *mucous plug* (not really a plug but thick mucus produced in the cervix), *bloody show* (an unfortunately named and blood-tinged mucous discharge), increasing frequency of Braxton-Hicks contractions, and diarrhea. But nothing is a sure sign. Loss of the mucous plug or bloody show may occur hours, days, or weeks before labor, or in some cases, not at all. This unpredictability may add to your anxiety, but it also makes the whole process more exciting.

WARNING

Vigorously rubbing or massaging the nipples can cause contractions, but it shouldn't be performed at home because it can lead to hyperstimulation of the uterus (that is, too-frequent contractions), which isn't healthy for you or your baby. It's not a sure thing, in any case, because as soon as you stop the nipple stimulation, the contractions usually also stop.

Using perineal massage

In the past few years, *perineal massage* has generated a great deal of interest. This process involves using an oil or cream on the *perineum* (the area between the vagina and the rectum) and massaging the area in preparation for childbirth. Although studies suggest that this practice decreases the need for *episiotomies* (cutting the perineum to allow room for the baby to pass during childbirth — see Book 2, Chapter 5) or lacerations, the number of cases in which it has made a clear difference isn't very large. There's no harm in trying it, though. If you think perineal massage may help and it's comfortable for you, go right ahead.

The Third Trimester

Getting Ready to Head to the Hospital

You're so close to delivery now that it's a good idea to make sure you're ready to walk out the door and head for the hospital. You probably won't want to stop to pack a suitcase at the last minute, nor will you have time to stop off at the store to shop for a car seat. Getting these must-do items off your pre-delivery checklist now will free you up to concentrate on the important things, like that 437th daily trip to the bathroom.

Packing your suitcase

Many women find it comforting to know that their bag is packed for the trip to the hospital or birthing center. Having your bag ready allows you to concentrate on watching for signs of labor and helps keep you from worrying about being prepared.

TIP

You may want to have a few things on hand while you're in labor, including the following:

>> **A camera:** Don't forget to charge the batteries and get extra memory cards.

>> **A cellphone or calling card:** Bring along your address book with home, work, and cell numbers.

>> **Insurance information:** Don't forget your card. (This one is actually a "must bring.")

>> **Socks:** Your feet will probably get cold, so plan ahead.

>> **Glasses:** They may be less trouble than contact lenses during labor.

>> **A snack for your partner or coach:** You don't want your partner to leave you for a trip to the hospital cafeteria.

>> **Hard candies or lollipops:** You may have to go for some time without eating or drinking.

>> **Something your partner can use to massage your back during labor:** Some people find that a tennis ball, a narrow paint roller, or a lightweight rolling pin works well.

>> **A CD or MP3 player, if you find music relaxing:** Don't forget to bring your favorite CDs.

>> **Change for parking meters, telephones, or vending machines:** You never know when someone may need some quarters (hopefully not your practitioner).

TIP

After delivery, some additional items can help make your life easier, more comfortable, or more fun:

>> A post-delivery snack for yourself

>> Champagne for a post-delivery toast, if you like

>> Modern, stick-on sanitary napkins

>> Sturdy cotton underwear that you won't mind staining

>> A bathrobe and nightgown

>> Toiletries

>> Extra-large shoes that will accommodate your swollen feet

>> Loose, comfortable clothes to go home in

>> Clothes for your baby — or babies! — to go home in

>> An infant car seat

Determining who's coming to the hospital

Before the time comes to head to the hospital, take a moment and think about whom you want to accompany you. These days, many hospitals allow more than one family member or friend in the labor and delivery room to offer continuous labor support. You may want to consider having some of the following people in your room during delivery:

>> **The baby's father or your partner:** This is an obvious choice.

>> **Your parents:** Some women choose to have one or both of their parents with them.

>> **Your sister or a close friend:** Either may provide the support you need.

>> **A doula:** Some women hire a *doula,* a woman with extensive experience with birth who provides emotional and physical support throughout labor. The following are some doula referral organizations that you may find helpful:

- Doulas of North America (DONA); phone 888-788-DONA; website www.dona.org

- toLabor; phone 804-320-0607; website www.tolabor.com

The Third Trimester

REMEMBER

Continuous labor support refers to the constant, nonmedical care given to a woman in labor. It involves emotional support and encouragement to both the patient and her partner, attention to physical comforts (massage, assistance with positioning and grooming), and, often, providing information and explanations of various procedures and events. Advantages to continuous labor support may include a shorter labor, less need for a cesarean section, less need for pain relief, and a more positive childbirth experience.

Some women with other children may want them to be present during the delivery to share the full family experience. However, you should consider the maturity of the children (or other family members) and whether it would be an emotionally satisfying or unnerving situation for them. Although many labors proceed completely smoothly and without any complications, others may be stressful or more difficult. Keep this in mind when you're considering whom to bring with you to the delivery.

Choosing — and using — a car seat

Buying a car seat for your baby is one of the most important but confusing purchases you'll make. You have many choices, so staying informed about what to look for is important. Basically, you can choose from two types available for newborns:

>> **Infant-only seat:** Designed for babies who are under 1 year of age or weigh less than 20 pounds, this car seat is smaller and more lightweight than the alternative and should be used only in a rear-facing position. (A seat that faces the rear is essential for newborns, because it supports the child's back, neck, and head during a car accident.) This type of seat is also more convenient because it's lightweight and can also be used as an infant carrier, feeding chair, or rocker.

>> **Convertible or infant-toddler seat:** Car seats of this type are usually larger than infant-only car seats. You use them in a rear-facing position until your baby reaches a certain age and weight — typically 1 or 2 years of age or about 20–30 pounds, but check your state's car seat laws to make sure you're up to date. (Go to the Governors Highway Safety Association website to see laws by state: www.ghsa.org/html/stateinfo/laws/childsafety_laws.html.) Some models have weight limits as high as 30 to 32 pounds for rear-facing use. The advantage of this type of seat is that you make only one purchase instead of buying both an infant seat and then a convertible seat after the age of 1.

When shopping, look for a model that's simple to use. Also, pay attention to price — the higher-priced seats aren't necessarily better. If you choose a convertible seat, try it out in your car to make sure it fits both backward and forward before you throw away the receipt. Also, check out whether the car seat is easy to install — you shouldn't need to be a mechanical engineer to properly install your baby's car seat.

The following considerations are also important when choosing a car seat:

>> A five-point safety harness with straps that adjust from the front

>> Plenty of head and neck support

>> An easy-to-clean seat

After you've made your selection, you may want to practice buckling the seat into your car before taking your baby out for her first ride. Remember that your baby should ride in a semi-reclined position (at about a 45-degree angle), with the straps snugly against her body.

TIP

If you want to cover your baby, buckle the harness first and then put a blanket over her. A blanket under the harness or even bulky clothing like a snowsuit may make the harness too loose. Often, firefighters can help install and educate parents on proper installation and proper buckling of infants into car seats.

If your baby is a preemie, ask your doctor if the baby needs to be tested in her car seat before discharge. Premature babies are at a greater risk for periods of *apnea* (absent breathing) or depressed heart rate in a car seat. You may need to use rolled-up towels or diapers on either side of the baby's head to help keep her head and neck from slumping.

Recognizing Causes for Concern

During the final weeks and months of pregnancy, you see your practitioner more often than before. Still, certain questions and problems may arise between visits. Everything starts to heat up during the later stages of the third trimester, with both the baby and your body preparing for delivery. Here are some of the key things that may lead you to call your doctor.

Bleeding

WARNING

If you experience any significant bleeding, let your practitioner know immediately. Some third-trimester bleeding is harmless to you and your baby, but sometimes it has serious implications. Getting evaluated to be sure everything is fine makes sense. Possible causes of third-trimester bleeding include the following:

>> **Preterm labor:** This is defined as having contractions and changes in the cervix before you're 37 weeks along.

>> **Inflammation or irritation of the cervix or the harmless bleeding of a superficial blood vessel on the cervix:** Either of these can occur after intercourse or after a pelvic exam.

>> **Placenta previa or a low-lying placenta:** See Book 6, Chapter 2.

>> **Placental separation or abruption:** See Book 6, Chapter 2.

>> **Bloody show:** This show is usually less than the amount of blood you would see during a normal menstrual period, and it's often mixed with mucus. See Book 2, Chapter 4.

Breech presentation

A baby is in a so-called *breech* position when her buttocks or legs are down, closest to the cervix. Breech presentation happens in 3 to 4 percent of all singleton deliveries. A woman's risk of having a breech baby decreases the further along she goes in her pregnancy. (The incidence is 24 percent at 18 to 22 weeks but only 8 percent at 28 to 30 weeks. By 34 weeks, it's down to 7 percent, and by 38 to 40 weeks, 3 percent.)

If your doctor determines your baby is in a breech position during your third trimester, she'll discuss your options, including vaginal breech delivery (which is rarely done these days), external cephalic version (turning the baby), or cesarean section. See Book 6, Chapter 2 for details about handling breech presentation.

Decreased amniotic fluid volume

The medical term for decreased amniotic fluid volume is *oligohydramnios*. (It also used to be called *dry birth*.) It may be found on a routine ultrasound, or your doctor may suspect it just by feeling your uterus. This condition can occur in association with intrauterine growth restriction (see the later section "Fetal growth problems"), preterm rupture of the membranes, or other conditions, or the cause may not be identifiable.

Usually, a mild decrease in amniotic fluid isn't a major cause for concern; however, your practitioner begins to monitor you more closely — with nonstress tests and ultrasound exams — to make sure no problem arises. If you're very close to your due date, your practitioner may want to deliver the baby. On the other hand, if you're only 30 weeks along, the best option may be increased rest and close observation. Of course, the management of the problem also depends on its cause. See Book 6, Chapter 2 for details on problems with amniotic fluid.

Decreased fetal movement

WARNING

If you're not feeling the amount of fetal movement you're accustomed to, let your doctor know. Fetal movement is one of the most important things to pay attention to as you near your due date (see the section "Movin' and shakin': Fetal movements" earlier in this chapter).

Fetal growth problems

You may find out at a routine prenatal visit that your practitioner thinks your uterus is measuring either too big or too small. This finding isn't cause for immediate alarm. Often in this situation, your practitioner suggests that you have an ultrasound exam to get a better idea of how big the baby is. Ultrasound is used to measure parts of the baby — the head's size, the abdomen's circumference, and the thighbone's length. Your practitioner then plugs these measurements into a mathematical equation that gives the estimated fetal weight (EFW). That estimate is then entered on a curve plotting the baby's age in weeks against weight, which represents the average growth of thousands of fetuses at each gestational age.

Your practitioner can check to see where your baby's weight falls on the curve and thus tell which percentile the baby is in. If the baby's weight is anywhere between the 10th and the 90th percentiles, the weight is considered normal. Remember, not every baby is at the 50th percentile, so the 20th percentile is still normal and no reason to worry.

REMEMBER

Keep in mind that although ultrasound is an excellent tool for assessing fetal growth, it isn't perfect. Judging the baby's weight by an ultrasound exam isn't the same as putting the baby on a scale. Weight estimates can vary by as much as 10 to 20 percent in the third trimester due to variations in body composition. So if your baby is outside the normal range, don't worry.

If your baby measures very large (*macrosomia*), your practitioner may suggest you have another glucose screen to check for gestational diabetes (see Book 6, Chapter 3). If your baby measures especially small (*intrauterine growth restriction*), your doctor may suggest you be followed more closely — that you undergo nonstress tests and repeat ultrasound exams to keep an eye on fetal growth. For information on problems with fetal growth and how to manage them, head to Book 6, Chapter 2.

The Third Trimester

Leaking amniotic fluid

If you notice your underwear is wet, several explanations are possible. It may be a little urine, vaginal discharge, the release of the mucous plug in the cervix, or actual leakage of amniotic fluid (also known as *rupture of the membranes*). Often, you can tell what it is by examining the fluid. Mucous discharge tends to be thick and globby, whereas vaginal discharge is whitish and smooth. Urine has a characteristic odor and doesn't flow continuously without your effort. Amniotic fluid, on the other hand, is normally clear and watery and often is lost in spurts. Sometimes you have a big gush of water when membranes rupture, but if the membrane has only a small hole, the leakage may be scant.

If you think your water might be broken, avoid intercourse, douching, soaking in a bath, or swimming until it's ruled out by your physician.

WARNING

If you leak what you think may be amniotic fluid, call your practitioner right away or go to your hospital for evaluation. If you aren't preterm and the amniotic fluid is clear, leaking fluid isn't an emergency; however, most practitioners want you to let them know so that they can tell you what to do. If the fluid is bloody or greenish-brown, be sure to let your practitioner know. Greenish fluid may mean the baby has had a bowel movement (meconium) inside the uterus. Most of the time, such an event doesn't indicate a problem, but sometimes it means the baby is being stressed. Your practitioner makes sure the baby is okay by monitoring the baby's heartbeat (usually by performing a nonstress test).

Preeclampsia

In *preeclampsia,* a condition unique to pregnancy, high blood pressure is associated with the spilling of protein into the urine and sometimes swelling (*edema*) in the hands, face, and legs. Preeclampsia (also called *toxemia* or *pregnancy-induced hypertension*) isn't uncommon; it occurs in 6 to 8 percent of all pregnancies. It can range from being very mild to being a serious medical condition. Book 6, Chapter 2 provides you with the signs and symptoms of preeclampsia.

Preeclampsia usually comes on gradually. Your practitioner may at first notice only a slight elevation in your blood pressure. She may then tell you to rest more, to lie on your side as much as possible, and to come in for more frequent visits. But occasionally, preeclampsia happens suddenly.

Preterm labor

The technical definition of *preterm labor* is when a woman begins to have contractions and changes in her cervix before she's 37 weeks along. Many women have contractions but no cervical change — in which case it isn't real preterm labor. However, in order to find out whether your cervix is changing, you need to be examined. In addition, your practitioner determines how often you're contracting by placing you on a uterine contraction monitor (like the one used to perform a nonstress test — see the "Nonstress test [NST]" section earlier in this chapter).

The contractions associated with preterm labor are regular, persistent, and often uncomfortable. They usually start out feeling like bad menstrual cramps. (Braxton-Hicks contractions, in contrast, aren't regular or persistent, and they usually aren't uncomfortable.) Preterm labor may also be associated with increased mucous discharge, bleeding, or leakage of amniotic fluid.

Diagnosing preterm labor as early as possible is important. Medications aimed at arresting premature labor work best if the cervix is dilated less than 3 centimeters. If labor occurs after 35 weeks, your practitioner probably won't try to stop your contractions except in rare circumstances (such as poorly controlled diabetes).

WARNING

If you find that you're having regular, uncomfortable, persistent contractions (more than five or six in an hour) and you're not yet 35 to 36 weeks pregnant, call your practitioner. The only way to tell whether you're experiencing real preterm labor is to be examined. Also, if you think your membranes have ruptured (your water has broken) or if you're having any bleeding, call your practitioner right away. See Book 6, Chapter 2 for more-detailed coverage on preterm labor.

When the baby is late

For nearly 40 weeks, you think that your baby is going to come on a certain date. But in fact, only about 5 percent of women actually deliver on their due dates. Eighty-two percent deliver between 37 and 42 weeks, which used to be considered "full-term." Five-and-a-half percent deliver even later, and the rest (12.5 percent) are preterm deliveries.

At one time, what were thought to be post-term pregnancies were often simply a reflection of incorrectly estimated due dates. But today, with the widespread use of ultrasound, the due dates are pretty accurate. An ultrasound performed during the first trimester is especially accurate, usually within three to four days. A third-trimester ultrasound, in contrast, may be off by two to three weeks.

Many practitioners advise that labor be induced if the pregnancy reaches 42 weeks. If your pregnancy goes on any longer, the baby is likely to still be fine, but greater health risks are possible. See Book 2, Chapter 4 for details.

FOR PARTNERS: GETTING DOWN TO THE WIRE

Your partner may begin to feel uncomfortable because of all the changes in her body — and because of her sheer size. Many women have trouble sleeping late in pregnancy, which only makes it harder for them to tolerate their discomfort. As you did during the first and second trimesters, take on more of the day-to-day household duties and give your partner the time she needs to rest. Consider treating her to a day at her favorite salon, or send her out for something else that makes her feel special. She deserves to feel good about herself and the changes her body is going through. And things will go easier for both of you if you can find a way to help her accept her pregnant body, relax, and take things a little easier.

Later in the third trimester, naturally, both of you start to focus on labor and delivery. You may have a million questions: Will the baby be okay? Do I really want to be in the delivery room? How will my partner tolerate labor? How will I tolerate labor? Will I get queasy during the delivery? Psychologically, childbirth can be a real challenge for the partner. You care about the course of events very much, but you're clearly not in the driver's seat, and this situation may make you feel anxious.

At the same time, imminent parenthood faces you head-on. And the onset of this new responsibility may cause still more anxiety and more questions: Will I be able to provide for my family? Will I be a good parent? Can I figure out how to change a diaper? How will I know how to handle a fragile newborn? These questions are all normal. Again, they're probably very similar to the questions running through your partner's head. Communication is everything. Most couples find they can talk each other through their respective panic attacks.

Chapter 4

Honey, I Think I'm in Labor!

Despite the incredible advances that have been made in science and medicine, no one really knows what causes labor to begin. Labor may be triggered by a combination of stimuli generated by the mother, the baby, and the placenta. Or labor may begin because of rising levels of steroid-like substances in the mother or other biochemical substances produced by the baby. Because no one knows exactly how labor starts, no one can pinpoint exactly when it will occur.

This chapter helps you recognize the signs of labor and tells you what to expect at each of the three stages of labor. It also addresses such important issues as labor induction, pain management, how your baby's health is monitored, and alternative birthing methods.

Knowing When Labor Is Real — and When It Isn't

Being unsure whether you're really in labor is actually fairly common. Even a woman expecting her third or fourth child doesn't always know when she's genuinely in labor. This section helps you better identify your own labor (but you still may find yourself calling your practitioner several times or even making many trips to the hospital or birthing center, only to find out that what you think is labor really isn't).

You may experience some of the early symptoms of labor before labor actually begins. Instead of indicating that you're in labor, these symptoms suggest that labor may occur fairly soon. Some women experience these labor-like symptoms for days or weeks, and others experience them only for several hours. Most of the time, going into labor isn't as dramatic as it's portrayed on sitcoms, and women very rarely lack the time they need to get to the hospital before they deliver.

TIP

If you think you're in active labor, don't run to the hospital right away. Instead, telephone your practitioner first.

Noticing changes before labor begins

As you near the end of your pregnancy, you may recognize certain changes as your body prepares for the big event. You may notice all these symptoms, or you may not notice any of them. Sometimes the changes begin weeks before labor starts, and sometimes they begin only days before:

>> **Bloody show:** As changes in your cervix take place, you may expel some mucous discharge mixed with blood from your vagina. The blood comes from small, broken capillaries in your cervix.

>> **Diarrhea:** Usually a few days before labor, your body releases *prostaglandins,* which are substances that help the uterus contract and may cause diarrhea.

>> **Dropping and engagement:** Especially in women who are giving birth for the first time, the fetus often drops into the pelvis several weeks before labor (see Book 2, Chapter 3). You may feel increased pressure on your vagina and sharp pains radiating to your vagina. You also may notice that your whole uterus is lower in your belly and that you're suddenly more comfortable and can breathe more easily.

>> **Increase in Braxton-Hicks contractions:** You may notice an increase in the frequency and strength of Braxton-Hicks contractions (see Book 2, Chapter 3). These contractions may become somewhat uncomfortable, even if they don't grow any stronger or more frequent. Some women experience strong Braxton-Hicks contractions for weeks before labor begins.

>> **Mucous discharge:** You may secrete a thick mucous discharge known as the *mucous plug.* During your pregnancy, this substance plugs your cervix, protecting your uterus from infection. As your cervix starts to thin out *(efface)* and dilate in preparation for delivery, the plug may wash out. Don't worry; losing your plug doesn't mean you're prone to infection.

TIP

CONTRACTION OR NOT?

A *contraction* occurs when your uterus's muscle tightens and pushes the baby toward the cervix. Usually, contractions are uncomfortable and therefore unmistakable. But many women worry that they won't know they're having contractions. You can tell whether you're experiencing contractions by using a quick and easy trick.

With your fingertips, touch your cheek and then your forehead. Finally, touch the top part of your abdomen, through which you can feel the top part of your uterus (the *fundus*). A relaxed uterus feels soft, like your cheek, and a contracting uterus feels hard, like your forehead. This exercise is also good to try if you think you may be in preterm labor (see Book 6, Chapter 2 for more information).

Discerning false labor from true labor

Distinguishing true labor from false labor isn't always easy. But a few general characteristics can help you determine whether the symptoms you're experiencing mean you're in labor.

In general, you're in false labor if your contractions

» Are irregular and don't increase in frequency

» Disappear for any reason but especially when you change position, walk, or rest

» Are not particularly uncomfortable

» Occur only in your lower abdomen

» Don't become increasingly uncomfortable

On the other hand, you're more likely to be in actual labor if your contractions

» Grow steadily more frequent, intense, and uncomfortable

» Last approximately 40 to 60 seconds

» Don't go away when you change position, walk, or rest

» Occur along with leakage of fluid (due to rupture of the membranes)

» Make normal talking difficult or impossible

>> Stretch across your upper abdomen or are located in your back, radiating to your front

Sometimes the only way you can know for sure whether you're in labor is by seeing your practitioner or going to the hospital. When you arrive at the hospital, your doctor, a nurse, a midwife, or a resident physician performs a pelvic exam to determine whether you're in labor. The practitioner also may hook you up to a monitor to see how often you're contracting and to see how the fetal heart responds. Sometimes you find out right away whether you're truly in labor. But the practitioner may need to keep you under observation for several hours to see whether the situation is changing.

You're considered to be in labor if you're having regular contractions and your cervix is changing fairly rapidly — effacing, dilating, or both. Sometimes women walk around for weeks with a partially dilated or effaced cervix but aren't considered to be in labor because these changes are occurring over weeks instead of hours.

Deciding when to call your practitioner

If you think you're in labor, call your practitioner. Don't be embarrassed if he tells you you're probably *not* in labor — it happens to many women. Timing your contractions for several hours before you call (to see whether they're getting closer together) is a good idea because your practitioner can use this information to help determine whether you're in true labor. If your contractions are occurring every five to ten minutes and they're uncomfortable, definitely call. If you're less than 37 weeks along and feeling persistent contractions, don't sit for hours counting their frequency — call your practitioner immediately.

WARNING

Call your practitioner if any of the following apply to you:

>> Your contractions are coming closer together, and they're becoming increasingly uncomfortable.

>> You have ruptured membranes. When your water breaks, a small amount of watery fluid may leak out, or it may be a big gush. If the fluid is green, brown, or red, let your practitioner know right away.

Meconium (your baby's first bowel movement) usually happens after the baby is born, but 2 to 20 percent of babies pass meconium during labor, most commonly if they're born past their due date. Passing meconium doesn't necessarily indicate anything is wrong, but it can be associated with fetal stress.

>> You have bright red heavy bleeding (more than a heavy menstrual period) or are passing clots, in which case you should go to the hospital immediately (after calling your practitioner).

>> You're not feeling an adequate amount of fetal movement (see Book 2, Chapter 3 for more information).

>> You have constant, severe abdominal pain with no relief between contractions.

>> You feel a fetal part or umbilical cord in your vagina. In this case, go to the hospital right away!

Checking for labor with an internal exam

When a practitioner is trying to determine whether you're in labor, he performs an internal exam to look for several things:

>> **Dilation:** Your cervix is closed for most of your pregnancy but may gradually start to dilate during the last couple of weeks, especially if you've had a baby before. After active labor begins, the rate of cervical dilation speeds up, and the cervix dilates to 10 centimeters by the end of the first stage of labor. Often, you're considered to be in active labor when your cervix is about 4 centimeters dilated or 100 percent effaced.

>> **Effacement:** *Effacement* is a thinning out or shortening of the cervix, which happens during labor. Your cervix goes from being thick (uneffaced) to 100 percent effaced (see Figure 4-1).

FIGURE 4-1:
During cervical effacement, the cervix progresses from an uneffaced state to 100 percent effaced and partially dilated.

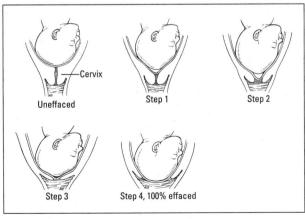

Illustration by Kathryn Born, MA

>> **Station:** When you're in labor, the practitioner uses the term *station* to describe how far your baby's head (or other presenting part) has descended in the birth canal in relation to the *ischial spines,* a bony landmark in your pelvis (see Book 2, Chapter 3 for more information).

>> **Position:** When labor begins, the baby typically starts out facing to the left or right side. As labor progresses, he rotates until his head is face-down, and he comes out looking at the floor. Occasionally, the baby rotates to the opposite position and comes out sunny-side up, looking at the ceiling.

Getting Admitted to the Hospital

Whether you're in labor, being induced, or having a cesarean delivery, you need to be admitted to the hospital's labor floor. If you're preregistered (ask your practitioner about the process), your records are already on the labor floor when you arrive, and a hospital unit number is assigned to you. When you arrive at the hospital or birthing center, you go through an admission process and are assigned to a room.

Settling into your hospital room

Although each hospital or birthing center has its own system, getting settled in usually follows this routine after you get to your room:

>> A nurse asks you to change into a gown.

>> A nurse asks you questions about your pregnancy, your general health, your obstetrical history, and when you last ate. If you think your water has broken or you're leaking fluid, let your nurse know.

>> A nurse, midwife, resident, or other practitioner performs an internal exam to see how far along in labor you are.

>> Your contractions and the fetal heart rate are monitored.

>> A nurse may draw your blood and start an IV *(intravenous)* line in your arm (for delivering fluids and, possibly, medications).

>> You're asked to sign a consent form for routine hospital care, delivery, and possibly cesarean section. (You sign the consent form when you're admitted in case you need an emergency cesarean during labor and you don't have time to sign consent forms.) Signing a consent form doesn't mean you're limiting your care options.

SUPPORTING YOUR PARTNER DURING LABOR

Women in labor need lots of support. Your partner needs to hear that she's doing well, that things are progressing as they should, and that she really can do this. Even if her mother, sister, doula, and five of her dearest friends are with her, she needs *you.* Support means different things to different women, though, and your job is to figure out what your partner needs while in labor and do it.

Your partner may not be in a talkative mood during labor, so asking her what she wants you to do may get you kicked out of the room. This is one time in her life when she wants you to think for yourself and take action. Take the lead by offering choices. Ask her whether she wants

- A back rub

- A massage

- A hand to hold

- You to sit behind her and support her back

- An epidural

- You to kick her mom out of the room

- Ice chips

- To get in the tub

- Any of the other labor options you discussed before today

TIP

You may want to hand over any valuables you have with you to your partner or another family member (or simply leave them at home).

Checking out the accommodations

Some women go through labor in the same room in which they deliver the baby, and others are moved to a different room for delivery. Most hospital rooms include some standard features, so the room you're placed in probably includes the following:

>> **Bed:** In a room used for both labor and delivery (also known as a *birthing room*), the bed is specially designed to come apart and be turned into a

delivery table. Some hospitals have rooms where you labor, deliver, and even remain for your postpartum recovery. These rooms are called *LDR* (labor, delivery, and recovery) *rooms* or *LDRP rooms* (the *p* stands for *postpartum*).

>> **Doppler/stethoscope:** Your practitioner or nurse uses these portable tools to listen periodically to the fetal heartbeat instead of using the continuous fetal monitor.

>> **Fetal monitor:** This machine has two attachments, one to monitor the baby's heart rate and one to monitor your contractions. The fetal monitor generates a *fetal heart tracing,* which is a paper record of how the baby's heart rate rises and falls in relation to your contractions.

>> **Infant warmer:** This device has a heat lamp to keep the newborn's body temperature from dropping.

>> **IV line:** This tube is connected to a bag of *saline* (salt water) containing a glucose mixture to keep you properly hydrated. It also provides access for medications in case you need pain control or have an emergency.

>> **Rocking chair or recliner:** The extra chair is for your partner, your coach, or another family member.

Monitoring Your Baby

While you're in labor, your practitioner keeps an eye on your baby in a number of ways to make sure he's tolerating the whole process well. Most hospitals and most practitioners advise monitoring the baby's heart rate during labor. Although some low-risk patients may require only intermittent monitoring, other patients are better off with continuous monitoring. Sometimes knowing whether continuous monitoring makes sense isn't possible until you're in labor and your practitioner can see how the baby is responding. This section outlines how your practitioner may monitor your baby.

Fetal heart monitoring

Labor puts stress on both you and the baby. *Fetal heart monitoring* provides a way to make sure that the baby is handling the stress. Monitoring can be done in several ways.

External monitoring

Electronic fetal heart monitoring uses either two belts or a wide elastic band placed around the abdomen. A device attached to the belt or under the band uses an ultrasound-Doppler technique to pick up the fetal heartbeat. A second device uses a gauge to pick up the contractions. An external contraction monitor can show the frequency and duration of contractions, but it can't provide information about how strong they are. An external fetal heart monitor gives information about the fetus's response to contractions and records *variability* — that is, periodic changes in heart rate that help determine how the baby is tolerating the labor process.

You may hear your practitioner use the following terms to describe the fetal heartbeat:

>> **Normal baseline heart rate:** About 110 to 160 beats per minute.

>> **Bradycardia:** A decrease in the fetal heart rate from baseline to below 110 beats per minute that lasts for more than ten minutes.

>> **Tachycardia:** An increase in the fetal heart rate to above 160 beats per minute for more than ten minutes.

>> **Accelerations:** Brief increases above baseline in the fetal heart rate, often after a fetal movement. Accelerations are a reassuring sign.

>> **Decelerations:** These are intermittent decreases below the baseline fetal heart rate. The significance of decelerations depends on their frequency, how far the heart rate drops, and when they occur in relation to contractions. Decelerations are classified as early, variable, or late, according to when they occur in relation to contractions.

There tends to be a large variability in the interpretation of fetal heart rate tracings. For this reason, the National Institute of Child Health and Human Development created a three-tier system for interpreting fetal heart rate tracings:

>> **Category 1:** Normal tracing — predicting normal fetal acid-base status

You can take heart when fetal heart monitoring indicates the following:

● A normal baseline heart rate of 110 to 160 beats per minute

● An absence of late or variable decelerations

● Moderate fetal heart rate variability (fluctuations of the fetal heart rate) of about 6 to 25 beats per minute above and below baseline

>> **Category 2:** Indeterminate tracing — requires closer observation and possible treatment (fluids, oxygen, change in position, and so forth)

>> **Category 3:** Abnormal tracing — predicting abnormal fetal acid-base status at the moment

Internal monitoring

Your practitioner uses an internal fetal heart monitor when your baby needs closer observation than is possible with external monitoring. Your practitioner may be concerned about how your baby is tolerating labor, or she may simply be having difficulty picking up the heart rate externally — if, for example, you're having more than one baby. The monitor is placed during an internal exam. It's passed through the cervix via a flexible plastic tube. This procedure is no more uncomfortable than a pelvic exam. The tiny electrode is then attached to the baby's scalp.

An internal monitor for contractions (called an *internal pressure transducer,* or IPT) is sometimes used to better assess how strong the contractions are. The monitor consists of thin, flexible, fluid-filled tubing, which is inserted between the fetal head and the uterine wall during an internal exam. Sometimes, this same device is used to infuse saline into the uterus — if very little amniotic fluid is present or if the fetal heart tracing indicates the umbilical cord is being compressed.

Other tests of fetal health

If the information from the fetal monitor raises concerns or is ambiguous, your practitioner can perform other tests to help determine how to proceed with your labor.

Some practitioners, and some mothers, prefer not to monitor. But most doctors believe that monitoring is very useful and that the benefits of monitoring outweigh the risk that monitoring will lead to an unnecessary cesarean delivery.

Labor admission test

This test involves performing electronic fetal heart rate monitoring for about 20 to 30 minutes upon admission to the labor and delivery floor. It's a good way of initially assessing fetal well-being and may be helpful in quickly identifying those rare occasions where the fetus needs quick delivery.

Scalp pH

If your practitioner is concerned about how well the baby is tolerating labor, she may want to perform a *scalp pH test.* This involves sampling a small amount of the baby's blood through a little prick of his scalp and measuring the pH, which reflects how well the baby is doing during labor. This test requires that the cervix be dilated enough to access the fetal scalp. Many labor floors no longer have the machinery to perform this test because the machines require a lot of maintenance and quality control.

Scalp stimulation

Scalp stimulation is an easy test to see how the fetus is doing. The practitioner simply tickles the baby's scalp during an internal exam. If this touch causes the fetal heart rate to increase, the baby is usually doing fine.

Fetal pulse oximetry

Another potential way of assessing fetal well-being is by measuring fetal oxygen saturation. This can be measured in a variety of ways, including using a device that attaches to the fetal scalp or a probe that sits inside the mother's vagina. However, at this time, there isn't good data to clarify whether fetal pulse oximetry improves newborn outcome beyond regular fetal heart rate monitoring.

Nudging Things Along: Labor Induction

To *induce* labor means to cause it to begin before it starts on its own. Induction may be a necessity (due to some obstetric, medical, or fetal complications) or elective (performed for the convenience of the patient or her practitioner).

Medically indicated induction

An induction is *indicated* (is a medical necessity) when the risks of continuing the pregnancy are greater — for the mother or the baby — than the risks of early delivery.

Problems with the mother's health that may warrant induction include

» Preeclampsia (see Book 6, Chapter 2 for information)

» The presence of certain diseases, such as diabetes (see Book 6, Chapter 3) or cholestasis (see Book 2, Chapter 3), which may improve after delivery

» An infection in the amniotic fluid, such as chorioamnionitis

Potential risks to the baby's health that may warrant induction include

» Pregnancy well past the due date; because this can increase the risk of certain complications, most practitioners induce labor after the 41st or 42nd week

» Ruptured membranes before labor has started, a situation that may place the baby at risk for developing an infection

>> Intrauterine growth restriction (see Book 6, Chapter 2)

>> Suspected *macrosomia* (fetus weighing more than 8 pounds, 13 ounces)

>> Rh incompatibility with complications (see Book 6, Chapter 2)

>> Decreased amniotic fluid *(oligohydramnios)*

>> Tests of fetal well-being indicating the fetus may not be thriving in the uterus

Elective induction

Although some women like the idea of a planned delivery, others prefer labor to occur spontaneously. Some practitioners gladly perform elective inductions, and others are opposed to the whole concept of it. A woman may choose to undergo an elective induction for several reasons, including the following:

>> To enable her to make arrangements for her other children, her work, or her partner's work; or for the convenience of other family members, who will know exactly which day she's going into labor

>> To ensure that a particular physician in a group practice, with whom she's developed a special relationship, delivers her baby

>> To deliver when the maximum number of labor floor personnel or other specialists are present if she's at risk for certain neonatal or labor complications

>> To reduce anxiety after a history of poor pregnancy outcomes (such as a previous full-term fetal death) by delivering earlier than she naturally would

>> To make sure she'll get to the hospital on time if she lives far away and has a history of rapid deliveries

Some studies in medical literature suggest elective induction of labor may lead to an increase in cesarean deliveries. If the cervix is neither dilated nor effaced, or if the fetal head isn't engaged in the pelvis, the risk of a cesarean delivery is probably higher. But if all conditions are favorable for induction, the risk of cesarean may not be increased at all. However, the length of time the patient spends in the hospital is likely to increase slightly when labor is induced.

REMEMBER

If an elected induction of labor is planned, it should not be performed at less than 39 weeks along in the pregnancy. Delivery before this time should be medically indicated. If you're considering elective induction of labor, you and your partner should fully understand that you may stand a slightly increased risk of needing a cesarean delivery. If both the expectant parents and the practitioner involved understand these risks, elective induction of labor can be appropriate for personal, medical, geographical, or psychological reasons.

Inducing labor

The way in which labor is induced depends on the condition of the cervix. If your cervix isn't favorable, or *ripe* (thinned out, soft, and dilated), your practitioner may use various medications and techniques to ripen it. Occasionally, ripening alone may put you right into labor.

TECHNICAL STUFF

One of the most common agents used for cervical ripening is a form of prostaglandin that helps to soften the cervix and may cause contractions, too. A commonly used ripening agent is misoprostol, which is a prostaglandin E1 analog. It comes as a small tablet that's inserted into the vagina. An alternative is a prostaglandin E2, which comes as a vaginal insert (Cervidil). Other devices that can mechanically dilate the cervix are also used. Laminaria are small sticks that, when inserted into the cervix, absorb water and expand the cervix. Another good alternative is a catheter, or small tube with an inflatable balloon on the end that is also inserted into the cervix and inflated. Typically once the cervix is dilated, the balloon catheter falls out.

WARNING

Some recent information in medical literature indicates that the risk of uterine rupture is higher in women who have had a cesarean section in the past and are having labor induced. The risk of this potentially serious complication seems to be highest if the patient is given a prostaglandin for induction. For this reason, many practitioners prefer not to induce with prostaglandins and instead prefer to use a balloon catheter.

If your cervix isn't yet ripe and you require induction, you're likely to be admitted to the hospital in the evening and given medications to ripen the cervix at bedtime. Then your practitioner can administer *oxytocin* (a synthetic hormone similar to one that your body naturally releases during labor) to induce labor in the morning.

If your cervix is already ripe, you're likely to be admitted in the morning. Labor is then induced either by administering oxytocin intravenously or by rupturing your membranes (often called *breaking your water*). The doctor performs an *amniotomy*, or rupturing of the membranes, with a small plastic hook during an internal examination. This procedure usually isn't painful.

Your practitioner then instructs your nurse to administer oxytocin (usually known by its brand name, Pitocin) through an IV, and a special pump carefully adjusts and controls the dosage. Oxytocin is a hormone that causes the uterus to contract. It can be used to start labor for induction or speed up labor that started on its own. You begin with very little medication, and the level of medication increases at regular intervals until you have adequate contractions. Sometimes labor starts within a few hours after the induction is started, but it may take much longer. Occasionally, it may take as long as two days to really get things going.

REMEMBER

A common misconception is that oxytocin makes labor more painful. It doesn't. Oxytocin is similar to the hormone that your body naturally releases during labor, and it's administered in about the same doses that your body would produce to cause normal labor.

Augmenting labor

Doctors can use oxytocin to augment labor that is already happening. If your contractions are inadequate or if labor is taking an unusually long time, your practitioner may use oxytocin to help move things along. Again, the contractions produced as a result of this augmentation are no stronger and no more painful than contractions occurring during a spontaneous labor.

Getting the Big Picture: Stages and Characteristics of Labor

Each woman's labor is, in some ways, unique. An individual woman's experience may even vary from pregnancy to pregnancy. Anyone who delivers babies knows all too well that labor can always surprise you. A doctor may expect one woman to deliver quickly and find that her labor takes a long time, while another woman, whom he thinks will take forever, may deliver very rapidly. Still, in the vast majority of pregnant women, labor progresses in a predictable pattern. It passes through easily discernible stages at a fairly standard rate.

If you're going through your first delivery, the entire labor process is likely to last between 12 and 14 hours. For deliveries after the first one, labor is usually shorter (about 8 hours). Labor is divided into three stages, described in this chapter and in Book 2, Chapter 5.

Tracking your progress through labor

Your practitioner can track your progress through labor by performing internal exams every few hours. How easily you progress through labor is measured by how quickly your cervix dilates and how smoothly the fetus descends downward through the pelvis and birth canal. By plotting cervical dilation and fetal station along a graph (see the earlier section "Discerning false labor from true labor" for more information), practitioners can measure the progress of labor objectively. Doctors become concerned over the progress of labor if it's too slow or if the cervix stops dilating and the fetus doesn't descend. They have a shorthand system for describing the variables that determine how easily a woman makes her way through labor: the three *P*s (passenger, pelvis, and power):

>> Passenger — the baby's size and position

>> Pelvis — the pelvis's size

>> Power — the contractions' strength

Your practitioner must pay attention to all these factors, because if labor doesn't progress normally, it may be a sign that the baby would be better off delivered with assistance — with forceps or vacuum, or by cesarean delivery.

The first stage

The first stage of labor occurs from the onset of true labor to full dilation of the cervix. This stage is by far the longest (taking an average of 11 hours for a first child and 7 hours for subsequent births). It is divided into three phases: the early (latent) phase, the active phase, and the transition phase. Each phase has its own unique characteristics.

Early or latent phase

During the early phase of the first stage of labor, contractions occur every 5 to 20 minutes in the beginning and then increase in frequency until they're less than 5 minutes apart. The contractions last between 30 and 45 seconds at first, but as this phase continues, they work up to 60 to 90 seconds in length. During the early phase, your cervix gradually dilates to about 5 to 6 centimeters and becomes 100 percent effaced.

The entire early phase of the first stage of labor lasts an average of 6 to 7 hours in a first birth and 4 to 5 hours for subsequent births, although recent data shows that this may in fact be longer. Often, the exact length of labor is unpredictable because knowing when labor actually begins is difficult.

In the beginning of the early phase, your contractions may feel like menstrual cramps, with or without back pain. Your membranes may rupture, and you may have a bloody show (see the earlier section "Noticing changes before labor begins"). If you've been admitted to the hospital, your doctor may use a small plastic hook to rupture your membranes in order to help things along.

Early on in this phase, you may be most comfortable at home. You can try resting or sleeping, or you may want to stay active. Some women find they have an overwhelming desire to clean or perform some other household chores. If you're hungry, eat a light meal (soup, juice, or toast, for example), not a heavy one — in case you later need anesthesia to deal with labor complications. You may want to time your contractions, but you don't need to obsess about it.

WARNING

If you start to become more uncomfortable, the contractions occur with more frequency or intensity, your membranes rupture (your water breaks), or you have vaginal bleeding, call your practitioner or go to your hospital.

TIP

Many women find walking around makes them more comfortable and distracts them from the pain during the early part of labor. Others prefer to rest in bed. Ask your practitioner whether your hospital has any restrictions on walking during labor.

Active phase

The active phase of the first stage of labor is usually shorter and more predictable than the early phase. For a first child, it usually lasts about 2 to 3 hours, on average. For subsequent babies, it lasts about 1½ to 2 or more hours. Contractions occur every 3 to 5 minutes in this phase, and they last about 45 to 60 seconds. Your cervix dilates from 5 or 6 centimeters to a full 10 centimeters.

You may feel increasing discomfort or pain during this phase and maybe a back-ache as well. Some women experience more pain in the back than in the front, a condition known as *back labor.* This may be a sign that the baby is facing toward your front rather than toward your spine.

By this time, you're likely already in the hospital or birthing center. Some patients prefer to rest in bed; others would rather walk around. Do whatever makes you comfortable, unless your practitioner asks that you stay in bed to be monitored closely. Now is the time to practice the breathing and relaxation techniques you may have learned in childbirth classes.

TIP

If you need pain relief, let your practitioner know (for more information, see the later section "Handling Labor Pain"). Your partner may help ease your pain by massaging your back, perhaps by using a tennis ball or rolling pin.

Seeing an end in sight!

In addition to intense contractions, you may notice an increase in bloody show and increased pressure, especially on your rectum, as the baby's head descends. During this last part of the first stage of labor, you may feel as if you have to have a bowel movement. Don't worry; this sensation is a good sign and indicates that the fetus is heading in the right direction.

LABOR CURVES

Until recently, practitioners relied on something called a *Friedman Curve* to assess a woman's progress in labor. This was based on now-historic data from the 1950s, when Dr. Friedman evaluated the course of labor of 500 women having their first child. Based on this original information, active labor occurred when a woman dilated to 3 to 4 centimeters, and the minimum rate of cervical dilation during the active phase was 1.2 cm/hour for first births and 1.5 cm/hour for subsequent births. It now seems that labor actually takes longer.

Dr. Zhang and his co-researchers evaluated data from a comprehensive study called the Consortium of Safe Labor. They looked at information on more than 60,000 women with singleton pregnancies in spontaneous labor who delivered vaginally with normal newborn outcomes. This study was sponsored by the National Institute of Child Health and Development (NICHD). Zhang's labor curve shows that more than half the women did not dilate at greater than 1 cm/hour until reaching 5 to 6 centimeters. It seems that the normal rate of cervical change from 3 to 6 centimeters is much slower than previously thought. After reaching 6 centimeters, cervical dilation is more rapid.

REMEMBER

If you feel the urge to push, let your practitioner know. You may be fully dilated, but try not to push until your practitioner tells you to do so. Pushing before you're fully dilated can slow the labor process or tear your cervix.

TIP

Try to practice breathing exercises and relaxation techniques, if they work for you. When you want pain medication or an epidural anesthetic, let your practitioner know. She decides what pain relief options are best for you based on how far along in labor you are and other factors related to you and your baby's health.

TIP

Partners, women aren't responsible for anything they say during labor, but you are, so don't get upset over any suggestions your partner makes about your anatomy or her comments on your ancestry. And she doesn't really mean what she said about your mother, either. And because pain makes people say things they don't mean and may not even remember, don't file away her remarks for another day. Vocalizing the pain in this way is both healthy and normal. Because you're not in pain, you don't get the same privileges, so save the snappy retorts for another time.

Potential problems during labor's first stage

Most women experience labor's first stage without any problems. But if a problem arises, the following info will prepare you to handle it with a clear, focused mind:

>> **Prolonged latent phase:** The latent or early phase of labor is considered prolonged if it lasts more than 20 hours in a woman having her first child or more than 14 hours in someone who has delivered a previous child. Your practitioner may not be able to determine when labor actually starts, so knowing for sure when labor becomes prolonged isn't always easy, either.

When a practitioner determines that labor is taking too long, he responds in one of two ways.

- One approach is to use medication, such as a sedative, to help you relax. Labor may then subside (which means that it was false labor all along), or active labor may begin.

- The other approach is to try to move labor along by performing an *amniotomy* (rupturing the membranes or breaking your water) or by administering oxytocin (Pitocin). Both procedures are covered in more detail earlier in this chapter.

>> **Protraction disorders:** Protraction disorders can occur if the cervix dilates too slowly or if the baby's head doesn't descend at a normal rate. If you're having your first baby, the upper limit of time to dilate, according to this recent data, means than it can take up to 6 hours to progress from 4 to 5 centimeters and more than 3 hours to progress from 5 to 6 centimeters, regardless of parity. After that, the average and upper limit to dilate 1 cm/hour is shown in Table 4-1.

Protraction disorders may be caused by *cephalopelvic disproportion,* or CPD, which is the term for a poor fit between the baby's head and the mother's birth canal. Protraction disorders may also occur because the baby's head is in an unfavorable position or because the number or intensity of contractions is inadequate. In both cases, many practitioners try administering oxytocin to improve labor progress.

>> **Arrest disorders:** Arrest disorders occur if the cervix stops dilating or if the baby's head stops descending for more than two hours during active labor. Arrest disorders are often associated with CPD, but an infusion of oxytocin may solve the problem. If oxytocin doesn't alleviate the arrest disorder, you may need a cesarean section. Typically, arrest of labor is diagnosed when the cervix is at least 6 centimeters dilated and membranes are ruptured and when no cervical change occurs for at least four hours with adequate contractions and six hours with inadequate contractions.

TABLE 4-1 **Average and 95th Percentile (Extreme Upper End of Normal) for Patients in Active Labor, Based on Zhang Labor Curves**

Change in Cervix	First Birth Average Hours and (95th%)	Subsequent Births Average Hours and (95th%)
From 6 to 7 cm	0.6 (2.2)	0.5 (1.9)
From 7 to 8 cm	0.5 (1.6)	0.4 (1.3)
From 8 to 9 cm	0.5 (1.4)	0.3 (1.0)
From 9 to 10 cm	0.5 (1.8)	0.3 (0.9)

The second stage

Labor's second stage begins when you're fully dilated (at 10 centimeters) and ends with your baby's delivery. This part is the "pushing" stage and takes about one hour for a first child and 30 to 40 minutes for subsequent births. The second stage may be longer if you have an epidural. Book 2, Chapter 5 describes the second stage in detail.

The third stage

The third stage occurs from the time of delivery of the baby to delivery of the placenta — usually less than 20 minutes for all deliveries. For details on this stage, go to Book 2, Chapter 5.

Handling Labor Pain

During labor's first stage, pain is caused by contractions of the uterus and dilation of the cervix. The pain may feel like severe menstrual cramps at first. But in labor's second stage, the stretching of the birth canal as the baby passes through it adds a different kind of pain — often a feeling of great pressure on the lower pelvis or rectum. But none of this pain needs to be excruciating, thanks to well-practiced breathing and relaxation exercises and, in many cases, modern anesthesia.

Most practitioners acknowledge that even for women who have diligently attended childbirth classes, labor is inherently painful. The degree of pain — and the willingness and ability to tolerate it — varies from woman to woman. Some women choose to deal with the pain on their own or with the help of breathing and distraction techniques mastered in childbirth classes — and that's a perfectly acceptable choice. Many other women want medication to help them deal with the pain, no matter how well prepared they are.

REMEMBER

Don't feel that you're in any way falling short of being a perfect mother or that your pregnancy isn't "natural" if you need medication to help with labor pain. Everyone responds to pain differently, both emotionally *and* physiologically, so even if your best friend, your sister, or your mother got through labor with little or no pain medication, you aren't weak if you choose to use it. Look at it this way: Women who are in excruciating pain usually don't breathe regularly. They also tense their muscles, and, by doing so, they may only prolong labor.

Today doctors generally administer medication in two different ways to help you deal with labor pain: *systemically* — that is, by injection either into a blood vessel (intravenously) or into a muscle (intramuscularly) — or *regionally*, with the use of an epidural or other local anesthesia.

Systemic medications

The most common medications used systemically are relatives of the narcotic morphine — drugs such as meperidine (brand name Demerol), fentanyl (Sublimaze), butorphanal (Stadol), and nalbuphine (Nubain). These medications can be given every two to four hours as needed, either intravenously or intramuscularly.

REMEMBER

Any medication you take (even when you're not pregnant) has side effects, and pain relievers used during labor are no exception, although your doctor will do what he can to reduce these side effects, often by combining medications. Nausea, vomiting, drowsiness, and a drop in your blood pressure are the main side effects for the mother. The degree to which the fetus or newborn is also affected depends on how close to the time of delivery the medication is given. If a large dose is given within two hours prior to delivery, the newborn may be sleepy or groggy. In rare cases, his breathing may be weak. If this problem is significant, your doctor or the baby's doctor can give a medication that immediately reverses or counteracts the pain medication. No evidence suggests that these medications, when given in appropriate doses and with proper monitoring, have any effect on the progress of labor or on the rate of cesarean deliveries.

Regional anesthetics

Systemic medications are distributed via the bloodstream to all parts of the body. Yet most of the pain of labor and delivery is concentrated in the uterus, vagina, and rectum, so regional anesthesia is sometimes used to deliver pain medication to those specific areas. Medications used in regional anesthesia can be a local anesthetic (like lidocaine), a narcotic (such as those in the preceding section), or a combination of the two. Commonly used techniques for administering regional pain relief include epidural and spinal anesthesia and caudal, saddle, and pudendal blocks. The following sections go into more detail on these techniques.

Epidural anesthesia

When it comes to relieving labor pain, there is nothing like an epidural. Epidural anesthesia is perhaps the most popular form of labor pain relief. Almost universally, women who've had it say, "Why didn't I get this earlier?" or "Why was I hesitant about this?" An anesthesiologist with special training in epidural catheter placement must administer an epidural, so epidurals may not be available in every hospital. This is definitely something you want to find out ahead of time so there are no surprises on the day (or night) of the big event!

TECHNICAL STUFF

With an epidural, a tiny, flexible, plastic catheter is inserted through a needle into your lower back and threaded into the space above the membrane covering the spinal cord. Before inserting the needle, the anesthesiologist numbs your skin with a local anesthetic. While the needle is going in, you may feel a brief tingling sensation in your legs, but the process really isn't painful for most women. After the catheter is in place, medication can be sent through it to numb the nerves coming from the lower part of the spine — nerves that go to the uterus, vagina, and perineum (the area between the vagina and anus). The catheter (not the needle) stays in place throughout labor in case you need what's called a *top-up* dose of the anesthetic to get you through the rest of labor and delivery.

A major advantage of epidural anesthesia is that it uses smaller doses of pain medication. However, because your sensory nerves run very close to your motor nerves, large doses of anesthetic can temporarily affect your ability to move your legs during labor.

The amount and type of medication you need can be adjusted according to the stage of labor you're in. During the first stage, pain relief focuses on uterine contractions, but during the second (pushing) stage, pain relief focuses on the vagina and perineum, which are distended by the baby passing through. Epidurals can also make repairing a tear, or *episiotomy,* much more tolerable.

Years ago, anesthesiologists wouldn't give epidurals during early labor because it confined patients to their beds for the remainder of their labor. Recently, however, *walking epidurals* — the kind that allow you to walk around, because they use medications that have little or no effect on motor function — have become more popular for this often painful stage of labor. Some anesthesiologists, however, question the effectiveness of this type of epidural in relieving pain.

Epidurals can also relieve pain in cesarean deliveries, although different medications in different doses are used. In fact, epidurals are very popular for cesareans because they enable the mother to be awake during delivery and to experience her child's birth. In cases in which cesarean delivery is an emergency or when the mother has blood-clotting problems, however, an epidural may not be possible.

Doctors once thought epidurals, especially if placed too early, prolonged labor and increased the need for forceps, vacuum-assisted, or cesarean delivery. For this reason, many practitioners were reluctant to recommend epidurals to their patients. Most doctors today accept that these problems are negligible when an experienced anesthesiologist places the epidural after labor is well-established and that the benefit outweighs the risk.

A MENU OF EPIDURAL TECHNIQUES

The method used to administer an epidural is usually determined by the anesthesiologist, based on his expertise, his individual preferences, and your specific situation (such as how far along you are in labor or any medical conditions you may have). The various techniques by which an epidural can be administered include the following:

- **Intermittent epidural bolus dosing** was the standard way of administering epidural anesthesia for many years. With this technique, intermittent doses of local anesthesia are given through the catheter. Injections are either timed to the woman's complaints of pain or set at specific intervals. The disadvantage of this method is that often pain is felt as the medication wears off, and more intervention by the anesthesiologist is required.

- **Continuous epidural infusions** provide continuous infusion of pain medicine, which provides a smooth and constant relief from pain. If needed, the dosing can be changed, and extra medication can be given.

- **Patient-controlled epidural analgesia (PCEA)** differs from the continuous infusion method in that you're the one who controls the amount of medication given. Some anesthesiologists use this technique alone, whereas others prefer a combination of continuous infusion with the patient-controlled method.

- **Combined spinal-epidural analgesia** gives a dose in the spinal area for immediate pain relief (within five to ten minutes) and, at the same time, places a catheter in the epidural space for continuous infusion.

- **Walking epidural** describes a technique of administering pain relief that doesn't interfere with motor function. The truth is that, for various reasons, 40 to 80 percent of women don't actually walk during labor, anyway!

Sometimes the epidural takes away the sensation you feel when your bladder is full, so you may need a catheter to empty your bladder. In some cases, the epidural may block motor nerves to the point where you have difficulty pushing. You also may experience a rapid drop in blood pressure that can lead to a temporary drop in the baby's heart rate.

Overall, pain control simply makes the whole experience of labor and delivery much more enjoyable for the mother and her partner (and the person doing the delivery, too!).

Spinal anesthesia

Spinal anesthesia is similar to an epidural except that the medication is injected into the space *under* the membrane covering the spinal cord rather than above it. This technique is often used for cesarean delivery, especially when a cesarean is needed suddenly and no epidural was placed during labor. The information in the preceding section about epidurals (regarding the amount of medication needed and the risks involved) applies to spinal anesthesia, too.

Caudal and saddle blocks

Caudal and *saddle blocks* involve placing the medications very low in the spinal canal, so they affect only those pain nerves going to the vagina and perineum. These methods have a more rapid onset of pain relief, but the medication wears off sooner.

Pudendal block

Your doctor can place a *pudendal block* by injecting an anesthetic inside the vagina, in the area next to the pudendal nerves. This technique numbs part of the vagina and the perineum, but it does nothing to relieve the pain from contractions.

General anesthesia

When you have general anesthesia, you're made fully unconscious by an anesthesiologist using a variety of medications. Doctors almost never use this technique for labor anymore, and this technique is only rarely used for cesarean deliveries because it's associated with a higher risk of complications. General anesthesia obviously also causes you to sleep through your baby's delivery. But if, in a cesarean delivery, you have a clotting problem that rules out placing a needle into your spinal column or if the cesarean is an emergency and there isn't enough time to place an epidural, general anesthesia should be used.

Considering alternative forms of labor-pain management

Whereas systemic medications or various anesthetic techniques are aimed at eliminating the physical sensation of pain, alternative or nonpharmacologic methods are directed toward preventing the suffering associated with labor pain. These approaches to pain management emphasize labor pain as a normal side effect of the normal process of labor. Women are given reassurance, encouragement, and guidance to help them build self-confidence and maintain a sense of control and well-being. Many hospitals offer some of these techniques, although other techniques require special training and may not be available in all birthing facilities:

» **Continuous labor support:** This refers to nonmedical care given to a laboring woman, often by a doula or trained professional (see Book 2, Chapter 3 for information).

» **Maternal movement and positioning:** Sometimes walking or changing positions can alleviate some of the pain associated with labor. Your caregiver or nurse may suggest different positions to try.

» **The Birth Ball:** The Birth Ball is a large inflated exercise ball used to help in movement and relaxation during labor. During labor, you can sit or lean against the ball, which provides stability and soft support. The ball also increases the number of positions you can find for comfort.

» **Touch and massage:** These techniques provide encouragement, reassurance, and a sense of love, and they may be used to enhance relaxation and decrease pain.

» **Acupuncture and acupressure:** Acupuncture involves the placement of needles at various points on the body, whereas acupressure (or Shiatsu) refers to the placement of pressure with fingers or small beads at acupuncture points. In some studies, acupuncture use during labor was associated with more relaxation but no difference in pain intensity.

» **Hypnosis:** Usually hypnosis during labor involves self-hypnosis, where the woman herself is taught to induce the hypnotic state. Studies have shown that the use of hypnosis does lead to less use of pain medication and epidural anesthesia.

» **Transcutaneous Electrical Nerve Stimulation (TENS):** This technique involves the transmission of electrical impulses from a hand-held generator to the skin through surface electrodes. During labor, the electrodes are placed near the spine, and the woman controls the intensity of the current through a dial. TENS causes a buzzing sensation that may reduce awareness of contraction pain. Most studies have not shown a real reduction in pain, but some do suggest less use of pain medication and increased satisfaction.

>> **Intradermal water injections:** This technique involves injecting a small amount of sterile water into four locations on the lower back. This has been shown to reduce severe back pain for 45 to 90 minutes, but it doesn't seem to help the abdominal pain associated with labor.

>> **Application of heat and cold:** Often this is a matter of personal preference, as no scientific data suggests that one is better for pain relief than the other.

>> **Music and audioanalgesia:** The idea behind this method is that music, white noise, or environmental sounds may help to decrease the perception of pain. Although not clearly beneficial for pain relief, it may help to increase pain tolerance via mood elevation or help the woman to breathe more rhythmically (heavy metal is probably not the best choice, though!).

>> **Aromatherapy:** The use of aromatherapy appears to be on the rise. In one study, about half of the women felt it was helpful in reducing pain, anxiety, and nausea while improving their sense of well-being.

Chapter 5

Special Delivery: Bringing Your Baby into the World

When you're nearing the end of the second stage of labor, you're very close to the point of delivery. Now is the time you've been waiting and preparing yourself for. Keep in mind that you don't have to worry too much ahead of time. You *can* prepare yourself — by taking childbirth classes and by reading this book, for example. And remember that your practitioner and her assistants in the delivery room will guide you through the process. Accept and rely on their help. Trust in yourself, too, and let this natural process move along one step at a time.

Basically, babies are delivered in one of three ways: through the birth canal by your pushing, through the birth canal with a little assistance (that is, using forceps or a vacuum extractor), or by cesarean delivery. The method that's right for you depends on many factors, including your medical history, the baby's condition, and your pelvis's size relative to your baby's size. Don't feel overwhelmed. This chapter gives you the lowdown on all three.

Having a Vaginal Delivery

Most expectant mothers spend a great deal of time during the 40 weeks of pregnancy thinking ahead to the actual delivery. If you're having a baby for the first time, it may seem pretty scary. Even if you've had a child before, worrying a bit until you see your beautiful baby is normal. A little knowledge goes a long way, though, and being informed and prepared for all possibilities is always helpful.

REMEMBER

The most common method of delivery is, of course, a vaginal delivery. (Figure 5-1 gives you an overview of the process.) Most likely, you'll experience what doctors call a *spontaneous vaginal delivery,* which means that it occurs as a result of your pushing efforts and proceeds without a great deal of intervention. If you do need a little help, it may come in the form of forceps or a vacuum extractor. A delivery requiring the use of one of these tools to help pull the baby out is called an *operative vaginal delivery.* We cover both courses of events in this chapter.

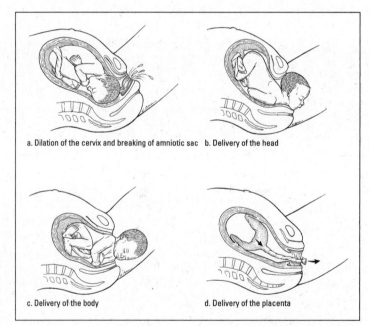

a. Dilation of the cervix and breaking of amniotic sac   b. Delivery of the head

c. Delivery of the body   d. Delivery of the placenta

FIGURE 5-1:
An overview
of the delivery
process.

Illustration by Kathryn Born, MA

During the first stage of labor, your cervix dilates and your membranes rupture. When your cervix is *fully dilated* (open to 10 centimeters), you reach the end of the first stage of labor and are ready to enter the second stage, in which you push your baby through the birth canal (vagina) and actually deliver the baby. At the end of the first stage, you may feel an overwhelming sensation of pressure on your rectum. You may feel as if you need to have a bowel movement. This sensation is likely to be greatest during contractions. Your baby's head descending in the birth canal and putting pressure on neighboring internal organs is causing this sensation.

If you have an *epidural* (a type of regional anesthesia used to take away the pain of labor — see Book 2, Chapter 4), you may not feel this pressure, or the feeling may be less intense. If you do feel it, let your nurse or practitioner know because it's probably a sign that your cervix is getting close to being fully dilated and that it may be time for you to push. Your nurse or doctor performs an internal exam to confirm that your cervix is fully dilated. If it is, she tells you to start pushing.

REMEMBER

Whether your nurse, doctor, or midwife is actually coaching you during pushing varies from hospital to hospital and from practitioner to practitioner. The important factor is that someone is with you to help you through this stage of labor.

Occasionally, you may be fully dilated when the fetal head is still relatively high up in the pelvis. In this case, your practitioner may want you to wait until the contractions cause the head to descend more before you start to push.

Pushing the baby out

Pushing generally takes 30 to 90 minutes (though sometimes it takes as long as three hours), depending on the baby's position and size, whether you have an epidural, and whether you've had children before. (If this isn't your first delivery, your cervix may begin to dilate weeks before your due date, and after you're fully dilated, you may push only once or twice to deliver!) Your nurse or practitioner gives you specific instructions on how to push.

While you're pushing, your baby moves farther along his downward course. Women often begin pushing as soon as the baby's head has descended into the pelvis. How long you push depends on how far down the head is when you start pushing and how efficient you are at it. Sometimes it takes a while to get the hang of it. After you deliver the head, your doctor may tell you to stop pushing so that she can suction some fluid out of the baby's mouth and also feel to see if the umbilical cord is around the baby's neck. After that, you'll push one or two more times to deliver the rest of the baby.

You have several possible positions in which to push (Figure 5-2 shows three that can help):

>> **Lithotomy position:** In this position, which is the most common, you lean back and pull your flexed knees to your chest. At the same time, you bend

your neck and try to touch your chin to your chest. The idea is to get your body to form a *C*. The position isn't the most flattering, but it does help to align the uterus and pelvis in a position that makes delivery relatively easy.

>> **Squatting position:** An advantage of squatting is that you have gravity working with you. A disadvantage is that you may be too tired to hold the position for very long, and any monitoring equipment or an intravenous line you may have can be cumbersome.

>> **Knee-chest position:** The knee-chest position is one in which you push while on all fours. This position is sometimes helpful if the baby's head is rotated in the birth canal in such a way that makes pushing the baby out in the lithotomy or squatting position difficult. The knee-chest position may be awkward for some women and difficult to stay in for very long.

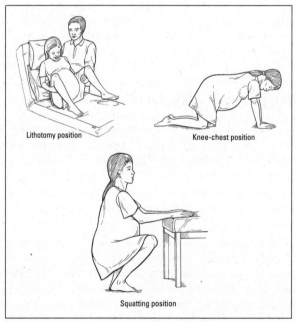

Lithotomy position

Knee-chest position

Squatting position

FIGURE 5-2:
Positions you can assume in childbirth.

Illustration by Kathryn Born, MA

TIP

Finding the one position that feels and works best for you may take a bit of experimentation. If you find that you're not making progress, try changing positions.

When you start to feel a contraction, your nurse or doctor usually tells you to take a deep, cleansing breath. After that, you inhale deeply again, hold in the air, and push like crazy. Focus the push toward your rectum and *perineum* (the area between the vagina and the rectum), trying not to tense up the muscles of your vagina or rectum. Push like you're having a bowel movement. Don't worry or be embarrassed if you pass stool while you're pushing. (If it happens, a nurse quickly cleans the perineum.) It's the rule rather than the exception, and all the people helping to take care of you have seen it many times before. In fact, passing stool is a sign that you're pushing correctly, so congratulate yourself. Trying to hold it in only impedes your efforts to push the baby out.

Hold each push for about ten seconds. Many nurses count to ten or ask your coach to count to ten to help you judge the time. After the count of ten, quickly release the breath you have been holding, take in another deep breath, and push again for another ten seconds, exactly as before. You usually push about three times with each contraction, depending on the length of the contraction.

Between contractions, try your best to relax and rest so that you can get ready for the next one. If it's okay with your practitioner, your coach may give you some ice chips or pat your forehead with a damp, cool cloth.

After your baby gets far enough down the birth canal, the top of the head becomes visible during your pushing efforts. This first glimpse is called *crowning* because your practitioner can see the crown of the baby's head. Some labor rooms have mirrors so that you, too, can see the head crowning, but many women have no desire to look. (Don't feel bad or somehow inadequate if you don't want to — you're busy enough.) After the contraction, the baby's head may again disappear back up into the birth canal. This retraction is normal. With each push, the baby comes down a little farther and recedes a little less afterward.

TO WATCH OR NOT TO WATCH

Some partners want to see everything that's happening during childbirth; others feel uncomfortable even being in the delivery room. Likewise, some women want their partners to witness everything, and others prefer that their partners not see them in this situation.

However you feel about it, communicate your feelings to your partner so that you can make each other feel as comfortable as possible. The last thing you need is for you or your partner to be embarrassed during a time that should be one of joy and happiness.

Getting an episiotomy

Just before birth, the baby's head distends the perineum and stretches the skin around the vagina. As the baby's head comes through the vagina's opening, it may tear the tissues in the back, or *posterior,* part of the vaginal opening, sometimes even to the point that the tear extends into the rectum. To minimize tearing of the surrounding skin and perineal muscles, your practitioner may make an *episiotomy* — a cut in the posterior part of the vaginal opening large enough to allow the baby's head to come through with minimal tearing or to provide extra room for delivery. Although an episiotomy may decrease the likelihood of a severe tear, it doesn't guarantee that you won't get one (that is, the cut made for the episiotomy may tear open even further as the baby's head or shoulders are delivered).

Your practitioner doesn't know whether you need an episiotomy until the head is almost out. Some doctors routinely make an episiotomy, and others wait to see whether it's necessary. Episiotomies are more common in women having their first baby than in those who have delivered before because the perineum stretches more easily after a previous birth. Tell your practitioner if you have strong wishes regarding receiving an episiotomy. Keep in mind, though, that some natural tears can be worse than an episiotomy.

The type of episiotomy made depends on your body, on the position of the baby's head, and on your practitioner's judgment. Practitioners can choose from two main types of episiotomies:

» **Median:** Straight down from the vagina toward the anus

» **Mediolateral:** Angled away from the anus

A local anesthetic can numb the area if you haven't had an epidural.

A median episiotomy may be less uncomfortable later on, and it may heal more easily. (See Book 2, Chapter 7 for coverage of the care and healing of an episiotomy.) However, a median episiotomy has a slightly greater chance of extending to the rectum. A mediolateral episiotomy, on the other hand, may be more uncomfortable later on and take longer to heal, but it has less chance of extending to the rectum when the baby's head passes through.

Most tears or lacerations that occur during delivery are in the perineum or are extensions of an episiotomy, which is also in that area. Occasionally, especially when the baby is exceptionally large or you have an operative vaginal delivery, lacerations can occur in other areas, such as the cervix, on the vagina's walls, the labia, or the tissue around the urethra. Your practitioner examines the birth canal carefully after delivery and sews up any lacerations that need to be repaired.

"DO I REALLY NEED AN EPISIOTOMY?"

The answer to this question depends on many factors, including the point of view of your practitioner. It's an issue of frequent debate among people who deliver babies. And as you may already know, it's also a big topic of discussion among pregnant women. Many practitioners believe that repairing a controlled cut in the perineum is easier than repairing any uncontrolled tear through the skin and perineal muscles that may occur without an episiotomy. The same people usually contend that episiotomies heal better, too. Although a doctor may see the layers of tissue in a cut better than in a tear, medical professionals aren't sure that makes any major difference. Compounding the issue is the fact that it's difficult to tell before labor whether the patient will need an episiotomy.

During delivery, the baby's head stretches the vagina's opening when the mother pushes. Sometimes the birth canal stretches enough that the baby's head doesn't need the extra room that an episiotomy provides. Then again, sometimes the birth canal doesn't. If you can "hold" the head at the perineum to let additional stretching occur, you may help matters. But holding the head there is easier said than done because of the incredible pressure that the baby's head exerts. One potential advantage of epidurals is that they allow for a slower delivery of the head and therefore reduce the chances that you'll need an episiotomy.

These lacerations usually heal very quickly and almost never cause long-term problems. Don't worry about having the stitches removed — most doctors use the type of sutures that dissolve on their own.

Handling prolonged second-stage labor

If you're having your first child and you remain in the second stage of labor for more than two hours (or three hours if you have an epidural), the labor is considered prolonged. If you're having your second or subsequent child, a second stage nearing one hour (or two hours if you have an epidural) is also considered prolonged.

A prolonged second stage may be due to inadequate contractions or to *cephalopelvic disproportion,* which is a poor fit between the baby's head and the mother's birth canal (see Book 2, Chapter 4). Sometimes, the baby's head is in a position that blocks further descent. Oxytocin (Pitocin) may help, or your practitioner may try to rotate the baby's head. You may also try changing your position to push more effectively. Sometimes forceps do the trick if the baby's head is low enough in the birth canal (see the later section "Assisting Nature: Operative Vaginal Delivery"). If all else fails, your doctor may recommend a cesarean delivery.

The big moment: Delivering your baby

When the baby's head remains visible between contractions, your nurse helps get you into position to deliver. If you're laboring in a birthing room, all she needs to do is to remove the platform at the foot of your bed and set up padded leg supports. If you need to be moved to a delivery room (more like an operating room), your nurse moves you and all your monitors to a stretcher. Whether you deliver in a birthing room or a delivery room depends both on the facility where you have your baby and on any risk factors you may have.

When you're in position to deliver, you still have to keep pushing with each of your contractions. Your doctor or nurse cleans your perineum, usually with an iodine solution, and places drapes over your legs to keep the area as clean as possible for the newborn. As you're pushing, your perineum is getting more and more stretched out. Whether you need an episiotomy is usually determined in these final moments.

With each push, the baby's head descends farther and farther until finally it comes out of the birth canal. After the baby's head delivers, your practitioner tells you to stop pushing so that she can suction secretions from the baby's mouth and nose before the rest of the body comes out.

TIP

To stop pushing at this point can be difficult because of the intense pressure in your perineal area; panting (breathe as if you're blowing out tiny candles!) may make it a little easier not to push. If you have an epidural, you may not feel this intense pressure.

Your practitioner also checks at this point to see whether the umbilical cord is wrapped around the baby's neck. A *nuchal cord*, as it's called, is actually quite common and very rarely a cause for worry. Your practitioner simply removes the loop from around the baby's neck before delivering the rest of the baby.

Finally, your practitioner instructs you to push again to deliver the baby's body. Because the head is typically the widest part, delivery of the body is usually easier. After your baby has made it fully into the world, her mouth and nose are suctioned again.

Normally, after the baby's head delivers, the shoulders and body follow easily. Occasionally, though, the baby's shoulders may be stuck behind the mother's pubic bone, which makes delivery of the rest of the baby more difficult. This situation is known as *shoulder dystocia*. If you have this problem, your practitioner can perform various maneuvers designed to dislodge the shoulders and deliver the baby. These methods include the following:

>> Applying pressure directly above your pubic bone to push away the entrapped shoulder

>> Flexing your knees back to allow more room for delivery

>> Rotating the baby's shoulders manually

>> Delivering the posterior arm of the baby first

Although shoulder dystocia can occur in women with no risk factors, certain characteristics make this condition more likely:

>> Very large babies

>> Gestational diabetes

>> Prolonged labor

>> A history of large babies or babies with shoulder dystocia

Delivering the placenta

After the baby is born, the third stage of delivery begins — the delivery of the placenta, also known as the *afterbirth* (refer to Figure 5-1). This stage lasts only about 5 to 15 minutes. You still have contractions, but they're much less intense. These contractions help separate the placenta from the uterus's wall. After this separation occurs and the placenta reaches the vagina's opening, your practitioner may ask you to give one more gentle push. Many women, exhilarated by and exhausted from the delivery, pay little attention to this part of the process and later on don't even remember it.

Repairing your perineum

After the placenta is out, your practitioner inspects your cervix, vagina, and perineum for tears or damage and then repairs (with stitches) the episiotomy or any tears. (If you didn't have an epidural and you have sensation in your perineum, your practitioner may use a local anesthetic to numb the area before repairing it.)

After the practitioner finishes with the repairs, a nurse cleans your perineal area, removes your legs from the leg supports, and gives you warm blankets. You may also continue to feel mild contractions; these contractions are normal and actually help to minimize bleeding.

Assisting Nature: Operative Vaginal Delivery

If the baby's head is low enough in the birth canal and your practitioner feels that the baby needs to be delivered immediately or that you can't deliver the baby vaginally without some added help, she may recommend the use of forceps or a vacuum extractor to assist. Using either of these instruments is called an *operative vaginal delivery*. Such a delivery may be appropriate to use when

>> You've pushed for a long time, and you're too tired to continue pushing hard enough to deliver.

>> You've pushed for some time, and your practitioner thinks you won't deliver vaginally unless you have this type of help.

>> The baby's heart rate pattern indicates a need to deliver the baby quickly.

>> The baby's position is making it very difficult for you to push it out on your own.

Figure 5-3 shows *forceps*, two smooth, curved, spatula-like instruments that are placed on the sides of the baby's head to help guide it through the outer part of the birth canal. The *vacuum extractor* is a suction cup that is placed on the top of the baby's head, to which suction is applied to allow your practitioner to gently pull the baby through the birth canal.

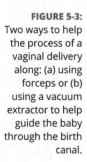
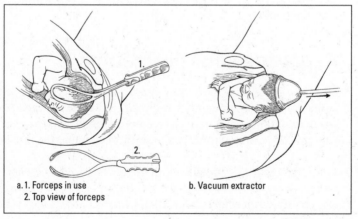

FIGURE 5-3: Two ways to help the process of a vaginal delivery along: (a) using forceps or (b) using a vacuum extractor to help guide the baby through the birth canal.

a. 1. Forceps in use
2. Top view of forceps

b. Vacuum extractor

Illustration by Kathryn Born, MA

Both techniques are safe for you and the baby if the baby is far enough down in the birth canal and the instruments are used appropriately. In fact, these techniques can often help women avoid cesarean delivery (but not always — see the next section). The decision to use forceps or a vacuum extractor often depends on your practitioner's judgment and experience and the baby's position and station.

If you haven't had an epidural, you may need extra local anesthesia for a forceps or vacuum delivery, and most practitioners perform an episiotomy to make extra room. After the forceps or vacuum is applied, the practitioner asks you to continue to push until the head emerges. The forceps or vacuum extractor is then removed, and the rest of the baby is delivered with your pushing.

If forceps are used, very often the baby is born with marks on her head where the forceps were applied. If this happens to your baby, remember that it's typical and that the marks disappear within a few days. A vacuum extractor may cause the baby to be born with a round, raised area on the top of the head where the extractor was applied. This mark, too, goes away in a few days.

Having a Cesarean Delivery

Many patients wonder whether they'll need a cesarean. Sometimes your doctor knows the answer before labor even begins — if you have placenta previa (see Book 2, Chapter 2), for example, or if the baby is in a *breech* or *transverse lie* (that is, the baby is lying sideways within the uterus rather than head-down). But most of the time, neither you nor your doctor can know whether you'll need a cesarean until you see how your labor progresses and how your baby tolerates labor.

Because a cesarean is a surgical procedure, a doctor performs a cesarean delivery in an operating room under sterile conditions. A nurse inserts an intravenous line in the patient's arm and a catheter in the bladder. After a nurse or nurse's assistant scrubs the patient's abdomen with antiseptic solution, a nurse places sterile sheets over the patient's belly. One of the sheets is elevated to create a screen so that the expectant parents don't have to watch the procedure. (Although childbirth is usually an experience shared by both parents, a cesarean delivery is still a surgical operation. Most doctors feel that the procedure isn't something that expectant parents should watch because it involves scalpels, bleeding, and exposure of internal body tissue that's normally not seen, which is disturbing to many people.)

Many hospitals allow the coach or partner to be in the operating room during a cesarean delivery, but this decision depends on the nature of the delivery and on hospital policy. If the cesarean is an emergency, the doctors and nurses are moving quickly to ensure the safety of both the mother and the baby, which may make it necessary for the partner or coach to wait elsewhere.

The exact place on the woman's abdomen where the incision is made depends on the reason she's having the cesarean. Most often, it is low, just above the pubic bone, in a transverse direction (perpendicular to the torso). This cut is known as a *Pfannenstiel incision* or, more commonly, a bikini cut. Less often, the incision is vertical, along the midline of the abdomen.

TECHNICAL STUFF

After the doctor makes the skin incision, she separates the abdominal muscles and opens the inner lining of the abdominal cavity, also called the *peritoneal cavity*, to expose the uterus. She then makes an incision in the uterus itself, through which the infant and placenta are delivered. The incision in the uterus can also be either transverse (most common) or vertical (sometimes called a *classical incision*), depending again on the reason for the cesarean and previous abdominal surgery. After delivery, the uterus and abdominal wall are closed with sutures, layer by layer. A cesarean delivery takes 30 to 90 minutes to perform.

Understanding anesthesia

The most common forms of anesthesia used for cesarean deliveries are epidural and spinal (see Book 2, Chapter 4 for more information on anesthesia). Both kinds of anesthesia numb you from mid-chest to toes but also allow you to remain awake so that you can experience your child's birth. You may feel some tugging and pulling during the operation, but you don't feel pain. Sometimes the anesthesiologist injects a slow-release pain medication into the epidural or spinal catheter before removing it in order to prevent or greatly minimize pain *after* the operation.

If the baby has to be delivered in an emergency and there's no time to place an epidural or spinal, general anesthesia may be needed. In that case, you're asleep during the cesarean and totally unaware of the procedure. Also, general anesthesia may be needed in some cases because of complications in pregnancy that make it unwise to place epidurals or spinals.

Looking at reasons for cesarean delivery

Your doctor may perform a cesarean delivery for many reasons, but all are about delivering the infant in the safest, healthiest way possible while also maintaining the mother's well-being. A cesarean delivery can be either planned ahead of labor (*elective*), unplanned during labor (when the doctor determines that delivering the baby vaginally isn't safe), or done as an emergency (if the mother's or the baby's health is in immediate jeopardy).

UNCOVERING CESAREAN'S ROOTS

Cesarean delivery, in which the baby is born through an incision in the mother's abdomen, is hardly a new medical innovation. Cases have been documented since the beginning of recorded history. In fact, many famous works of medieval and Renaissance art depict abdominal deliveries.

The origin of the term *cesarean section* is a subject of some controversy. Julius Caesar, it turns out, probably wasn't delivered this way, according to *Cesarean Delivery,* a history written by physicians Steve Clark and Jeffrey Phelan (published by Chapman & Hall). In those days, it was rare for the mother to survive the procedure. Yet Caesar's mother survived her delivery and was depicted in Renaissance art that recounted the life of Caesar as an adult.

One theory is that the name comes from the *Lex Cesare,* the laws of the ancient Roman emperors. One of those laws mandated that any woman who died while she was pregnant be delivered by an abdominal incision so that the infant could be baptized. This rule later became canon law of the Catholic Church. A third possible explanation for the term *cesarean* is its relationship to the Latin term *cadere,* which means *to cut.* The term *section* also implies surgical cutting, so if *cadere* is indeed the origin of *cesarean,* then *cesarean section* is redundant. In modern obstetrics, the phrase is *cesarean delivery* or *cesarean birth.* Still, many people continue to call the operation a cesarean section or *c-section.*

REMEMBER

If your practitioner feels that you need a cesarean delivery, she'll discuss with you why it is needed. If your cesarean is elective or proposed because your labor isn't progressing normally, you and your partner have time to ask questions. In cases in which the baby is in a breech position, you and your practitioner may consider together the pros and cons of having either an elective cesarean delivery or a vaginal breech delivery (refer to Book 6, Chapter 2). Both carry some risks, and often your practitioner asks you which risks are most acceptable to you. If the decision to perform a cesarean is due to a last-minute emergency, the discussion between you and your doctor may happen quickly, while you're being wheeled to the operating room.

REMEMBER

If things seem hurried or rushed when you're on your way to the operating room for an emergency cesarean, don't panic. Doctors and nurses are trained to handle these kinds of emergencies.

Your practitioner may suggest that you have a cesarean delivery for one of many reasons. The following lists describe the most common ones.

Reasons for elective, or planned, cesarean delivery:

» The baby is in an abnormal position (breech or transverse).

» You have placenta previa (see Book 6, Chapter 2).

» You've had extensive prior surgery on the uterus, including previous cesarean deliveries or removal of uterine fibroids. (See Book 6, Chapter 1 for information on vaginal births after cesarean delivery.)

» You're delivering triplets or more.

Reasons for unplanned but nonemergency cesarean delivery:

» The baby is too large in relation to your pelvis to be delivered safely through the vagina — a condition known as *cephalopelvic disproportion (CPD)* — or the position of the baby's head makes vaginal delivery unlikely.

» Signs indicate that the baby isn't tolerating labor.

» Maternal medical conditions, such as severe cardiac disease, preclude safe vaginal delivery.

» Normal labor comes to a standstill.

Reasons for emergency cesarean delivery:

» Bleeding is excessive.

» The baby's umbilical cord pushes through the cervix when the membranes rupture.

» There's prolonged slowing of the baby's heart rate.

Other than the fact that the baby and placenta are delivered through an incision in the uterus rather than through the vagina, for the baby, there's not much difference between cesarean and vaginal delivery. Babies delivered by a cesarean before labor usually don't have cone-shaped heads, but they may if you're in labor for a long time before having a cesarean. As the baby is trying to make its way through the vaginal canal, the head often molds, forming a cone-shape as it squeezes through. Sometimes, the early formation of swelling, leading to a cone-head shape and occurring way before the pushing stage, may be a sign that the baby isn't fitting through. (For more on cone-shaped heads, see Book 2, Chapter 6.)

REMEMBER

Women who have labored for a long time only to find they need a cesarean delivery are sometimes understandably disappointed. This reaction is natural. If it happens to you, keep in mind that what is ultimately most important is your safety and your baby's safety. Having a cesarean delivery doesn't mean that you are a failure in any way or that you didn't try hard enough. Roughly 20 to 30 percent of women need a cesarean delivery for a variety of reasons. Practitioners stick to basic guidelines when monitoring progress through labor, and those guidelines are all about giving you and your baby the best chance for a normal, healthy outcome.

All surgical procedures involve risks, and cesarean delivery is no exception. Fortunately, these problems aren't common. The main risks of cesarean delivery are

>> Excessive bleeding, rarely to the point of needing a blood transfusion

>> Development of an infection in the uterus, bladder, or skin incision

>> Injury to the bladder, bowel, or adjacent organs

>> Development of blood clots in the legs or pelvis after the operation

Recovering from a cesarean delivery

After the surgery is finished, you're taken to a recovery area, where you stay for a few hours until the hospital staff can make sure that your condition is stable. Often, you can see and hold your baby during this time.

The recovery time from a cesarean delivery is usually longer than from a vaginal delivery because the procedure is a surgical one. Typically, you stay in the hospital for two to four days — sometimes longer, if complications arise. Check out Book 2, Chapter 7 for details on recovering from a cesarean delivery.

DEBUNKING MYTHS OF CESAREAN RATES

Some women choose their practitioner or the hospital where they're going to deliver based on the number of cesarean deliveries (as a percentage of total deliveries) that the practitioner, group, or hospital has done. However, that number is meaningless, unless you also know the demographics of the practice or hospital. For example, a maternal–fetal medicine specialist who predominantly cares for older women, women with many medical problems, or women carrying twins or more is expected to have a higher cesarean rate than a doctor or midwife who takes care of young, healthy women. The important issue isn't the cesarean delivery rate but whether the cesareans were done for appropriate reasons.

Congratulations! You Did It!

Women may experience any and every kind of emotion after their babies are born. The spectrum of feelings is truly infinite. Most of the time, you're completely overcome with joy when your long-awaited baby finally is born. You may be incredibly relieved to see that your baby appears healthy and obviously okay. If your baby requires extra medical attention for some reason and you can't hold her right away, you may be upset or, at the very least, disappointed. Just remember that very soon you'll have her to hold and enjoy for the rest of your life. Some women feel too scared or overwhelmed to care for their baby right away. Don't feel guilty about any such feelings — they, and most others, are completely normal. Just take one moment at a time. You've come through a phenomenal event.

Shaking after delivery

Almost immediately after delivery, most women start to shake uncontrollably. Your partner may think that you're cold and offer you a blanket. Blankets do help some women, but you aren't shivering because you're cold. The cause of this phenomenon is unclear, but it's nearly universal — even among women who've had cesarean deliveries. Some women feel nervous about holding their babies because they're shaking so much. If you feel this way, let your partner or your nurse hold your baby until you feel up to it.

REMEMBER

Don't be concerned at all about this shaking. It usually goes away within a few hours after delivery.

Understanding postpartum bleeding

After delivery — either vaginal or cesarean — your uterus begins to contract in order to squeeze the blood vessels closed and thus slow down bleeding. If the uterus doesn't contract normally, excessive bleeding may occur. This condition is known as *uterine atony*. It can happen when you have multiple babies (twins or more), if you have some infection in the uterus, or if some placental tissue remains inside the uterus after the placenta is delivered. Then again, in some cases, excessive bleeding happens for no apparent cause. If it happens to you, your doctor or nurse may first massage your uterus to get it to contract. If massage doesn't solve the problem, you may be given one of several medications that promote contracting, like oxytocin, methergine, or hemabate.

If you have some placental material remaining in your uterus, it may need to be removed by reaching inside the uterus or by a *D&C (dilation and curettage)*, which involves scraping the uterus's lining with an instrument. The vast majority of the time, the bleeding stops without a problem. However, if it doesn't stop with these medications and procedures, your doctor will discuss other forms of treatment with you.

Hearing your baby's first cry

Shortly after delivery, your baby takes her first breath and begins to cry. This crying is what expands your baby's lungs and helps clear deeper secretions. In contrast to the stereotype, most practitioners don't spank a baby after she's born but instead use some other method to stimulate crying and breathing — rubbing the baby's back vigorously, for example, or tapping the bottom of the feet. Don't be surprised if your baby doesn't cry the very second she's born. Often, several seconds, if not minutes, pass before the baby starts making that lovely sound!

Checking your baby's condition

All babies are evaluated by the Apgar score, named for Dr. Virginia Apgar, who devised it in 1952. This score is a useful way of quickly assessing the baby's initial condition to see whether she needs special medical attention. Five factors are measured:

>> Heart rate

>> Respiratory effort

>> Muscle tone

>> Presence of reflexes

>> Color

Each parameter is given a score of 0, 1, or 2, with 2 being the highest.

The Apgar score is calculated twice, at both one and five minutes following birth. The parameters are added up. The lowest score is a 0 (very rare), and the highest, a 10. An Apgar score of 6 or above is perfectly fine. Because some of the characteristics are partially dependent on the infant's gestational age, premature babies frequently get lower scores. Factors such as maternal sedation also can affect a baby's score.

Many new parents anxiously await the results of their child's Apgar score. In fact, an Apgar score taken one minute after the baby is born indicates whether the baby needs some resuscitative measures but is not useful in predicting long-term health. An Apgar score taken five minutes later can indicate whether resuscitative measures have been effective. Occasionally, a very low five-minute Apgar score may reflect decreased oxygenation to the baby, but it correlates poorly with future health. The purpose of the Apgar score is merely to help your doctor or pediatrician identify babies who may need a little extra attention in the very early newborn period. It certainly is no indication of whether your baby will get into Harvard or Yale.

Cutting the cord

After the baby is actually delivered, the next step is to clamp and cut the umbilical cord. Some practitioners may offer your labor coach the opportunity to cut the cord — but your partner is under no obligation to do so. If having the opportunity to cut the cord is something you feel strongly about, let your practitioner know ahead of time.

At the time of this writing, there has been a lot of discussion about the risks and benefits of delayed cord clamping. The idea is that by delaying the clamping of the cord by two or three minutes, you can give your baby more blood that is stored within the cord and placenta. Recent data based on an analysis of about 15 different studies showed a significant benefit in premature infants. For these preemies, delayed cord clamping showed lower rates of transfusion for anemia, lower rates of a complication called *necrotizing enterocolitis,* and lower rates of intraventricular hemorrhage (known as IVH, a potentially serious complication in very preterm babies). Although the levels of bilirubin (a breakdown product of hemoglobin, which in high levels can cause problems) were higher, there was no greater need to treat these babies with phototherapy (a way of breaking down bilirubin).

In contrast, in full-term babies, the studies did show that although hemoglobin levels were higher in the immediate newborn period and there was less iron deficiency at 3 and 6 months, there was a 40 percent increase in the need for phototherapy for high bilirubin levels and jaundice. Therefore, the decision to perform delayed cord clamping should be individualized. There doesn't seem to be large proven benefits in term infants, and there are some significant risks, so at this time it isn't routinely performed. However, in premature infants, the decrease in the risk of IVH is compelling and should be considered.

After cutting the cord, your practitioner either lays your baby on your abdomen or gives the baby to your labor nurse to put under an infant warmer. The choice depends on your baby's condition, your doctor's or nurse's standard practice, and the institutional policy where you're delivering. (See more on newborn care in Book 2, Chapter 6.)

Banking cord blood and tissue

Cord blood is blood that is left in the umbilical cord and placenta after birth. Recently, couples have had the option of collecting this blood through a private or public bank. The rationale for collecting the cord blood is that it contains blood-forming stem cells, which may be used to treat some disorders of the blood or immune system and even for complications associated with certain cancer treatments. Very recently, some facilities started storing umbilical cord tissue, which contains stem cells that may be used for the treatment of other conditions.

You may store cord blood for public or private use:

>> **Public cord banks** store umbilical cord blood that is available for anyone who needs it. There is no charge for collection and storage. You don't, however, have control over your child's own cord blood. Public cord banking is not available in all, or even many, institutions.

>> **Private cord banks** store your blood specifically for your own use. The blood may be used to treat your child or other relatives. There's an annual fee for storage of the blood and often a charge for collecting the blood.

There are some important things to know about cord blood cells. If a baby is born with a genetic disorder, the practitioner can't use the baby's own stem cells for treatment because they have the same genes that caused the disorder in the first place. Also, if a child gets leukemia, you can't use that child's own stem cells for treatment. However, stem cells from a healthy child can be used to treat another child's leukemia.

Many couples ask whether it's worth paying the money to bank their child's cord blood. The chance that the cord blood will actually be needed to treat your child or a relative is low, about 1 in 2,700. However, that number may change as research on treating various conditions advances. The cord stem cells are not miracle cells, and they can't treat all conditions. It also isn't known how long the cells will last. If you do decide to store the umbilical cord blood privately, you should find out the specific fees and ask what would happen if the company were to go out of business.

Finding out about new uses for your placenta

The placenta is an amazing organ that provides nutrients and oxygen to your baby and provides for elimination of waste from your fetus. It's rich in hormones and protein. Some couples ask if they can take their placenta home — you'd need to discuss this with your doctor or find out from the hospital.

TECHNICAL STUFF

Some potential uses of the placenta (not necessarily scientifically proven) are as follows:

» **Cultural norms:** Some cultures advocate eating the placenta for nutritional as well as cultural significance. Others believe that eating the placenta can ward off postpartum depression.

» **For use in beauty products:** Many companies sell skin treatments containing extracts of animal placenta. Don't be surprised at ads claiming anti-aging properties and the elimination of dark spots! Placentas have also been found in hair products that claim to strengthen hair. Many of these products use cow or sheep placentas. Believe it or not, horse placenta is thought to heal sports injuries.

Of course, if you've had any complications, such as preeclampsia or a baby measuring small, or you delivered prematurely, your placenta should be sent to pathology for scientific evaluation.

Chapter 6

Hello, World! Meeting Your Newborn

For almost 40 weeks, you and your baby have been in one body, and if you're like most women, you've focused on staying healthy to help your baby grow — and on preparing to deliver your baby safely. Now suddenly, your baby is out in the world, and you finally get to take your first real look at her. You may find that in some ways, your baby's appearance surprises you. Newborns typically look a little funny. Remember that many superficial aspects of your baby's appearance — the cone-shaped head, the blotches, and especially the white, pasty goo — will soon disappear.

This chapter gives you an idea of what to expect when you first meet your little darling and explains the role of the hospital and the pediatrician who visits your baby in the first hours or days.

Looking at Your Bundle of Joy

Immediately after delivery, your practitioner puts your baby on your belly or hands her over to a nurse for some judicious cleansing and toweling off before putting the baby in your arms.

In the first moments after your baby is born, you may be overwhelmed by feelings of love. The shock and relief of it all may daze you. Most likely, you also think that your baby is the most beautiful thing you've ever seen. Then again, maybe you don't. Contrary to the fairy tales you see on TV soap operas, *I Love Lucy* reruns, and cartoons, babies don't always come out clean and smelling like a spring shower. Your baby is far more likely to be covered with some of your blood, amniotic fluid, and white goo known as *vernix*. Her skin may be blotchy, and she may even have a few bruises from delivery. So you may need to keep an open mind when assessing her appearance right off the bat.

REMEMBER

Feeling a little hesitant at first or overwhelmed at the sight of your new baby actually isn't uncommon. Often it takes a few days before you establish a true connection or bond with your baby. If you're feeling a little detached, don't worry. As reality sets in and you get to know your baby, you'll feel much better.

Soon, you notice other features about your new baby's appearance, from her little stump of an umbilical cord to the amazingly long fingernails and toenails. And you observe her first behaviors, from the initial cry to the way she startles at loud noises. This section goes over many of your newborn's characteristics.

Varnished in vernix

A thick, white, waxy substance typically covers a newborn baby from head to toe. The formal name for this substance is *vernix caseosa*, a phrase with Latin roots meaning "cheesy varnish." Vernix is a mixture of cells that have sloughed off the baby's skin and debris from the amniotic fluid.

Experts have several theories about this substance. Some doctors believe that vernix acts as an emollient to protect the tender fetal skin from the dryness that may result from living within a bag of amniotic fluid. Others believe that the vernix acts as a lubricant to help the baby slide through the birth canal. Some babies have more vernix than others; some have none at all. The amount isn't significant. If your baby passed meconium while inside the uterus (see Book 2, Chapter 3), the vernix may look a little greenish.

Regardless of what it looks like, most of the vernix usually comes off when the nurses dry off your baby. There's no reason to leave the vernix on the baby's skin. Any vernix that doesn't come off in the drying process is usually absorbed within the first 24 hours.

The shape of the head

Caput succedaneum — more commonly called *caput* — refers to a circular area of swelling on the baby's head, located at the spot that pushed against the cervix's opening during delivery. The exact location of the swelling varies, depending on the position that the baby's head was in. The swollen area can range in size from only a few millimeters in diameter to several centimeters (a few inches). Caput generally goes kaput within 24 to 48 hours after birth.

Babies who are born headfirst (*vertex*) often go through a process known as *molding.* This molding occurs because throughout labor, as the baby descends gradually through the birth canal, she "fits" her way along (see Figure 6-1). In fact, your practitioner may tell you that he can feel the baby's head molding to the canal even before the baby is born. Molding doesn't cause any harm. The bones and soft tissues in the baby's head are designed to allow this molding to happen. The result is often a baby with a cone-shaped head (see Figure 6-2). By 24 hours after delivery, the molding usually disappears, and the baby's head appears round and smooth.

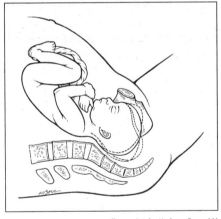

FIGURE 6-1:
A baby's head is often molded as it descends through the birth canal.

Illustration by Kathryn Born, MA

Some women, particularly those who have had children before or who had rapid labor, have babies with no molding. Also, babies born in the breech presentation or by cesarean may not have molding.

Sometimes, during the passage through the birth canal, a baby's ears can also fold down into strange positions. The same thing can happen with the baby's nose, so that at first, it may appear *asymmetric*, or pushed to one side, but these features are no reason to rush your baby to a plastic surgeon. These minor oddities are temporary and disappear during the first few days.

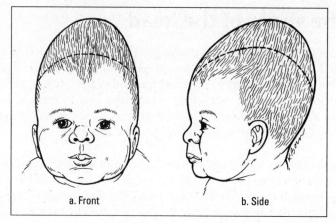

FIGURE 6-2:
The cone shape
usually goes
away after about
24 hours.

a. Front   b. Side

Illustration by Kathryn Born, MA

Black and blue marks

Quite often, babies are born with black and blue marks on their heads from the labor and delivery process. These marks usually happen because the forces of labor put so much pressure on the baby's scalp. They can also be the result of a forceps or vacuum delivery. A bruise doesn't indicate that anything harmful has occurred; it's merely a reflection of how vigorous the labor process can be. Most black and blue marks go away within the first few days of life.

Blotches, patches, and more

Most people think of newborn skin as blemish-free — the very definition of perfection — but newborns have all kinds of spots and markings. Most disappear within a matter of days or weeks. Some of the most common newborn skin conditions include the following:

>> **Dry skin:** Some babies, particularly those who are born late, have an outer layer of skin that looks shriveled like a raisin and peels off easily shortly after birth. You can use lotion or baby oil, if needed, as a moisturizer.

>> **Hemangiomas:** A type of reddish spot, known as a *hemangioma,* may not appear until a week or so after delivery. It can be almost any size, large or small, and can occur anywhere on the infant's body. Although the majority of these spots go away in early childhood, some persist. You can treat the spots that become bothersome (because of their appearance). Discuss treatment options, if needed, with your pediatrician.

>> **Mongolian spots:** Bluish-gray patches of skin on the lower back, buttocks, and thighs are especially common in Asian, Southern European, and

African-American infants. These patches are sometimes called *Mongolian spots*. They often disappear in early childhood.

>> **Neonatal acne:** Some babies are born with tiny white or red pimples around the nose, lips, and cheeks, and some babies develop them weeks or months later. These bumps are completely normal and are sometimes called *neonatal acne* or *milia*. No need to rush to the dermatologist, though. The little bumps disappear in time.

>> **Red spots:** Reddish discoloration on the skin, whether very deep and dark or light and hardly noticeable, is very common in newborns. Most of these discolorations go away or fade, but some may persist as birthmarks. One type of discoloration in particular, *erythema taxicum,* can be extensive. It looks like bad hives, and it comes and goes over the baby's first few days of life.

>> **Stork bites:** You may notice small ruptured blood vessels around your baby's nose and eyes or on the back of the neck. These marks are commonly known as *stork bites* or *angel kisses*. They're common in newborns, and they also disappear after a while, although it sometimes takes weeks or months.

Baby hair

Some babies enter the world totally bald, whereas others come out looking like they need a haircut. The amount of hair present at birth doesn't necessarily predict what the baby's hair will look like later on. Most often, newborn hair thins out and is replaced by new hair. Different babies grow hair at different rates; some have relatively little hair even at a year of age, whereas others already need a trip to the beauty salon.

REMEMBER

Often, a soft, fine layer of dark hair, which can be especially prominent on the forehead, shoulders, and back, covers babies' bodies. This hair is called *lanugo* and is quite normal. Lanugo is most common in preterm babies and in infants of mothers who have diabetes. It falls out within several weeks of life.

Extremities

Newborn babies often assume a position similar to the one that they became familiar with inside the uterus, the so-called *fetal position.* You may notice that your baby likes to be curled up a bit, with her arms and legs bent and fingers balled into a fist.

Watch out for those nails, though! Newborn fingernails and toenails may be surprisingly long and sharp. Many hospitals dress newborn babies in little shirts with mitten-like attachments to cover the hands so that the babies can't scratch themselves. To minimize this risk, keep the nails relatively short. Pick up a pair of baby nail scissors or clippers from your local drugstore.

TIP

A good time to trim fingernails and toenails is when your baby is fast asleep and oblivious to what you're doing.

Eyes and ears

At birth, a baby's vision is quite limited. Newborns can see an object only if it's close; they see things best at a distance of about 7 to 8 inches away. They also respond to light and appear to be interested in bright objects.

All newborn babies have dark blue or brown eyes, regardless of what color of eyes the parents have. By the age of 4 months, baby eye color changes to the permanent hue. Right after birth, the whites of your baby's eyes may have a bluish tint. This tint is normal and disappears in time.

Often, a newborn's eyes appear a little swollen or puffy. The whole delivery process causes this puffiness; it's perfectly normal, and it quickly subsides. Some puffiness may also be due to an antibiotic ointment put in the eyes after birth (see the later section "Caring for your baby's eyes").

Babies are fully able to hear from the moment they're born, which is why you may notice that your baby reacts with a startled motion to loud or sudden noises. Newborns also can distinguish various tastes and smells.

Genitalia and breasts

Babies are often born with a swollen or puffy scrotum or labia. The breasts also may appear slightly enlarged. Maternal hormones that cross the placenta cause this swelling. Sometimes, high maternal hormone levels even cause female babies to secrete a whitish or pinkish discharge from the breasts (known as *witch's milk*) or from the vagina (like a period). Like so many newborn characteristics, these secretions are both normal and transient; they go away within a few weeks after birth.

The umbilical cord

The stump of your baby's umbilical cord probably has a little piece of plastic attached to it. After delivery, your practitioner closes the cord with a small plastic clamp and then cuts it. Usually, your practitioner removes this clamp before you take the baby home. Then the umbilical cord stump quickly dries up and shrivels so that it looks like a hard, dark cord. Within one to three weeks, the stump usually falls off. Don't try to pull it off.

TIP

To keep the stump clean, you can dip a cotton swab in water, alcohol, or peroxide and clean around the base. However, some pediatricians think this cleaning is unnecessary — unless a lot of goopy stuff is around the base.

Newborn size

In general, newborn babies weigh about 6 to 8 pounds (about 2,700 to 3,600 grams) and measure 18 to 22 inches (46 to 56 centimeters) long. The exact size depends on the baby's gestational age (the number of weeks the pregnancy lasted), genetics, and many other factors, such as whether the mother had diabetes, whether she smoked, and how healthy her diet was during pregnancy.

REMEMBER

You may notice that your baby's head seems disproportionately large compared to her body. This feature is true of all newborns. Your baby can't hold up her head and needs time to develop muscles strong enough to hold it up without assistance. You also may notice soft spots on the back and top of your baby's head. These are *fontanelles,* areas where the baby's skull bones meet. Fontanelles allow for the rapid growth of the baby's brain. The back spot (posterior fontanelle) usually closes within a few months, but the anterior or top fontanelle (the one most typically called the *soft spot*) usually remains until the baby is 10 months to 1 year old.

Seeing how your baby breathes

Often, the baby starts to cry spontaneously shortly after delivery, but not every baby cries right away. A full-throated cry is music to the ears of the hospital staff because they know that the cry triggers the baby's first breathing efforts. Healthy breathing can begin without a loud cry, however, and some babies give only a little whimper. Some babies have normal respiration even if they don't wail at high decibels.

If your baby is slow to start breathing spontaneously, you may notice the doctor, nurse, or midwife stimulating your baby by rubbing her back, drying her off, or tapping her feet. Contrary to the stereotype portrayed in old movies, your practitioner is unlikely to turn your baby upside down and give her a little spank on the behind to elicit that first cry.

During pregnancy, a fetus receives oxygen through the placenta. After delivery, the baby takes over respiratory function by using her own lungs. While the baby is in the womb, a special fluid bathes your baby's lungs, and this fluid is often pushed out during delivery. Sometimes, however, a baby needs extra time and help — in the form of suctioning or stimuli — to expel all the fluid in the lungs.

REMEMBER

You may notice that your baby breathes differently than you do. Most babies breathe 30 to 40 times a minute. A newborn's respiratory rate also can increase with physical activity. Newborns breathe through their noses rather than their mouths. This great natural adaptation enables them to breathe while nursing or bottle-feeding.

You may also think that your baby's belly looks unusually large and protuberant, but it's just a normal new baby's belly. The fact that the belly rises up and down quite noticeably during breathing and gets somewhat distended as the baby starts to swallow some air only enhances the effect. This movement is also normal because babies use their diaphragms to breathe, not their chest muscles, as older children and adults usually do.

Knowing What to Expect in the Hospital

After your nurse and practitioner are assured that your baby is fine (usually determined by an Apgar test — see Book 2, Chapter 5 for details), the hospital staff starts cleaning the baby and helping her make a comfortable transition to life outside the womb. Like butterflies emerging from their cocoons, newborns must adjust to a new state of being in various ways. Suddenly, and for the first time, they can breathe on their own and see the wide world around them. This section points out what happens next in the hospital to ensure that your baby is warm, safe, and healthy.

BRACELETS ARE FOR SECURITY, NOT A FASHION STATEMENT

At the hospital, your baby wears an identification bracelet to identify her as yours. All hospitals also require that the mother wear a bracelet with the baby's ID number on it. (Many hospitals now also require every new partner to wear an ID band.) Each time the staff brings the baby to the mother, the staff member reads off the numbers to ensure that the right baby is given to the right mother. Most hospitals also take additional security measures to prevent any mix-ups and to prevent unauthorized individuals from gaining access to the nursery. Many nurseries are locked, and all are closely supervised.

Preparing baby for life outside the womb

A lot happens in the few hours immediately after your baby is born. She has made a pretty significant change and has a lot to adjust to. The medical staff takes immediate action to give her the best start in life.

Keeping your baby warm and dry

Because body temperature drops rapidly after birth, keeping your new baby warm and dry is important. If newborns become cold, their oxygen requirements increase. For this reason, a nurse dries the baby off, places her in a warmer or warmed bassinet, and then watches her temperature closely. Often the nurse wraps or swaddles her in a blanket and puts a little hat on her to reduce the loss of heat from the head. When the baby gets to the nursery, a nurse usually dresses her in a little shirt and then wraps her again in a blanket.

Caring for your baby's eyes

Most hospital staffs routinely place an antibiotic ointment into a newborn's eyes to lower the chance that she'll develop an infection from passage through the vagina of a mother who has chlamydia or gonorrhea. The ointment doesn't appear to be bothersome to babies and is completely absorbed within a few hours.

REMEMBER

Some parents worry that the ointment may blur the baby's vision and thus hinder parent–child bonding. You don't have any reason to be concerned about possible blurring, however. Babies don't see clearly in any case (see the "Eyes and ears" section earlier in this chapter).

Boosting vitamin K

Most hospitals give newborns an injection of vitamin K to decrease the risk of serious bleeding. Vitamin K is important in the body's production of substances that help the blood clot. This nutrient doesn't pass through the placenta to a baby very easily, however, and newborn livers, because they're immature, produce very little of it. So babies are typically low in this nutrient. Giving the baby vitamin K is an important preventive measure.

Making tracks: Baby's footprints

Most likely, a nurse takes your baby's footprints shortly after she is born to make a permanent record of identity. (The unique ridges that form on a baby's feet are actually present several months before birth.) Some hospitals give you a copy of your baby's footprints for your scrapbook. Although most hospitals still use this technique of identification, not all do.

Vaccinating for hepatitis B

Many hospitals now routinely start the vaccination process against hepatitis B for newborn babies, whereas others prefer that a pediatrician administer the first of the three shots after the baby is discharged from the hospital. (The last two are given over the course of the next six months.) Wherever your baby receives the vaccine, this shot is an important tool to reduce her chances of contracting hepatitis B later in life.

Understanding baby's developing digestive system

Most babies wet their diapers six to ten times a day by the time they're one week old. The frequency of bowel movements depends on whether you bottle- or breastfeed. Typically, a breast-fed baby has two or more bowel movements per day, whereas a formula-fed baby has only one or two per day.

Don't be surprised if your baby's first stool looks like thick, sticky, black tar — that's normal. It's called *meconium.* Ninety percent of newborns pass their first stool within the first 24 hours, and almost all the rest do so by 36 hours. Later on, the color of the stools lightens, and the texture becomes more normal. A formula-fed baby typically has semi-formed, yellow-green stools, whereas a breast-fed baby has looser, more granular, yellowish stools.

REMEMBER

Most newborns urinate within the first few hours after birth, but some don't urinate until the second day. The passage of meconium and urine is an important sign that your baby's gastrointestinal and urinary tracts are functioning well.

Considering circumcision

Circumcision is the surgical removal of the foreskin of a male infant's penis. Parents of boy babies must decide whether they want their son to have this procedure performed. The decision to have a circumcision may involve cultural and religious considerations as well as personal preferences. More than half of newborn boys in the United States are circumcised, but in many other countries, circumcision is rarely performed. The frequency of circumcision in the United States is on the decline, as new information is emerging that challenges the medical arguments for performing the procedure.

Doctors once thought that circumcision helped reduce the incidence of penile cancer, that it prevented infections, and that it reduced the incidence of changes in the appearance of a penis related to a tight foreskin. However, these advantages haven't proved to be true. In fact, the American Academy of Pediatrics has issued a formal statement that existing evidence is not sufficient to recommend routine circumcision. That said, there is some data that shows that circumcision may decrease the risk of a male infant contracting a urinary tract infection or the risk of a male contracting HIV from an infected female partner. Some possible complications associated with circumcision include bleeding, infection, and scarring. Circumcision based on cultural or religious views is still relatively common. The decision, of course, is one that both parents should be comfortable with.

Some people feel that circumcision is beneficial for hygienic reasons. For example, some uncircumcised males build up a thick white discharge called *smegma* under the foreskin, which may lead to a bad odor or infection. However, a boy can be taught to wash his penis and prevent this from happening.

If you decide to circumcise your son, your obstetrician or pediatrician performs the procedure within a day or two after your son is born — as long as he is healthy, full-term (or nearly full-term), and without any congenital abnormalities that would cause your doctor not to do the procedure. For some Jewish and Muslim families, male circumcision is part of their religious practice. Jewish families often have a ceremonial circumcision after the baby is discharged from the hospital, performed by a *mohel.*

Many hospitals offer injectable anesthetics or an anesthetic cream that doctors apply to the baby's penis prior to the procedure. The emphasis on pain medication is a humane and important medical advance, prompted by studies that show that newborns do indeed react to the pain and stress associated with circumcision. Just doing comforting things like swaddling the baby, giving him sugary fluid by mouth, and administering Tylenol are not enough to decrease the pain associated with circumcision, although they can help reduce the stress level. Good options for real pain management, or *analgesia,* include a topical anesthetic cream (EMLA cream); a nerve block called a *dorsal nerve block,* which reduces pain sensation to the area; or a *subcutaneous ring block,* again acting as a block to pain sensation.

After circumcision, the doctor wraps the baby's penis in petroleum jelly–soaked gauze. When this gauze falls off after about four hours, the top of the penis may look reddish and slightly swollen.

TIP

If the gauze doesn't fall off, don't pull at it. Squeeze warm water over the gauze to help it loosen. In the first few days, clean the area with warm water and keep it dry. After each diaper change, apply an antibacterial ointment or petroleum jelly until the penis heals.

WARNING

The penis is usually completely healed within one week. During this time, you may notice a crusty substance at the tip; this substance is normal and goes away with time. But if the penis looks unusually swollen and discolored or if your baby has a fever, call your pediatrician.

Hello, World! Meeting Your Newborn

Spending time in the neonatal intensive care unit

During the hospital stay after delivery, most newborns room with their mothers or stay at least part of the time in the regular hospital nursery — sometimes called the *well-baby nursery*. But sometimes newborns need the kind of extra attention they can get only in a *neonatal intensive care unit* — sometimes called a *special care nursery*. Within such a nursery, you may find a special area for critical care, where one-on-one nursing, sophisticated monitors, breathing machines, and so on are available. You may also find the so-called *step-down area*, for babies who aren't yet ready to go to the well-baby nursery but don't need critical, one-on-one care.

If your pediatrician thinks that your baby needs care in the neonatal intensive care unit, it doesn't automatically mean that something is wrong. Often, doctors place babies in special care nurseries for a short while just for observation — for any number of reasons. Here are some of the most common reasons (this list is far from inclusive):

>> The baby was born prematurely.

>> The baby doesn't weigh quite enough to make the birth weight cutoff established by your particular hospital.

>> The baby may need antibiotics — for example, because the mother had a fever during labor or because she had a prolonged rupture of membranes prior to delivery.

>> The baby's breathing seems somewhat labored. This reason is a relatively common one for putting a baby under observation for a short period of time.

>> The baby has a fever or had a seizure.

>> The baby is anemic.

>> The baby was born with certain congenital abnormalities.

>> The baby requires surgery.

Checking In: Baby's First Doctor Visit

Before or after delivery, someone from the hospital asks for your pediatrician's name. Your pediatrician should be someone who is authorized to work at the hospital where you delivered but may or may not be the same pediatrician you plan to use after you leave the hospital. If you live some distance from the hospital and have selected a pediatrician close to your home who doesn't have privileges at the hospital where you deliver, you still need another pediatrician to care for your baby during the hospital stay. Depending on the time you deliver, the pediatrician may see the baby on the same day, or he may see the baby the next day.

When the pediatrician examines your baby, he checks the baby's general appearance, listens for heart murmurs, feels the *fontanelles* (the openings in the baby's skull where the various bones come together), looks at the extremities, checks the hips, and generally makes sure that the baby is in good condition. The pediatrician orders a variety of standard blood tests and newborn screening tests. The specific screens that are required vary from state to state but often include tests for thyroid disease, *PKU* (a condition in which a person has trouble metabolizing some amino acids), and other inherited metabolic disorders. The results of these screening tests usually don't come back until after you take your baby home. The pediatrician gives you the results at your baby's first office visit. If any of the tests come back positive, the state also notifies you by mail. Upon discharge, be sure to ask the pediatrician when your baby should be seen again.

Considering heart rate and circulatory changes

Remember how your practitioner checked the fetal heart rate during prenatal visits? You may have noticed then how fast the beat was. In utero, the baby's heart rate is, on average, 120 to 160 beats per minute, and this heart rate pattern continues during the newborn period. Your baby's heart rate also can increase with physical activity and slow down when she sleeps.

TECHNICAL STUFF

After your baby is born, important changes in circulation occur. In utero, because a fetus doesn't use the lungs to breathe, a structure called the *ductus arteriosus* shunts away much of the blood from the lungs. Normally, this shunt closes on the first day of life. Sometimes, a murmur is heard in the first days after the baby is born, which indicates changes in blood flow. This murmur, which is called a PDA (for *patent ductus arteriosus*), is usually normal and nothing to worry about. However, some heart murmurs may require further investigation — specifically, by having a special sonogram, or *echocardiogram,* of the baby's heart. Even when a cardiologist finds murmurs due to small structural problems (like a small hole in the heart's septum), many murmurs go away on their own. If your baby is diagnosed with a murmur, discuss it thoroughly with the baby's pediatrician or a pediatric cardiologist who specializes in these conditions.

Looking at weight changes

Most newborns lose weight during their first few days of life — usually about 10 percent of their body weight — which, of course, if she weighs only 7 or 8 pounds (3,200 or 3,600 grams), amounts to less than a pound (454 grams). This phenomenon is completely normal and is usually caused by fluid loss from urine, feces, and sweat. During the first few days of life, the typical infant takes in very little food or water to replace this weight loss. Preterm babies lose more weight than full-term babies, and it may take them longer to regain their weight. In contrast, babies who are small for their gestational age may gain weight more rapidly. Generally, most newborns regain their birth weight by the tenth day of life. By the age of 5 months, they're likely to double their birth weight. By the end of the first year, they triple it.

For Partners: Home at Last — with the New Family

In the hospital, the primary focus is on the patients — in the case of childbirth, the mother and her baby. But the hospital stay is usually short, and as soon as Mom and baby come home, the partner is expected to join them on center stage. In fact, you're likely to find yourself in a starring role.

If pregnancy, labor, and delivery weren't enough to jolt you into the realization that your life is changing forever, getting home from the hospital with your new family certainly does. You and your partner now have a new set of responsibilities.

Long gone are the days when it was normal for men to assume that the mother would take on those responsibilities all by herself. Men can help change diapers (they even have changing tables in men's restrooms these days), feed the baby, shop, and do household chores. Even if your partner is breastfeeding, you can sometimes feed the baby breast milk she has pumped and put into a bottle. In fact, parents may want to prepare bottles this way regularly because feeding the baby is an important and highly satisfying way to bond.

Your partner is going to need at least six weeks to get back to her pre-pregnancy shape — probably longer. During the first couple of months, she may be exhausted. She's recovering from labor and delivery, after all. And chances are good that both you and she are somewhat sleep-deprived. Conditions like these make it easy for anyone to lose patience from time to time or to lose his or her temper more often than usual. Simply being aware of the fact that you're operating under special circumstances for a while is helpful. See that your partner has time for rest — and try to take naps yourself.

In a stressful (even if very joyful) situation such as having a new baby, sex may not be a huge priority. Give yourself and your partner the time you both need to adjust your sex drives. Even after your partner's practitioner gives her the go-ahead to resume sex (usually about six weeks after delivery) and you're both ready, take things slow and easy at first. The tissue around your partner's vagina and *perineum* (the area between her vagina and rectum) may still be a little sore. And the fact that it has been some number of weeks or months since the two of you have had intercourse may add to the discomfort. Many couples find it useful to use a water-based lubricant for the first few times; some new mothers need to wait longer than six weeks after delivery before they're comfortable enough for sex.

Finally, don't be surprised if you feel unprepared for parenthood, lacking not only skills but also an understanding of what it takes to do a good job. Unlike cats, dogs, or jungle animals, humans aren't born with surefire instincts about how to be perfect parents. Both you and your partner need time to develop the skills it takes to handle babies — and children, and teenagers. Along the way, you often work by trial and error. Just realize and accept this situation. Talk about it with each other — often. And fasten your seat belts. You're in for an incredible adventure.

Chapter 7

Taking Care of Yourself after Delivery

According to the old adage, it takes nine months for a woman to make a baby and nine months for her body to return to normal afterward. In reality, the time it takes to recover from childbirth varies widely from woman to woman. But most of the changes that your body goes through during pregnancy revert to normal during the postpartum period — sometimes called the *puerperium* — which begins immediately after delivery of the placenta and lasts for six to eight weeks.

As you go through this period of change, you're likely to have many questions about what you can do to make the postpartum transition as easy as possible. In this chapter, you find out what life may be like as your body gets back into its old shape, as you begin to have sex again, and as you deal with all the physical and psychological challenges of new motherhood.

Recuperating from Delivery

The average hospital stay after an uncomplicated vaginal delivery is 24 to 48 hours. After a cesarean, you may stay in the hospital for two to four days. In some hospitals, you spend this recovery period in the same room in which you delivered. In others, you move to a separate postpartum unit. The nurses continue to monitor your vital signs (blood pressure, pulse, temperature, and breathing) and check your uterus to make sure that it's firm and well-contracted. Nurses (often the same ones taking care of you) also monitor your baby's vital signs. Your nurses can provide you with pain medication that your practitioner has prescribed, if you need it, and help you care for your tear or episiotomy if you have either one.

The following sections outline the ways your body begins to recuperate after a delivery and what you can expect.

Looking and feeling like a new mom

Only in movies and on TV do women throw on a sassy pre-pregnancy outfit and leave the hospital looking like they did before they even considered having a baby. Delivery takes a toll, and although most of the changes are fleeting, you'll notice that you look and feel different.

After delivery, your face may be swollen, very red, and possibly splotchy. Some women even have black marks under the eyes or broken blood vessels around their eyes and, all in all, look as though they've just been in a prize fight. All these characteristics are to be expected; pushing causes the rupture of tiny blood vessels in your face. Don't be alarmed. You'll look like your old self again in a few days. Also keep in mind that many women still look pregnant when they leave the hospital. Patients are often disappointed that they still have an enlarged abdomen after delivery.

You'll feel like yourself before long, but you're likely to experience *afterpains*, or contractions that persist sporadically after delivery. These pains are similar to the contractions you experienced during labor and delivery, and they gradually fade away within a few days. You may find the afterpains are more noticeable while you're breastfeeding.

Understanding postpartum bleeding

REMEMBER

Experiencing vaginal bleeding after delivery is completely normal, even if you had a cesarean delivery. Average blood loss after a vaginal delivery is about 500 cc, or 1 pint. After a cesarean, the average blood loss is twice that — about a liter, or a quart. In order to limit blood loss, many practitioners give medications to help keep the uterus contracted. When the uterus contracts, it squeezes shut the blood vessels from the placental bed to reduce bleeding. If your uterus doesn't seem to be contracting well, your doctor or nurse may massage your uterus, through your abdomen, to promote contractions.

The blood coming from your vagina, called *lochia*, may initially appear bright red and contain clots. Over time, it takes on a pinkish and later a brownish color. It gradually diminishes in volume, but the flow may persist for three to four weeks after delivery. You may notice that the amount of bleeding increases each time you breastfeed. This increase happens because the hormones that help produce breast milk also cause your uterus to contract, and this contraction squeezes out any blood or lochia in the uterus. For many women, the bleeding is heavier when they stand up after being in bed for a while. This extra bleeding happens simply because the blood pools in the uterus and vagina while you're lying down, and when you stand up, gravity draws it out. It's perfectly normal.

The best way to deal with postpartum bleeding is to use sanitary napkins, which come in varying thicknesses to accommodate whatever amount of bleeding you have. Don't use tampons, because they may promote infection during the time that your uterus is still recovering. Although the bleeding usually subsides after two weeks, some women experience bleeding for six to eight weeks. Occasionally, fragments of placental tissue stay within the uterus, and this condition can lead to extensive bleeding.

TIP

Traditionally, doctors told women not to take deep tub baths after delivery if they were still bleeding. Today, many practitioners say that tub baths are okay, and most feel that shallow baths — called *sitz baths* — are perfectly acceptable. If your practitioner says to avoid tub baths until your bleeding has subsided, she may be concerned that full baths will increase the chance of developing some infection inside your uterus. The trouble is that doctors really have no data on this topic — no studies demonstrate a risk from taking full baths. Ask your practitioner what she thinks you should do.

WARNING

Call the doctor in these instances:

>> If you have very heavy bleeding with clots that lasts for several weeks after your delivery

>> If your lochia takes on a foul odor, which may be a sign of infection

Dealing with perineal pain

The amount of pain or soreness you feel in your *perineum* (the area between the vagina and the rectum) depends largely on how difficult your delivery was. If your baby came out easily after only a couple of pushes and you have no episiotomy or lacerations, you probably feel little pain. If, on the other hand, you pushed for three hours and delivered a 10-pound budding linebacker, you're more likely to have perineal discomfort.

The pain you feel has several causes: The progression of the baby through the birth canal causes stretching and swelling of the surrounding tissues. Also, an episiotomy or tears in the perineum naturally hurt, just as an injury to any other part of your body would. The pain is worse during the first two days after delivery. After that, it rapidly improves and is usually nearly gone within a week.

Your perineum may be swollen, and if you had an episiotomy, you have stitches closing it up. Sometimes these stitches are visible on the outside, and sometimes they're buried underneath the skin.

REMEMBER

Many women are concerned about the stitches used to sew up their episiotomy or lacerations. These sutures aren't meant to be removed. They gradually dissolve over the next one to two weeks. They're strong enough to handle most activities, so don't worry that a sneeze, a difficult bowel movement, or lifting your 10-pound baby will cause the stitches to tear open.

WARNING

It's important to keep the perineal area clean to prevent an infection from developing. Such an infection is a rare complication, but call your doctor if you notice a foul-smelling discharge or increasing pain and tenderness in the area, especially if you have a fever higher than 100.4 degrees Fahrenheit.

Here are the best ways to care for your perineum as it recovers from your delivery:

>> Keep the perineal area clean. You may want to use a squirt bottle filled with warm water to help clean places that are difficult to reach.

>> Some women get relief from pain by taking a sitz bath. A *sitz bath* consists of soaking your bottom in a small amount of warm water. If you have a lot of swelling in the area, putting Epsom salts in the water may give you added relief.

>> You can buy various kinds of anesthetic sprays and pads that you can apply to the perineum to help ease the pain. Or you can soak gauze pads in witch hazel and apply them to the area. Some women find that chilling the witch hazel increases its effectiveness. Other women find that ointment or petroleum jelly is soothing, too. It keeps the skin moist and soft and prevents it from sticking to sanitary pads.

>> An ice pack applied to the perineum during the first 24 hours after delivery helps minimize swelling and discomfort.

>> Over-the-counter pain relievers — such as acetaminophen (Tylenol is a well-known example) or ibuprofen (such as Motrin or Advil) — or some prescribed pain medications further ease the pain. Taking these medications isn't a problem if you're breastfeeding.

>> Avoid standing for long periods of time, which can make the pain worse.

   You can relieve the gravitational pressure on your perineum from time to time by getting off your feet and lying down for a short while.

TIP

>> After a bowel movement, try not to contaminate the area with the toilet tissue you use to wipe yourself. Clean the area around the anus with a separate toilet tissue, and don't wipe from back to front. If the areas around the anus or the perineum are tender, try to just pat the area dry, instead of wiping. You may find that using baby wipes is really helpful, because they clean the area very well, don't shred, and are gentle on healing tissues.

>> Don't insert anything into your vagina (such as a tampon) for six weeks and don't douche.

>> Avoid intercourse for six weeks after delivery. Your doctor will see you for a routine postpartum checkup at the six-week mark. As long as you are well healed, sex should be okay at that time!

WARNING

If you're extremely uncomfortable, you may want to ask your doctor to prescribe pain medications. If you notice that your perineal area is very red or purple and tender, if you run a fever, or if you notice a foul-smelling discharge, let your practitioner know.

TIP

If you had any lacerations that extended near your rectum, you may want to take a stool softener (such as Colace), *not* a laxative, so that bowel movements aren't too terribly painful. At least make sure that you drink extra fluids and consume extra fiber in your diet so that your stool is soft. When you anticipate having a bowel movement, you may want to take a pain reliever ahead of time — acetaminophen (Tylenol), perhaps, or some other nonsteroidal anti-inflammatory agent, such as ibuprofen (Motrin or Advil).

Surviving swelling

REMEMBER

Immediately after delivery, especially after a vaginal delivery, you may discover that your entire body looks swollen. Don't freak out — this is normal. Many women develop swelling during the last few weeks of pregnancy, and this swelling often persists for a few days to a few weeks into the postpartum period. The intense pushing efforts required to deliver the baby may further cause your face and neck to swell, but this also goes away a few days after delivery. In general, it can take up to two weeks for the swelling to completely disappear.

Don't step on the scale the day after you deliver. You may find that you've actually gained weight from all the water you retain during delivery.

Many patients ask, "Isn't there something you can give me to help relieve the swelling, like a diuretic or something?" Prescribing medication usually isn't necessary because the swelling goes away on its own in a few days, when you're back up and around. Just be patient. You *will* have ankles again.

Coping with your bladder

When you were pregnant, you probably felt like all you did was pee, right? Now, after you've given birth, you may actually find urinating difficult immediately after delivery, or you may feel discomfort when you do urinate. This discomfort is a result of the way the bladder and urethra were compressed when the baby's head and body came through the vagina. The tissues around the opening to the urethra are often swollen after delivery, and this swelling can add to the discomfort.

Some women may need to be *catheterized* (a thin, flexible plastic tube is inserted through the urethra into the bladder) after delivery to help empty the bladder. The problem is sometimes worse if you have an epidural because the anesthesia can hang around in your system for several hours and temporarily make the bladder more difficult to empty. But your bladder regains its normal tone a few hours after delivery, so urinary discomfort is usually a short-lived problem.

If you feel a burning sensation primarily during urination, let your doctor or nurse know because it may be a sign that you're developing a urinary tract infection.

Some women experience the opposite problem: They find that they don't have good control over their bladder function — that they leak a little urine when they stand up or laugh or they have to run like a cheetah to make it to the john in time. If this incontinence happens to you, don't worry too much, because time usually solves the problem. In some cases, it may take a number of weeks to get things under control.

Kegel exercises may be useful if the problem persists (see the "Doing Kegel exercises" sidebar later in this chapter). Another good strategy is to make a conscious effort to go to the bathroom at regular intervals to empty your bladder before it becomes an emergency!

Battling the hemorrhoid blues

Most of your pushing efforts during delivery are focused toward the rectum, a fact that causes many women to develop *hemorrhoids* — dilated veins that pop out from the rectum. Unfortunately, having no problems with hemorrhoids before you go into labor is no guarantee that they won't appear after delivery. If you develop hemorrhoids during the last part of your pregnancy, they may get worse after delivery. At times, hemorrhoids can be more uncomfortable than an episiotomy, and they last a little longer. Turn to Book 2, Chapter 3 for tips on dealing with hemorrhoids.

REMEMBER

The good news is that the problem is usually temporary. Postpartum hemorrhoids typically go away within a few weeks. Sometimes they don't go away completely, but for the most part they aren't bothersome. They may not trouble you at all for a few months, and then they may be uncomfortable again for a few days and then get better again.

Consider taking a stool softener (such as Colace), and make sure you consume plenty of fluids and fiber. This way, bowel movements won't hurt so much and you won't have to push too hard (which makes hemorrhoids worse). Your hemorrhoids are likely to go away within one to two weeks.

Understanding postpartum bowel function

Many women find that they don't have a bowel movement for a few days after delivery. This lack of bowel function may be because you haven't eaten much or because epidurals and some other pain medications sometimes slow down the bowels a little. Your system may take a few days to return to normal.

REMEMBER

Many women are afraid of bearing down because they don't want to tear the stitches used to repair their episiotomy, so they try to avoid having a bowel movement altogether. But avoiding a bowel movement isn't a great idea. You have no reason to be afraid of tearing the stitches. Your episiotomy is repaired in several layers with strong sutures. Tearing the sutures is extremely difficult, especially by having a bowel movement.

Here are a few ways to make having a bowel movement easier:

>> Walk around the postpartum ward as much as you can. Walking improves circulation to the bowels and can help to eliminate any residual effects of the epidural.

>> Take a stool softener, such as Colace.

>> Try not to think about it too much. Things happen in time.

TIP

If you have hemorrhoids or a laceration that reaches back to the rectal area (see Book 2, Chapter 3), a bowel movement may be painful. You can reduce the discomfort by using a local anesthetic cream and by using a stool softener. Also, you may want to take a pain reliever shortly before you anticipate having a bowel movement.

Continuing to recover at home

By the time you're discharged from the hospital after a vaginal delivery, most of the acute pain is gone. After you get home, however, you can still expect some soreness. The main area of discomfort is around your perineum. No matter how easy your delivery may have been, this part of your body has undergone some real trauma, and it simply needs time to heal.

Try not to let the lingering discomfort associated with having just given birth frustrate you. Keep in mind what an amazing miracle your body has just been through. In addition to dealing with the soreness from delivery, you need to adjust to a new lifestyle — getting up at all hours of the night, changing diapers, and feeding your new baby.

Recovering from a Cesarean Delivery

The hospital stay after a cesarean delivery is generally a few days longer than after a vaginal delivery — usually three to four days in total. If you have a cesarean delivery, you're put on a stretcher immediately afterward and transported to the recovery room. You may even feel up to holding your baby during the trip. Just like any surgery, the first few days can be uncomfortable. Don't worry, though, because after the initial few days, most people recover quite easily.

Going to the recovery room

When you're in the recovery room, your nurse and anesthesiologist monitor your vital signs. The nurse periodically checks your abdomen to make sure that the uterus is firm and that the dressing over the incision is dry. Your nurse also checks for signs of excessive bleeding from the uterus. More than likely, you have a catheter in your bladder, and it stays in place for the first night so that you don't have to worry about getting up to go to the bathroom. You also have an intravenous (IV) line in place to receive fluids and any medications your doctor prescribes. If you had an epidural or spinal anesthetic, your legs may still seem a little numb or heavy. This feeling wears off in a few hours. If you had general anesthesia (that is, if you were put to sleep), you may feel a little groggy when you get to the recovery room. Just as with a vaginal delivery, you may experience some shaking (see Book 2, Chapter 5). If you're up to it and if you want to, you can breastfeed your baby while you're in the recovery room.

Most likely, you received pain medication in the operating room, and you may not need any more while you're in the recovery room. In some hospitals, if you have an epidural or spinal, your anesthesiologist injects a long-lasting medication into the catheter that keeps you almost pain-free for about 24 hours. If, however, your pain medication doesn't seem to be working, by all means, let your nurse know.

Taking it one step at a time

When your nurse and anesthesiologist are confident that your vital signs are stable and that you're recovering normally from the anesthesia, you're discharged from the recovery room — generally about one to three hours after delivery. You're transported on a stretcher to a hospital room, where you spend the rest of your recovery time.

The day of delivery

On the day of your cesarean, you should plan on just staying in bed. Thanks to your catheter, you don't need to worry about getting up to go to the bathroom. If you had your surgery early in the morning, you may feel like getting up later in the evening, if only to sit in a chair. Just be sure to check with your nurse first to see whether getting up is okay. When you get up the first time, make sure someone is there to help you.

Although some doctors still prefer that patients not have any food immediately after a cesarean, many doctors now allow women to eat and drink shortly after the surgery. If you feel queasy and nauseous, you're better off not eating. But if you feel hungry, drinking liquids and having small amounts of solid food is probably fine.

Like women who have had a vaginal delivery, expect some vaginal bleeding (lochia) after a cesarean. The bleeding may be quite heavy during the first few days after your surgery (see the earlier section "Understanding postpartum bleeding").

As far as care for the incision goes, many practitioners will remove the dressing on the first or second day after the cesarean. After the dressing is removed, you're usually able to shower. During the shower, don't rub the incision; just let the water run over it and pat it dry immediately after the shower. Some women's incisions are closed by sutures that will be reabsorbed over time with no need for removal, while others may be closed by staples, which do need to be removed.

Most women who have a cesarean delivery and have staples in their skin worry that removing the staples will hurt, but don't worry. Staple removal is a quick and painless procedure.

The day after

The first day after your surgery, your doctor is likely to encourage you to get out of bed and start to walk around. The first couple of times you get up to walk may be pretty uncomfortable — you may feel pain around the incision in your abdomen — so you may want to ask for a *top-up* dose of pain medication 20 minutes or so before getting up.

WARNING

Make sure someone is with you the first few times you get up to make sure you don't fall.

Depending on your fluid needs, your doctor may also discontinue your IV line. Most of the time, you're able to drink liquids on the first day, and many doctors also let you eat solid food.

Most likely, you have a bandage over your abdominal incision. Sometimes this bandage comes off on day one, but other times doctors prefer to leave it on longer.

Many women ask about *rooming in* — that is, having the baby stay in the room with them — after a cesarean delivery, especially after they've had a day or so to recover a bit from the procedure. Having the baby in the room with you is certainly fine if you feel up to it. But by no means should you feel that you have to. Keep in mind that you just had abdominal surgery, and you may not be physically able to attend to every single one of your baby's needs during the first few days afterward. The hospital nurses are there to help, so during this time, devote as much energy as possible to your own recovery. You'll be that much better able to care for your baby after you get home.

Understanding post-cesarean pain

You may feel a kind of burning pain at the site of your abdominal skin incision. This pain is worse when you get out of bed or change positions. Eventually, the burning diminishes to a sort of tingling sensation and is much improved within a week or two after surgery.

You may also feel pain from post-delivery uterine contractions — just as women who deliver vaginally do. Your doctor is likely to give you oxytocin (Pitocin) for the first few hours after your surgery to encourage contractions and thus minimize blood loss. Pain from contractions diminishes by the second day, although it may recur when you breastfeed because breastfeeding can trigger more contractions.

You may feel pain in tissues deep beneath your skin. In a cesarean, the physician must cut through several layers of tissue to reach the uterus. Each layer must then be repaired. And every one of the repaired incisions can generate pain. This pain usually takes one to two weeks to fade away. Many women say that they feel more pain on one side or the other, possibly because the stitches are a little tighter on one side. Whatever the reason, uneven pain is very common and nothing to worry about.

Many women say the worst pain of all is gas pain. The intestines accumulate a large amount of gas after a cesarean delivery, in part because of the way the intestines are manipulated during the surgery but also as a result of the medications — the anesthetics used during the operation and the painkillers given afterward. Gas pains typically begin on the second or third day after delivery and improve when you start to pass gas. Get up and walk around as much as possible, because doing so gets the gastrointestinal tract moving again.

If you have a cesarean delivery after going through labor for hours, you may have perineal pain — from pushing and from any number of internal exams — on top of everything else. This pain disappears soon after delivery.

Dealing with post-op pain

The amount of pain or discomfort experienced after a cesarean delivery varies from woman to woman, depending on the circumstances of her delivery and on her tolerance for pain. Your practitioner can prescribe pain medication, but she probably will specify that the medication shouldn't be given unless you ask for it. (Sometimes this is hospital policy.) So if you want the pain relief, ask for it — before your pain becomes excruciating.

Some hospitals offer a PCA (*patient-controlled analgesia*) pump, which is attached to your IV line. When you feel your pain increasing, you simply press a button on the pump to release a small amount of pain medication into your IV line. Because you receive the medication intravenously, you can feel its effects quickly, and by using the medication only when you feel you need it, you can often get by with much less medication in total. Don't worry about overdosing, because the pump has special settings that prevent you from getting too much medication.

Getting ready to go home

After surgery, you find that each day is noticeably easier and more comfortable than the one before. Over the course of three days, you gradually find it easier to get out of bed and walk around. You start to eat normally again. You're also able to shower — and many women find that first shower a truly big relief. But please keep in mind that you have just been through not only major surgery but also nine months of pregnancy! And you must recover from both.

The length of your hospital stay may be determined to some extent by what your insurance plan allows and what individual state laws mandate. And occasionally, a post-operative infection or some other complication necessitates a longer-than-usual hospital stay. But typically, you're ready to go home after about three days. Here are some indications that you may be ready to go home:

» You tolerate food and liquids without any problem.

» You urinate normally and without difficulty.

» Your bowels are on their way to recovering normal function.

» You have no signs of infection.

Continuing to recover at home

When you're discharged from the hospital after a cesarean delivery, you're well on your way down the road to recovery. However, getting back on your feet after a cesarean delivery takes longer than after a vaginal delivery, so take it easy for the first week or two after you return home. Keep the following pointers in mind as you recover.

Taking good care of yourself

Get the help you need from family and friends, if possible. If you can afford it, consider hiring a baby nurse for the first few weeks. (A baby nurse can be quite helpful for women who've had vaginal births, too.) Make sure, however, that any caregivers you recruit to help you have all their vaccinations up to date. Specifically, make sure that they've had a Tdap vaccine booster within the past ten years (see Book 1, Chapter 2). When you're on your own, try to keep the household chores you do to a minimum. Avoid running up and down stairs a lot. Devote your energy to taking care of your new baby and taking care of yourself. Pay attention, and your body will clearly let you know how much activity you can handle.

Some doctors recommend that you not drive a car for the first week or two. This restriction isn't because of the anesthesia you may have had — the anesthesia really doesn't affect your reflexes for more than a day or two after delivery. The problem is simply that any leftover pain you may be experiencing after delivery may make it difficult for you to quickly move your foot to the brake if you need to stop suddenly. When your pain is gone, you can safely resume driving.

Most doctors also advise you to postpone any abdominal exercises until after your six-week checkup so that the incisions in all the layers of your abdomen have time to heal completely.

Most women feel pretty much back to normal by the six-week point, but some need as long as three months to fully recover.

By the time you're home from the hospital, you should be able to eat normally. If you lost a great deal of blood during your surgery, however, you may want to ask your doctor whether you should take extra iron supplements.

Noticing changes in your scar

At first, the scar from your cesarean delivery looks reddish or pinkish. In time, it may turn a darker shade of purple or brown, depending to some extent on your skin color. Over the course of a year, the scar will fade and, eventually, assume a very pale color. If you have dark skin, it may be brownish. Most of the time, a cesarean scar is pencil-thin or even thinner. A scar from a cesarean delivery may look prominent immediately after the procedure, when the staples are still in place, but after they're removed and the scar has had several weeks to heal, you'll observe how it begins to fade into something far less obvious.

Many factors can affect the healing process and thus determine what the scar ultimately looks like. Some women are naturally prone to forming a thick type of scar, called a *keloid*. In these cases, doctors really can't do much to change the situation. Some over-the-counter products claim to help wounds heal, but none have proven to be beneficial.

REMEMBER

You may notice that the area around your incision becomes numb. This numbness occurs because in making the incision, your doctor cut through some of the nerves that transmit sensation in that area. The nerves do grow back, however, and in time the numbness turns into a mild tingling sensation and then returns to normal.

Some women notice a blood-tinged fluid discharge coming from the center or side of their incision. This drainage sometimes happens when blood and other fluids accumulate under the incision and then seep out. If only a small amount oozes out and the drainage then stops, it's okay. Applying a little pressure to this area with a clean bandage is a good idea.

WARNING

If you notice persistent blood-tinged or yellowish discharge from your incision, let your doctor know. Occasionally, the incision may open at the point where the drainage occurs. If so, your doctor may want you to take special measures to keep the opening clean so that it heals on its own.

Recognizing causes for concern

WARNING

Most women who have cesarean deliveries recover without any problems. In some cases, however, you may not heal quickly and smoothly. Call your doctor if you notice any of the following:

>> If pain from your incision or from your abdomen increases rather than decreases

>> If large amounts of blood or blood-tinged fluid drain from your incision

>> If you have a fever higher than 100.4 degrees Fahrenheit

>> If your incision begins to open up

>> If you notice any odor associated with the discharge from your incision

Going through More Postpartum Changes

Many aspects of postpartum life are the same whether you had a vaginal or a cesarean delivery. Now that you're no longer pregnant, your body begins shifting back to its pre-pregnancy state, and you're in for a number of changes. This section describes many of the common changes you may experience.

Sweating like a . . . new mom

REMEMBER

If you're managing to get any sleep at night despite having a new baby in the house, you may find that you wake up drenched in sweat. Even during the daytime, you may notice that you perspire significantly more than usual. This sweating is very common and is thought to have something to do with fluctuations in hormone levels that occur as your body returns to a nonpregnant state. It's very similar to the night sweats and hot flashes that menopausal women get due to a drop in estrogen levels. As long as the sweating isn't associated with a fever, it's not a problem. It will go away over the course of the next month or so.

Dealing with breast engorgement

A woman's breasts typically begin to *engorge,* or fill with milk, three to five days after she delivers her baby. You may be amazed to see how huge your breasts can really be! If you're breastfeeding, your baby lessens the problem for you as she gets the hang of nursing, figures out how to take in more milk, and establishes a pattern of feeding. (See Book 5 for more information about breastfeeding.)

TIP

If you're not breastfeeding, you may find that your breasts stay engorged for 24 to 48 hours (which can be quite painful), and then you begin to feel better. Wearing a tight-fitting supportive bra may make the process a little more comfortable. Applying ice packs or bags of frozen peas to your breasts helps the milk to "dry up," as does taking cold showers. Cold temperature causes the blood vessels in the breasts to constrict, lessening milk production, whereas warmth causes the blood vessels to dilate, promoting milk production. (Doctors no longer prescribe a medication to help a woman's milk dry up, because the drug they once used has been associated with some significant complications.)

Understanding hair loss

One of the stranger aspects of the postpartum return to normalcy is hair loss. A few weeks or months after delivery, most women notice that they're shedding like crazy. This shedding is normal, and it doesn't last long. Your hair is usually back to normal by nine months after delivery.

TECHNICAL STUFF

All hair follicles go through three phases of development: a *resting* phase, a so-called *transitional* phase, and a *shedding* phase. The elevated levels of estrogen that are present during pregnancy essentially freeze your hair in the resting phase. Within a few months after delivery, all that hair proceeds to the shedding phase. Suddenly, you notice large amounts of hair sticking in your brush or washing down the drain.

Chasing away the baby blues

Studies show that the vast majority of women — as many as 80 percent — suffer a bout of the blues during the first days and weeks after they deliver. Typically, you begin to feel a little down a few days after the birth, and you may continue to feel vague sadness, uncertainty, disappointment, and emotional discontent for a few weeks. Many women are surprised at the feeling; after all, they've looked forward to motherhood, and they feel sure that they're really thrilled about it.

No one knows for sure *why* women get the blues postpartum, but a few explanations are plausible. First, the shift in hormone levels that comes after delivery can affect mood. Also, when pregnancy ends, a mother must change her whole focus. After focusing on the birth for so many months, she suddenly finds that the big event is over, and she may feel almost a sense of loss. And face it — parenthood brings tremendous anxiety, especially for a first-time mother. Feeling overwhelmed by all the responsibility and all she needs to figure out about caring for a baby isn't unusual for a woman. Add in the physical discomfort — episiotomy repair, breast tenderness, hemorrhoids, fatigue, and the rest — and you begin to wonder how any new mother can avoid feeling a little blue.

REMEMBER

Fortunately, postpartum blues tend to fade away rather quickly, usually by about two to four weeks after the birth. Keep in mind that what you're feeling is extremely common and that it doesn't mean you don't love your child or that you won't be a fabulous parent.

TIP

If you find yourself suffering from the baby blues, remember that the feeling is as normal as pregnancy itself. And take heart: Those who have already grappled with the problem have found a number of ways to ease the blues. Consider this list of some of the best strategies:

>> **Try to get more sleep.** If the baby is napping, try to lie down and snooze. Lack of sleep compounds the problem of the baby blues. Everything is worse when you're physically fatigued. The amount of stress that you can handle when you've had your rest is much greater than if you hadn't slept enough.

>> **Accept other people's offers of help.** In most cases, you don't have to take care of your baby entirely by yourself. You're a great mom, even if you do let Aunt Suzie or Grandma Melba change a diaper or burp the baby.

>> **Talk about how you feel with other mothers, close family members, and friends.** Be open about it; let your partner, family members, and friends know how you feel, because you need love and support at this time. You're likely to find that they felt exactly as you do now. They can empathize with you and offer suggestions for how to cope.

>> **If possible, try to get some time to yourself.** Often, new parents are overwhelmed by the realization that their time is no longer their own. Get out of the house, if you can. Take a walk, read, watch a movie, or get some exercise. Have dinner with your partner or with a friend.

>> **Pamper yourself.** Try a manicure or pedicure, a trip to the hair salon, or a massage. Often the blues are exacerbated by the fact that your body still isn't back to what it used to be, and doing something that makes you feel beautiful may help.

WARNING

If you don't begin to feel better in three or four weeks, let your practitioner know. Some women go beyond the blues into full-blown postpartum depression. Check out the next section for information.

Recognizing postpartum depression

True *postpartum depression* isn't nearly as common as the blues, but it does affect more women than you may imagine. Between 10 and 15 percent of women develop depression within six months after they deliver. Symptoms include the following:

>> Severe unhappiness

>> Inability to enjoy being with the baby (or to enjoy life in general)

>> Lack of interest in caring for the baby

>> Insomnia

>> Weak appetite

>> Inability to function from day to day

>> Extreme anxiety or panic attacks

>> Thoughts of harming the baby or yourself

Although postpartum blues are usually mild and transient, full-blown depression can be severe and lasting. Despite the severity of the symptoms, postpartum depression often goes unrecognized, or the mother may attribute the problem to something else.

No one knows exactly why postpartum depression occurs, but certain characteristics put a woman at higher than normal risk. These risk factors include

>> History of postpartum depression

>> History of depression in general

>> Experience of anxiety before the birth

>> Life stress

>> Lack of a good support system

>> Marital dissatisfaction

>> An unplanned pregnancy

>> Unhappiness about the labor and delivery process

If you have postpartum blues and it doesn't go away after three or four weeks, if the feeling seems to be getting worse, or if you develop the blues more than two months after your delivery, discuss the situation with your doctor.

Treatment for postpartum depression includes counseling (group or individual psychotherapy), antidepressant medications, and, rarely, hospitalization. Recent studies have suggested that in some cases, taking small doses of estrogen under the tongue can help. Of course, follow this treatment only under your doctor's supervision. Your doctor may want to check to see whether you have postpartum thyroid disease, which can mask itself as depression or make your depression worse. Discuss all these with your doctor.

To get further information about how to handle postpartum depression, you may want to get in touch with one of the following resources:

>> **Postpartum Support International:** www.postpartum.net or call 1-800-944-4PPD.

>> **PPDMOMS.ORG:** www.1800ppdmoms.org or call 1-800-PPD-MOMS.

>> **March of Dimes:** Go to www.marchofdimes.com. Enter "postpartum depression" in the search field. There are numerous links to help you find the information that applies to your particular situation.

Checking your progress: The first postpartum doctor visit

Most practitioners ask their patients to come in for a checkup about six weeks after delivery if both the pregnancy and the birth were uncomplicated. If you had a cesarean or some complication, you may be asked to come in earlier.

During a postpartum checkup, your practitioner performs a complete exam (including a breast and vaginal exam) and obtains a PAP smear, if needed. In most cases, the six-week checkup suffices for your annual gynecological exam. Your practitioner probably also talks with you about your birth control options. Discuss the "spacing" of future children and other precautions before conceiving again — such as taking folic acid a few months beforehand and, if this pregnancy had complications, getting whatever special blood tests your practitioner may advise.

FOR PARTNERS: CHIPPING IN DURING THE RECOVERY PHASE

While your partner recovers, gets her hormones back together, and works into her new routine as a mom, she needs you to pick up the scut work around the house without being told what to do. Taking over the following list of chores makes for a happy mom, which means a happy baby — and a happy next six months for your new family:

- **Keep the house in order.** Because your partner is limited to lifting nothing heavier than a baby for the next six weeks, cleaning has just become your full responsibility. If you don't have time to clean every part of the house every day, ask your partner point-blank what tasks are most important to her, and then carry out her requests word for word. For example, if she wants the bathroom cleaned every day, then grab your toilet brush and get scrubbing. And when well-wishers come bearing a lot of stuff, try to keep the clutter under control. Mom is trapped indoors with a baby who's feeding around the clock, and feeling suffocated by balloons, flowers, and stuffed animals may only increase her anxiety. Make sure to find a new home for everything that comes into the house.

- **Assume laundry duty.** Laundering baby's things is a bit different from laundering your things. Wash brand-new infant clothes prior to first use to remove any chemicals or germs in the fabric. To avoid exposing your baby to dyes and chemicals that can irritate her delicate skin, wash baby clothes in dye- and chemical-free detergent. Be sure to treat stains. Rinse away or wipe off any detritus from the article of clothing or blanket, and spray on the treatment of your choice — prior to washing.

- **Become the gopher.** Grab the keys and get rolling, because driving duties are up to you for a while. Doctors recommend that women who have a vaginal birth don't drive for two weeks following delivery. That time could increase for a cesarean delivery; follow your partner's practitioner's instructions. Some suggest that she be able to pick up her foot and stomp on the ground without any abdominal pain before driving.

- **Take care of meals.** Whether you're the guy who likes to take charge in the kitchen or the type who routinely forgets to add the cheese packet to macaroni and cheese, making sure you and your partner are well-nourished is one of your most important roles. Breastfeeding women need to consume an additional 400 to 600 calories more than they would when eating a normal diet. New moms need to eat energy-packed, nutritious foods to help their bodies recover from labor and delivery. And with all the extra work you're doing on reduced sleep, you need these same foods too!

(continued)

Taking Care of Yourself after Delivery

(continued)

Tip: Because you'll be getting less sleep and doing more work around the house, you may not be eager to strap on the apron three times a day. To make the task easier on yourself, cook meals that you can eat multiple times or freeze for future consumption, such as easy-to-assemble casseroles or pots of soup. If time allows, this cooking can be a great nesting activity with your partner prior to delivery, too. And if friends and family ask you what they can do to help, ask them to bring you a meal in a freezer-safe storage container in lieu of flowers. Having prepared home-made meals on hand helps you avoid the temptation to order takeout or fast food, which is high in sodium and fat and not the most nutritious for mom and baby.

- **Call in backup, if necessary.** If you can't be home to help out during the early stages of parenthood, talk to your partner about the needs and desires she has while you're at work, and help her find the appropriate support from friends, family, and neighbors. Make chore lists for daytime helpers so your partner doesn't feel burdened by having to ask for help. If financially viable, hire a cleaning service. It will be the best gift you can give to your partner . . . and yourself.

Before you gratefully accept your parents' and your partner's parents' offers to visit and help, make sure your partner wants them around. All the advice and constant companionship from a parental figure may cause her more stress.

Returning to "Normal" Life

Your body typically needs six to eight weeks for the changes that you experience during pregnancy to disappear. After delivery, your body needs some time to get back in shape for your day-to-day activities, let alone for vigorous exercise or sex. This section focuses on what you can do to help make the transition easier.

Getting fit all over again

Making exercise a priority after delivery is important for every new mom. Fitness has many benefits for both your physical and emotional well-being. It can help your body recover from the stress of pregnancy, and it helps you feel more even-tempered and better about yourself. Resume your sports and workouts gradually. Over the course of two weeks, depending on how you feel, you can gradually increase your exercising until you're fully active again. Naturally, the amount of exercise you can handle depends on what kind of shape you were in before and during your pregnancy. Head to Book 4, Chapter 5 for information on how to get your body back.

After pregnancy, restoring strength to your abdominal muscles is especially important. In some women, pregnancy causes the abdominal or *rectus* muscles to separate a little, as shown in Figure 7-1. The medical term for this separation is *diastasis*. Do abdominal exercises to restore their strength and draw them together.

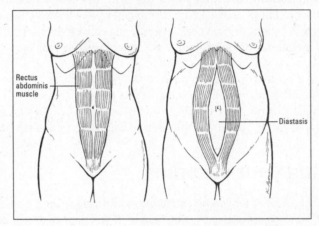

Rectus abdominis muscle

Diastasis

Illustration by Kathryn Born, MA

FIGURE 7-1:
After pregnancy, your abdominal muscles may be separated a bit, one side from the other.

TIP

Walking is great exercise for just about everyone. During the first two weeks after delivery, take it slow. But after that, you may find that long or brisk walks are enjoyable for both you and your baby — and a great form of exercise.

Losing the weight

You may feel like jumping onto a scale right after delivery to see how much weight you've lost. But take caution. Some women do lose a lot of weight quickly after delivery, but some actually gain weight from all the fluid retention. Rest assured that you'll soon weigh less than you did before you delivered — probably about 15 pounds less — but the loss may not register until a week or two after delivery. Most women need two to three months to get back to their normal weight, but, of course, the time varies according to how much weight you gain during pregnancy. If you gain 50 pounds (and have just one baby), don't expect to look fabulous in a bikini six weeks after you deliver. Sometimes a woman needs an entire year to get back into shape. A healthy diet and regular exercise help the weight come off.

TIP

Try to get as close to your pre-pregnancy weight — or your ideal body weight — as soon as is reasonably possible. You don't have to let a pregnancy turn into a permanent weight gain. If you let each successive pregnancy cause a little more accumulation, your health may suffer in the long run.

Pondering your postpartum diet

Any woman who's just had a baby needs to once again examine her diet. If you're breastfeeding, you want to ensure, as you did when you were pregnant, that you're eating a healthy combination of foods that provides both you and your baby with good nutrition and that you're also getting enough fluid. (For information about how to follow a balanced, nutritious diet, see Book 3.) Remember, the best approach to weight loss involves exercise plus a well-balanced diet that's low in fat and includes a mix of protein, carbs, fruits, and vegetables.

TIP

You may find that a program such as Weight Watchers (www.weightwatchers.com) offers the motivation and support you need to get your diet on track. Avoid diets that focus on rapid weight loss; instead look for ones designed to change your way of eating so you discover how to eat healthily and still lose weight.

Taking your vitamins

Regardless of whether you breastfeed, continue taking your prenatal vitamins for at least six to eight weeks after you deliver. If you do breastfeed, keep taking vitamins until you stop breastfeeding. Taking care of a new baby may make it hard for you to eat properly, and the childbirth experience may have left you anemic. If you lost a particularly large amount of blood during your delivery, your practitioner may suggest that you take iron supplements to help restore your blood count. Calcium is also very important for any woman, especially one who's breastfeeding, in order to maintain strong bones. A calcium supplement or extra calcium in your diet is a good idea.

Having sex again

If you're like most postpartum women, sex is the last thing on your mind. Many women find that their interest in sex declines considerably during the first weeks and months after pregnancy. But at some point, the fatigue and emotional stress of childbirth ease up, and your thoughts are likely to be more amorous again. For some women (and their lucky partners), the rebound occurs fairly quickly. For others, it may take 6 to 12 months.

The drastic hormonal shifts that occur after delivery directly affect your sex organs. The precipitous drop in estrogen leads to a loss of lubrication for your vagina and less engorgement of blood vessels as well. (Increased blood flow to the vagina is a key aspect of sexual arousal and orgasm.) For these reasons, intercourse after childbirth can be painful and sometimes not all that satisfying. With time, as hormone levels return to their pre-pregnancy norm, the problem tends to correct itself. In the meantime, using a lubricant sold specifically for this purpose helps.

DOING KEGEL EXERCISES

Kegel exercises are squeezing motions aimed at strengthening the muscles of the pelvic floor that surround the vagina and rectum. These muscles give support to the bladder, rectum, uterus, and vagina. Keeping them strong is key to reducing the adverse effects that pregnancy and delivery can have on this part of the body. If the pelvic floor muscles are very weak, your chances are greater of developing *urinary stress incontinence* (a leakage of urine when you cough, sneeze, laugh, or jump) or *prolapse* or *protrusion* of the rectum, vagina, and uterus (in which these organs begin to sag below the pelvic floor).

To perform these exercises, tighten the muscles around your vagina and rectum. When you're first doing Kegels, squeeze the muscles for as long as ten seconds and then release. Squeeze five to ten times per session, and try to do three to four sessions a day. Ultimately, you can build up to the point where you hold each squeeze for ten seconds and do 25 squeezes per session. Continue to do the Kegels four times a day. You can do them while you're sitting, standing, or lying down, and you can do them while you're doing something else — bathing, cooking, talking on the phone, watching television, driving your car, or standing in line at the grocery store.

Tip: Here's a simple way to find out what it feels like to do the exercises correctly: Sometime when you're urinating, try to stop the flow of urine midstream. Or insert a finger in your vagina and try to tighten the muscles around your finger. If you're doing Kegels correctly, your finger feels the squeeze. (Both of these techniques are simply ways of figuring out how to squeeze the muscles, not the way you normally practice the exercise.)

The exhaustion and stress of caring for an infant further reduces the desire for sex in some women. Your attention, and your partner's, too, is likely to be focused more on the baby than on the relationship between the parents. Set aside some time for the two of you to be alone together. This time together need not even include sex — just holding, hugging, and expressing feelings for each other.

Most doctors recommend that women refrain from intercourse for four to six weeks after the baby is born in order to give the vagina, uterus, and perineum time to heal and for the bleeding to subside. At your six-week follow-up doctor visit, you can ask your practitioner about resuming sex.

Choosing contraception

Many people believe that breastfeeding prevents a woman from becoming pregnant. Although breastfeeding usually delays the return of ovulation (and, thus, periods), some women who are nursing do ovulate — and do conceive again. You may not ovulate the entire time that you breastfeed, or you may start again as early as two months after delivery. And if you don't breastfeed, ovulation begins, on the average, ten weeks after delivery, although it has been reported to occur as early as four weeks. If you breastfeed for less than 28 days, your ovulation returns at the same time as it does for non-nursing women.

It's important to consider your options for birth control before you have sex again. Most women have a wide range of birth-control options regardless of whether they're breastfeeding. But some women have medical conditions that prevent them from using certain methods. Discuss your options with your practitioner at a postpartum visit.

3

All about Nutrition While Pregnant

Contents at a Glance

Chapter 1

Managing Your Eating Habits and Weight Gain

Eating the right foods while you're pregnant may not be as difficult as you think. Depending on what you ate before you started trying to get pregnant or before you got that positive pregnancy test, you may not need to make many changes after all. If you already gravitate toward fruits, vegetables, lean proteins, whole grains, and lowfat dairy, a healthy diet during pregnancy will be really easy for you to follow. Of course, if you survive on doughnuts, chips, and fast food, you may need to dig a bit deeper into changing those habits for the sake of your unborn child.

REMEMBER

Finding the right balance of calories is one of the many things that women wonder about when they get pregnant. You often hear people say, "Oh, you're pregnant. So now you can eat for two!" But that's not really the case. Just think about it for a minute. You're growing a little baby, not a full-sized adult. Yes, you do typically need to take in extra calories starting in your second trimester, but you certainly don't need to start eating double. Yet many women end up gaining too much weight, easily putting on 50 to 70 pounds during pregnancy by allowing themselves to eat whatever, whenever.

This chapter offers strategies to help you ensure that you're getting all the nutrients your body needs without gaining excess weight. And because how you eat can be a factor in your ability to manage your weight gain, this chapter offers advice on that, too.

Discovering How to Eat

People tend to focus most of their nutrition attention on what to eat or what not to eat. Not nearly enough attention goes toward *how* to eat. When you're pregnant, the key is to eat small quantities frequently throughout the day.

Eating frequent, small meals

In the first trimester, the goal of eating small amounts frequently is to prevent nausea by having a little bit of food in your stomach at all times (that way, your stomach doesn't have to go into acid overload). As your baby bump grows and you progress into your second and third trimesters, you'll find that your body literally has less room for your stomach! As a result, the baby may press on your stomach and the area where your esophagus meets your stomach, causing heartburn. If you have small amounts of food in your stomach, you're less likely to experience this reflux.

REMEMBER

The key to eating small amounts frequently is to enjoy a mix of smaller meals and regular snacks throughout the day. Now, before you start envisioning bags of chips and pints of ice cream in your snacking future, remember that the majority of your snacks need to contain the nutrients you and your little one need. Otherwise, you're just eating empty calories.

Keeping cravings in check

Another trick for keeping your eating in check is to avoid overindulging your cravings. You'll no doubt hear other women talk about cravings they had in pregnancy, and maybe you've already been experiencing them yourself. Although everything in pregnancy gets blamed on hormones, cravings are truly a case of hormones gone wild! Sometimes those hormones cause food aversions, and sometimes those hormones make it impossible to imagine living through another moment without one particular food. If you give in to every craving, you may end up putting on more pounds than you planned during your pregnancy. If you're determined to survive your cravings without experiencing excess weight gain, follow these tips:

>> **Eat a variety of foods throughout the day.** If you eat nothing but protein, you'll probably crave carbs. If you eat only carbs, you may find yourself craving a steak. Eat some carbs, protein, and fat at every meal and get a variety of grains, meats or meat alternatives, fruits, and veggies every day. Doing so helps you (and your baby) stay healthy! (See Chapter 2 in Book 3 for the lowdown on proper pregnancy nutrition.)

>> **Figure out how to distinguish between physical hunger and psychological hunger.** Ask yourself whether you're truly hungry or just bored, sad, happy, or stressed. If you're truly hungry, eat a snack or meal. If you're not, stall and distract yourself (see the next bullet).

>> **Stall and distract yourself if you aren't physically hungry.** Instead of giving in right away to a particular craving, buy yourself some time by engaging in another activity (call a friend or go for a walk, for example) to see if the craving goes away. A lot of times it does, but if you come back still wanting the particular food, then have it for your next meal or snack to satisfy the craving.

>> **Figure out what you really want, and choose the healthiest version of what you're craving.** If you're craving a strawberry milkshake, for example, ask yourself what you're really after. Are you craving the strawberries or the creamy, cold, sweet taste of the milkshake? Could you satisfy the craving with some fresh berries and whipped cream? What about a half cup of strawberry sorbet or lowfat ice cream? Would a strawberry-banana smoothie do the trick? Any of these options would be much lower in calories and/or have more nutritional value than the strawberry milkshake.

But don't substitute if no good substitute exists. For example, if you want pickles, eating a plain cucumber won't be very satisfying! Just eat the pickles and be done with the craving.

>> **Be aware of your portions, eat slowly, and enjoy every bite.** With foods like cake, ice cream, chocolate, cookies, chips, and other high-calorie foods, pay attention to the portions you eat. Place one serving on a plate and put the rest of the package away instead of plopping down on the couch with the entire container. Savor your food.

>> **Avoid trigger situations.** If your favorite doughnut shop is on the way home from work, take an alternate route to avoid craving doughnuts simply because you drove by the shop. Get rid of the candy jar at work. Ask your partner and those close to you to avoid tempting you unnecessarily.

>> **Rest up and pamper yourself.** When you're tired, you may crave food for energy. If you find yourself unusually tired or you're not getting the proper sleep at night, do everything you can to give yourself a break. Get a massage or pedicure, take a nap, or simply put your feet up with a good book or magazine. That way, you won't find yourself craving high-sugar, high-fat foods that'll just lead to energy crashes and excess weight gain later.

Gaining Weight Gradually

The best way to gain weight during your pregnancy is to gain it gradually. Doing so ensures your baby is getting good nutrition throughout the entire 40 weeks. The pounds you gain will distribute themselves in various tissues of your body, including fat and fluid, as well as your developing baby. (*Remember:* Gaining some fat deposits when you're pregnant is normal and actually necessary!)

REMEMBER

Gradual weight gain isn't linear weight gain. In other words, you may gain 3 pounds in one week and none for the next few weeks. As long as you're trending a steady weight gain, don't worry if you find that you gain more in one week and less in others. (Some women even lose a pound or two occasionally throughout their pregnancy.) As long as the overall trend is that you're gaining weight (slowly and steadily, of course), don't stress out about the exact number on the scale.

The amount of weight you should gain during your pregnancy is based on your pre-pregnancy weight status, or body mass index (BMI):

Body Mass Index	Recommended Weight Gain
Less than 18.5 (underweight)	28 to 40 pounds (12.5 to 18 kilograms)
18.5 to 24.9 (normal weight)	25 to 35 pounds (11.5 to 16 kilograms)
25 to 29.9 (overweight)	15 to 25 pounds (7 to 11.5 kilograms)
30 or more (obese)	15 pounds (7 kilograms) or less

Your healthcare provider can also help you establish weight-gain goals for each week, month, and/or trimester of your pregnancy. The following sections fill you in on what to do if you have trouble hitting that number.

TIP

To prevent excess weight gain and to keep your heart, lungs, and muscles strong, exercise throughout your pregnancy. In particular, aim for a mix of aerobic exercise, strength training, and yoga (see Book 4 for details).

ADDING UP THE NUMBERS

The pregnancy weight you gain isn't just the 6 to 8 pounds that your baby will weigh when he's born; it's also extra fat stores, blood, and body fluids that your baby needs to survive. The average weight gain is 27 to 30 pounds, and it breaks down like this:

- 7.5 for the baby

- 7 in fat stores that you need to sustain your pregnancy

- 4 in extra body fluids

- 3 to 4 in extra blood

- 2 in amniotic fluid

- 2 in the uterus

- 1 to 1.5 in the placenta

- 1 to 2 in the breasts

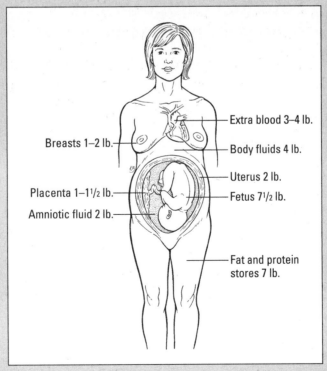

Illustration by Kathryn Born, MA

What to do when you're not gaining enough

Losing weight isn't uncommon during the first trimester, especially if you experience a lot of morning sickness. But if you get well into your second trimester without gaining much, if any, weight, your doctor will likely inquire more about your nutrition and exercise habits. He or she may even refer you to a registered dietitian (RD) for customized guidance.

WARNING

If you don't gain enough weight, your baby may not be getting the proper nutrients he needs to grow. The result can be a low-birth-weight infant or a premature delivery. Your baby may also be at risk of developmental delays if he doesn't get enough calories and nutrients in the womb.

Some women are afraid to gain weight during pregnancy for fear of not losing it afterward. If you're afraid of gaining weight to the point of restricting your calories to lower-than-recommended levels, seek out help from your doctor and a registered dietitian. Remember that if you're underweight before you even get pregnant, you likely need to gain a few more pounds than women who start their pregnancies at a normal weight.

Potential complications from gaining too much

Although a handful of pregnant women have trouble gaining enough weight, most are at a higher risk of going overboard and putting on too many pounds. Typically, that extra weight comes in the form of 20 or 30 extra pounds of fat, resulting in a total weight gain of 50 or 70 pounds over the course of the pregnancy. This extra weight isn't just a nightmare to get off after the baby is born; it can also lead to some serious health complications. Specifically, too much weight gain

>> May make it more difficult for your doctor to hear your baby's heartbeat and measure your uterus to plot your baby's growth

>> May lead to backaches, leg pain, and varicose veins — side effects that can persist even after you deliver your baby

>> Automatically puts you at a higher risk for medical conditions such as gestational diabetes, hypertension, and preeclampsia (you can find these conditions and the nutritional tactics for combating them in Book 3, Chapter 2)

>> Increases your risk of delivering your little one via cesarean delivery because your baby could grow too large to fit through the birth canal

Of course, the negative side effects aren't limited to pregnancy. More and more studies are showing the long-term impact of a mother's diet choices and weight gain during pregnancy on the weight status and health conditions of her children. Also, women who gain too much during pregnancy have a harder time getting the weight off after pregnancy, increasing their risk of many chronic diseases, specifically diabetes, heart disease, and certain cancers.

WARNING

If you started out your pregnancy overweight or obese, your doctor may not want you to gain *any* weight. Check with your doctor about his or her weight-gain recommendation and visit a registered dietitian for advice on how to meet that number the healthy way.

TECHNICAL STUFF

Some recent studies have shown better pregnancy outcomes when obese women maintained or even lost some weight while pregnant. That doesn't mean they were "dieting," per se, but they cleaned up their act from pre-pregnancy to include less junk and more nutrition, which resulted in fewer calories than their bodies were used to before. They filled up on nutritious foods and thus provided their babies with the nutrients they needed.

Avoiding the "pregnancy 50+"

In college, first-year students try to avoid gaining the "freshman 15." Now that you're expecting, your goal is to avoid gaining the "pregnancy 50" (or more).

REMEMBER

Without exercise, you need only about 300 extra calories per day to gain enough weight to feed and support your developing baby — not twice as many calories as you needed before you became pregnant. (Head to Book 3, Chapter 2 to see specific calorie requirements for each trimester and detailed nutrition advice.)

What happens to many pregnant women is that they follow the "eating for two" advice and see pregnancy as a time to eat whatever they want in whatever quantity feels good — and pregnancy can make you feel very hungry! They gain more than the weight of the baby, placenta, extra blood, and other essentials of pregnancy.

Follow these tips to get the extra calories and maintain a healthy weight:

>> **Go crazy with vegetables.** To maintain a healthy weight, eat all the vegetables you want. Eat your vegetables raw or cook them by grilling or steaming (frying adds fat and calories; boiling washes away many of the vegetable's nutrients). Don't add sauces, and use just a sprinkle of salt, if other herbs aren't flavorful enough.

Don't, however, overload on fruits. Pound for pound, fruits are much higher in calories than vegetables. Most fruits are full of vitamins and low in fat, but if you eat all the fruits you want until you're full, you'll probably exceed your required supply of calories for the day. Aim for four or five half-cup servings of fruit each day.

>> **Eat complex carbs that are high in fiber.** Look for high-fiber foods like lentils and beans, acorn squash, chia seeds, and steel-cut oats. Reduce your intake of foods that don't offer much nutritional benefit for their calories, such as white rice, potatoes, and white bread. See Book 3, Chapter 2 for more information on your need for carbohydrates.

>> **Drink plenty of water and skim milk.** Avoid sugary sodas, milkshakes, and other high-calorie drinks. Fruit juice offers many vitamins and minerals, but it's high in calories, so don't avoid fruit juice completely, but don't go overboard, either. Note that veggie smoothies and low-sodium vegetable juices (excess sodium can cause swelling during pregnancy) are far lower in calories than fruit juices and are full of vitamins.

TIP

Here are some other ways to avoid gaining more than your recommended weight range:

>> Eat small meals to keep yourself from consuming too many calories at one time (see the earlier section "Eating frequent, small meals" for details). Stop eating when you're satisfied, not full or stuffed.

>> Limit "junk" calories (as in the sugary, high-fat, and fried kind) because they neither fill you up nor provide the nourishment you and your baby need.

>> Stock your cabinets, purse, and desk drawers with nutritious foods so that you can satisfy your hunger the healthy way.

>> Bridge your hunger in between meals with frequent snacks that provide lasting energy. Choose snacks with plenty of fiber and protein.

>> Keep track of your calories by using apps like MyFitnessPal and Fooducate so that you can easily see when you've gone too high.

>> Avoid turning to food for emotional support or stress relief. Call a friend to talk it out or go for a walk to blow off some steam instead.

>> Join support groups for pregnant women who want to be healthy during their pregnancies. Meet to go for walks or do prenatal yoga, not to go out for ice cream.

>> Stay active and aim to get at least 30 minutes of moderate exercise each day. (Head to Book 4 for details on what exercises are safe during pregnancy.)

Thinking Ahead to Life Post-Delivery

Right now you're probably smiling as you imagine holding your precious baby in your arms for the first time. You may also want to think about how your life is going to change after your little one arrives.

For one thing, your body is going to need to recover, and it's going to need your help to do so. Also, eventually you'll need to think about shedding any lingering pregnancy pounds so that your body is in good shape — particularly if you want to have more kids. The following sections clue you in to the basics of post-delivery nutrition and the tricks to getting your pre-pregnancy body back. (Book 4, Chapter 5 has more detailed information on how to get your body back post pregnancy.)

Figuring out your body's post-pregnancy nutrition needs

Being pregnant obviously comes with specific nutrition requirements, but so does giving birth to your child and recovering from that birth. No matter how you end up delivering, your body will require energy and specific nutrients to heal itself. Eat protein foods (think meats, eggs, dairy, and beans) because they're essential for repairing your body. Include carbohydrates (especially whole grains that are high in fiber) because they're necessary for energy. Also incorporate some healthy fats (such as olive oil, nuts, and seeds) to provide important nutrients and additional energy for your body.

If you decide to breastfeed your baby, plan on eating pretty much the same foods you ate while pregnant throughout the length of time you choose to nurse. Of course, you may find that you need more calories while you're nursing than you did while you were pregnant; whether you do depends on how much milk you produce. *Note:* Nursing moms may lose some of their lingering pregnancy pounds fairly quickly due to their bodies' increased calorie needs and ability to use stored fat as energy to produce milk.

REMEMBER

If you're breastfeeding, drink plenty of fluids, get rest, and continue to take your prenatal vitamin because you can use the extra vitamins and minerals while nursing.

Getting back in shape

The key to post-pregnancy weight loss is to take it slow and steady, just as you did when gaining weight while you were pregnant. After all, you didn't gain all those pounds overnight, and they certainly won't come off that fast! As you get started, focus on eating smaller portions and leaving a few bites behind on your plate. Listen to your stomach when it tells your brain that it's satisfied and stop eating before you get overfull.

Don't give in to the temptation of starving yourself after pregnancy. You'll very likely be tired of carrying those extra pounds, but eating too little isn't good for you or your baby. Remember that your body is still recovering. If you're nursing, keep in mind that you need a good deal of calories to fuel milk production.

You may be surprised to find out that your pregnancy belly stays for a little while after delivery. The truth is much of your expanded stomach is actually your uterus, and it takes several weeks to shrink back to its normal size. Ignore anyone who tells you she wore her pre-pregnancy clothes home from the hospital, and make sure you hang on to your elastic-banded pregnancy pants for a little while longer (or live in comfy dresses).

As soon as you receive clearance from your doctor, which may take eight weeks or more if you have a cesarean (C-section) delivery, start adding exercise to your routine. Put your baby in the stroller and go for a walk, take a swim, pop in a yoga DVD, or attend a postnatal exercise class. Doing so will not only help you burn calories but also provide you with some much-needed stress relief and give you a nice boost of mood-elevating hormones. Book 4 has lots of exercise advice for pregnant women and those who've just given birth.

Chapter 2

Nourishing Your Bump: Proper Nutrition during Pregnancy

I f there's ever a time to eat right, it's during pregnancy. Why? Because the right mix of nutrients (everything that's nourishing your body, from protein and iron to fiber and water) helps keep you going strong and your baby growing steadily. This chapter gives you the nitty-gritty details of pregnancy nutrition. If you're a numbers person, you'll love this chapter because it specifies how many more calories you really need during pregnancy and shows you how to distribute those calories into the three major nutrients that make up your diet: carbohydrates, protein, and fat. If you're not a numbers person, just gloss over the numbers and pay attention to the foods recommended in this chapter.

Either way, you need to be aware that certain vitamin and mineral needs change when you're pregnant, whereas others don't change at all. Don't worry, though. This chapter tells you exactly which nutrients require your attention and which foods can provide you with them. It also covers fiber and hydration — the keys to smooth digestion — and reveals how to get the proper nutrients in your pregnancy diet if you're a vegetarian or facing unique circumstances like gestational diabetes and food allergies.

Eating for Baby and You: Balancing Calories Eaten and Calories Burned

Rule number one of pregnancy nutrition: Don't let anyone tell you (and don't tell yourself either!) that you're eating for two. Thankfully, your baby will never be as big as you while inhabiting your uterus. To think that you need to eat as many calories to support your baby as you need to support yourself is misguided. Eating for two may be a cute saying, but, in reality, eating for two won't make you look or feel cute!

You do need to consume some extra calories during the course of your pregnancy, but how many you consume varies according to the trimester you're in. (Also, depending on your size pre-pregnancy — whether you're petite or tall — you may need slightly more or less than the recommended numbers.) The following sections give you the specifics.

WARNING

Your weight status prior to pregnancy can dictate the number of calories you need. If you were overweight before you got pregnant, you may need fewer calories. If you were underweight, you may need to supplement the calorie numbers provided in this chapter with more calories to gain the proper amount of weight. Talk to your obstetrician (OB) to determine the approximate total amount of weight you can gain for a healthy pregnancy and the number of additional (or fewer) calories you need to consume to get there.

First trimester (weeks 1 through 13): Don't purposely take in extra calories

Even though the first trimester (weeks 1 through 13) is a time of incredible growth for your baby, she's still so small that her growth doesn't require any significant energy. So during these first few months, don't worry about purposely eating any more calories than you ate pre-pregnancy. No additional calories are required during the first trimester, and the total weight gain during this period is 1 to 4 pounds.

TIP

TRUST YOUR GUT

Don't start purposely eating extra calories as soon as you learn you're pregnant. Instead, follow your body's natural hunger cues.

What? Don't women need more calories while they're pregnant? Isn't it a mom-to-be's responsibility to ensure that she begins to stock up stores right away to ensure that she gets the nutrition she needs to support her pregnancy? How can she do that if she's not eating more?

After living as a pregnant woman for another month or so, you'll start to realize that this advice is simply brilliant. If you truly listen to your hormone-raging pregnant body, you will eat more when you need to eat more to support your pregnancy. Some days, you'll be nauseous and not eat much, but other days your appetite will be ravenous and you'll eat more. If you start at week 8 purposely trying to take in more calories every day, you'll likely gain too much in the first trimester, setting the stage for excess weight gain for the entire pregnancy.

REMEMBER

If food is the last thing on your mind because of nausea, take a deep breath and relax. Your pre-pregnancy nutrient stores will get you through this first trimester even if you aren't able to hold down much food. Just be sure to take your prenatal vitamin every day so you know you're getting enough folic acid. (For advice on dealing with nausea, refer to Book 1, Chapter 4.)

If you're not experiencing nausea, you may have the opposite problem — ravenous hunger! When hunger strikes, go with your instincts and eat, but eat foods that will fill you up and provide good nutrients. Avoid foods high in sugar and fat and focus instead on healthy foods.

Second trimester (weeks 14 through 27): Take in an extra 300 to 350 calories

The second trimester (weeks 14 through 27) is a time of incredible growth for your baby. She goes from weighing only about an ounce at the end of week 13 to weighing more than 2 pounds by the end of week 26. To support your little one's growth during this phase of pregnancy, you need to consume about 300 to 350 extra calories per day. If you're at a normal weight, look to gain approximately 1 pound per week; if you're overweight or obese, try to gain half a pound per week.

Nourishing Your Bump

You don't have to eat all 300 to 350 calories at one time. You can spread them out over the course of the day. Check out the following list for some great meal and snack ideas that'll give you the calories you need during your second trimester (the number of calories is in parentheses). Feel free to mix and match to make your own yummy combinations.

>> 1 large banana (120) + 1 large apple (95) + 30 pistachios (100)

>> 1 ounce whole-grain crackers (120) + 1 piece of string cheese (85) + ½ cup frozen yogurt (140)

>> 1 cup 1% cottage cheese (160) + 1 cup fresh sliced strawberries (50) + ½ cup edamame (95)

>> 1 cup fat-free milk (90) + 1 cup whole-grain cereal (175) + ½ cup blueberries (45)

>> Two slices whole-wheat toast (160) + 1 tablespoon almond butter (100) + 1 tablespoon raspberry preserves (55)

>> 1 ounce tortilla chips (140) + ¼ cup salsa (20) + ½ cup black beans (110) + 1 cup fresh pineapple chunks (80)

>> 6 ounces Concord grape juice (130) + ½ ounce dark chocolate (85) + 6 ounces nonfat fruited Greek yogurt (130)

>> 1 smoothie (310) made with ½ banana + ½ cup strawberries + ½ cup nonfat milk + 1 scoop protein powder + 1 tablespoon wheat germ

>> 1 frozen meal of your choice (about 300)

REMEMBER

Some days you'll be hungrier than others. Follow your hunger cues and eat more on the days when you're hungrier, but don't force yourself to eat on the days when you aren't. For most women, it all evens out. Besides, your doctor will let you know whether you're gaining too little or too much weight, so you can adjust your calories up or down as appropriate.

TIP

If you're so inclined, you can rely on the scale to tell you whether you're getting enough to eat (or too much, for that matter). Look at your average weight gain over the course of a few weeks to assess your progress. Turn to Book 3, Chapter 1 to see how much weight you should be gaining throughout your pregnancy.

THE SCIENCE BEHIND THOSE EXTRA CALORIES

Women need about 85,000 calories for the entire 40 weeks of pregnancy. If you do the math, those 85,000 calories break down to about 300 extra calories per day. However, studies vary, some estimating pregnant women need more calories and others estimating they need fewer calories.

One reason you need more calories when you're pregnant (at least in the second and third trimesters) is that your *resting metabolic rate* (RMR) increases. Your RMR is the number of calories you burn each day at rest. Your RMR increases with pregnancy because you burn more calories to grow another life. The other reason you need more calories is that you have to store fat and protein in your body throughout pregnancy.

While your RMR plays a large part in determining the number of calories you burn in a day, you can't forget about your daily physical activities. Some studies suggest that pregnant women don't need as many calories as many experts estimate because many women end up decreasing their physical activity during pregnancy. Whether that means exercising less intensely or simply sitting with your feet up more often, you may find yourself moving less than your pre-pregnancy self who kick-boxed her way to fitness and never sat down. As you work with your doctor to determine how many more calories you need, be sure to think about how much more or less you're moving during your pregnancy. Head to Book 4 for exercise information and tips.

Third trimester (weeks 28 through 40): Take in an extra 450 to 500 calories

During the third trimester, your baby gains about 4 more pounds. Because you're now carrying around even more weight than you were in the second trimester, you need to consume more calories so you have the energy to cart that extra weight around. Aim to eat about 450 to 500 more calories than you did pre-pregnancy (to gain about 1 pound a week if you're at a normal weight or half a pound per week if you're overweight or obese).

REMEMBER

Follow your hunger. Some days you'll be ravenous, and other days your appetite will subside. As long as you're gaining the proper weight, don't stress about eating exactly 450 to 500 extra calories per day.

Here are some ideas for how to get those extra 450 to 500 calories each day (the number of calories is in parentheses). Keep in mind that you can spread out the extra calories throughout the day. Mix and match foods from this list to create your own meals and snacks.

» ¼ cup hummus (100) + 1 cup fresh raw veggies (50) + 1 whole-grain pita pocket (120) + 1 ounce pasteurized feta cheese (75) + 1 cup chocolate soymilk (140)

» 2 Medjool dates (130) + 1 ounce (or 19 halves) pecans (195) + 1 ounce cheddar cheese (115) + 1 plum (30)

» 1 hard-boiled egg (75) + one 4-inch cinnamon raisin bagel (230) + 1 tablespoon peanut butter (95) + 4 ounces 100% pomegranate juice (80)

» 3 ounces salmon (175) + ½ cup quinoa (115) + 1 cup asparagus (40) + 1 table-spoon olive oil (120)

» 3 ounces lean strip steak (165) + 2 cups raw spinach (15) + 20 pine nuts (25) + 2 tablespoons Italian salad dressing (100) + 1 KIND or other fruit and nut nutri-tion bar (190)

» ½ cup garbanzo beans (130) + 1 mango (135) + 1 cup chocolate pudding (210)

» 6 ounces nonfat fruited Greek yogurt (130) + ½ cup granola (200) + 1 table-spoon honey (65) + 1 cup raspberries (65)

» ⅓ cup dry rolled oats (150) + 1 cup skim milk (90) + 1 ounce (or 14 halves) walnuts (185) + 1 large peach (70)

» ½ cup homemade tuna or chicken salad (200) + 1 cup grapes (65) + 15 almonds (105) + 1 SOYJOY or other soy protein nutrition bar (130)

» 2 mini Babybel or other round cheeses (140) + ½ cup barley (100) + 6 dried apricot halves (50) + 2 small chocolate chip cookies (160)

TIP

You can also get your extra 450 to 500 calories by eating larger portions at your meals, but adding some nutritious snacks in between meals is probably a better idea. Why? Because as the third trimester goes on, the sheer size of your belly may suppress your appetite or cause gastric reflux by pressing on your stomach. Limiting portions at meals and relying on snacks for added nutrients and energy can help you feel better overall.

Figuring Out Where Your Calories Should Come From

Of course, variety is the spice of life, and it should definitely be a part of your diet, whether you're pregnant or not. If you eat the same foods all the time, you get the same nutrients all the time. But if you vary your food choices, you get different nutrients in the foods you consume. But what should those foods be?

The majority of the extra calories you get while you're pregnant should come from three sources: carbohydrates, protein, and fat. The following sections explain why each of these nutrients is so important during pregnancy.

A FEW RULES ABOUT FOODS

Before you got pregnant, you may have thought that all you needed to stay away from during your pregnancy was alcohol and possibly caffeine. In reality, the list of taboo foods is a bit longer and includes the following:

- **Raw and undercooked beef, chicken, fish, and pork:** A meat thermometer can tell you for sure whether a particular meat has reached a safe temperature. (Book 3, Chapter 3 lists minimum safe temperatures.)

  When most people think of sushi, they think of raw fish. If you're a sushi fan, you may be heartbroken by the thought of not having it while you're pregnant. But take heart: You can have sushi — as long as it's not the raw tuna or salmon kind. Imitation crab (used in the California roll), real crab, shrimp, and eel are all cooked, so you can enjoy any of those in your sushi.

- **Runny eggs:** Eggs need to be cooked all the way through, whether they're in the skillet, a sauce, or a casserole. Cook (or order your eggs in a restaurant) scrambled well or over hard. If the white or yolk is still runny, send it back to the skillet to be cooked until firm. Egg casseroles should be cooked until they reach 160 degrees. Avoid sauces that contain raw eggs, such as hollandaise and béarnaise. And don't forget about raw cookie dough — no licking the spoon if there are raw eggs in the dough!

- **Unpasteurized milk and cheeses:** Avoid milk or cheese that claims to be *raw* or that doesn't say *pasteurized* on the label. You're free to eat any cheese (including soft cheeses) as long as it's been made with pasteurized milk.

For the full scoop on which foods to avoid completely and which to be cautious of during pregnancy, see Book 3, Chapter 3.

The United States Department of Agriculture (USDA) provides a guideline for the average person to follow for good nutrition. This guideline is called *MyPlate,* and it shows the proportion of calories that should come from each of the five food groups (grains, protein, vegetables, fruits, and dairy). You can see the MyPlate graphic and get specific recommendations for calories and portions based on your height, weight, age, and activity level by going to www.choosemyplate.gov.

The role nutrition plays in your baby's development is critical. In fact, some researchers suggest that the nutrients a developing fetus receives in the womb (and that a newborn receives in the first few weeks of life) are more critical than the nutrients received at any other time in life. That may seem quite shocking, but more and more evidence is connecting a woman's nutritional status during pregnancy to the health of her child, not just at birth but throughout that child's life.

Carbohydrates: Energy for the body

Carbohydrates (or *carbs,* as they're often called) are your body's (and your baby's) preferred source of energy, providing you with the glucose you need to keep your brain functioning. Some examples of carb-containing foods include grains (bread, cereal, oatmeal, and tortillas, just to name a few), fruits, vegetables, milk, desserts, and anything that contains sugar.

Without enough carbohydrates, your body has to break down other nutrients, like proteins and fats, for energy instead of letting them do what they're supposed to do in the body (see the next two sections for details). You can avoid this situation by making sure that anywhere from 45 to 65 percent of your daily calories come from carbs. A single gram of carbs contains 4 calories, so just multiply the grams of carbs in a food by 4 to figure out how many carb calories that food contains. (You can see how many carbs are in the foods you eat by looking for the phrase *Total carbohydrate* on the food label. Under the total carbohydrates, you usually also see the amount of fiber and sugar, in grams, that the food contains. Both fiber and sugar are part of the total carbohydrate number.)

An easier option is to keep track of the total grams of carbs you consume. If you take this approach, aim to eat between 225 and 325 grams (g) of carbs per day for an average 2,000-calorie intake. For fruits and veggies, you can skip the counts and just eat a lot of plants, especially the green, leafy kind.

The two categories of carbs are simple carbs and complex carbs. Simple carbs are sugars — not just table sugar but also the sugar found naturally in food, like fructose in fruit and lactose in milk. Complex carbs, also called starches, are long chains of sugars; they're found in foods like grains, rice, pasta, potatoes, and beans. Your body has to break down complex carbs into simple sugars for them to be absorbed from the digestive tract into the bloodstream. Focus on getting the majority of your carbohydrates as complex carbs.

TIP

Plan on having carbohydrates in the form of grains, fruits, and vegetables at every meal. Maintaining good energy means keeping your body fueled with its preferred energy source (you guessed it: carbs!) all day long.

Protein: Cell building and repair

REMEMBER

Protein is made up of *amino acids,* which are basically the building blocks of every cell in your body and in your developing baby's body. Aim to get 20 percent of your daily calories from protein (that's about 100 grams per day if you're eating a 2,000-calorie diet). A single gram of protein contains 4 calories. To figure out how many protein calories a food contains, simply multiply the grams-of-protein-per-serving info by 4. Of course, you can always eat more protein if you want, up to 35 percent of your daily calories (which amounts to 175 g if you're eating a 2,000-calorie diet).

Because a lot of protein-containing foods are fresh (think raw meat), they don't require a food label. That's nice for manufacturers but challenging for you when you're trying to keep track of your protein intake. Let Table 2-1 be your guide to how many grams of protein are in some common foods.

TABLE 2-1   ## Amount of Protein in Some Common Foods

Food	Amount of Protein
3 ounces lean cooked meat (poultry, pork, beef, and fish)	About 21 g (7 g/ounce)
6 ounces Greek yogurt	12–16 g
3 ounces firm tofu	9 g
1 cup lowfat milk	8 g
2 tablespoons peanut butter	8 g
½ cup black beans	7 g
6 ounces lowfat yogurt	5–7 g
1 large egg	6 g
1 ounce (or about 23) almonds	6 g
Most grain products (for example, a slice of bread, 1 ounce of cereal, or 2 ounces of dry pasta)	1–4 g per serving

Protein takes longer to digest than carbs, so eating protein keeps you full for a longer period of time than eating carbs. Always try to include protein at every meal. At breakfast, your protein source can be milk, eggs, or yogurt, and at lunch and dinner, it can be meat or meat alternatives. You can also get protein from your snacks by eating nuts and nut butters.

Fat: Nervous system development and function

REMEMBER

Even though you may be nervous about the weight you'll gain, pregnancy is *not* the time to go on a fat-free diet! Fat plays a key role in developing your baby's brain and keeping your brain and nervous system running smoothly. It's also an energy source for your body and helps keep you feeling fuller longer. Aim to get 20 to 35 percent of your calories from fat. Fat is more calorically dense than carbs and protein; a single fat gram contains 9 calories. Multiply the grams of fat in a food by 9 to figure out how many fat calories a food contains.

TIP

An easier way to track how many of your daily calories come from fat is to look for the *Calories from Fat* info on the Nutrition Facts panel. Another alternative is to track grams of fat. If you're eating a 2,000-calorie diet, you need to consume 45 to 78 g of fat per day.

Different fats have very different reactions in your body. So you need to be aware of what types of fats you're eating. Research has shown that certain fats are better for you than others. For example, saturated fat (butter, whole-fat dairy, and fatty meats) and trans fat (hydrogenated oils) have been shown to raise "bad" LDL cholesterol levels, leading to clogging of arteries and increased risk of heart disease. On the flip side, monounsaturated fats, like those found in olive oil and avocados, trigger less LDL cholesterol and more of the "good" HDL cholesterol. Polyunsaturated fats, like those found in vegetable oils and fish, are also beneficial. In fact, two specific types of polyunsaturated fats have a significant impact on brain development; for information on these fats, go to the later section "Omega-3 fatty acids."

WARNING

Limit your consumption of saturated fat to less than 22 g per day (that's 10 percent if you're consuming 2,000 calories a day) and try to avoid trans fat (like the kind found in hydrogenated oils and fried foods).

TIP

Not sure how to figure out how much fat you're getting? Just look for the *Total Fat* listing on the food label. The amounts of saturated fat and trans fat appear underneath that listing. Sometimes you also find the amounts of monounsaturated fat and polyunsaturated fat listed, but they don't have to be there.

Getting the Nutrients You Need

During pregnancy, you're literally forming a new life within your body — an act that requires more than just carbs, protein, and fat. Vitamins and minerals are also important members of the nutrition team, playing many different roles in the growth and development of your baby.

A supplement is one way to ensure you're getting the vitamins and minerals you and your little one need throughout your pregnancy. You find most, if not all, of the nutrients you need to supplement in a basic prenatal vitamin. Several brands of prenatal vitamins exist, including both over-the-counter and prescription varieties. A prescription prenatal isn't necessarily better, but your doctor may prescribe one for two reasons:

>> Women take pills better when they're prescribed rather than just recommended.

>> Some health insurance companies cover prescription prenatal vitamins, meaning that they may cost you less than the over-the-counter varieties.

In addition to a balanced diet, a regular multivitamin made with a women's formula (so it has extra folic acid and iron) may also get the job done. Women's multivitamins usually have all the essential nutrients for pregnancy, although they may not have as high of doses as the prenatal varieties. Prenatal vitamins also tend to have more iron and sometimes even the DHA omega-3 all in one place (see the later sections "Iron" and "Omega-3 fatty acids" for details).

TIP

Iron can cause nausea and constipation in some women. If you're one of them, skip the prenatal vitamin and at least take a separate folic acid supplement (with between 600 and 800 micrograms) or a general multivitamin with less iron.

Depending on your diet, you may also want to take extra calcium, iron, vitamin D, or DHA omega-3. Estimate how much of each nutrient you're getting in your diet and talk to your doctor about getting your blood values checked for certain nutrients, such as iron and vitamin D. Then supplement your diet with additional nutrients as needed.

REMEMBER

A supplement is just that — a *supplement* to your diet. In other words, don't eat junk and think the vitamins you're taking will be enough to keep you and your baby healthy. Nutritious food is still important!

Of course, because some nutrients are of special concern during pregnancy, you may want to take a closer look at them so you can really understand what they do for your growing baby, how much of them you need, and what you can eat to get them. The next sections provide these details.

Folate (folic acid)

Folate (the food form), also called *folic acid* (the supplement form), plays a key role in developing your baby's spinal cord early in pregnancy, but it's also an important nutrient to get later in pregnancy. Aim to get 600 micrograms (mcg) per day throughout your pregnancy. Your prenatal vitamin probably contains about this amount (check the label to make sure), but because vitamins are generally absorbed and utilized better through food than supplements, try to get it naturally in food, too.

You find folate in oranges (and orange juice), strawberries, avocados, beans (specifically black, garbanzo, kidney, navy, and pinto), black-eyed peas, lentils, nuts, dark-green leafy vegetables (like spinach, kale, and collards), asparagus, broccoli, and Brussels sprouts. You can also find folate-fortified grain products, such as flour and cereal.

Iron

Your daily iron needs practically double during pregnancy, from 18 to 27 milligrams (mg). This increase is due in large part to the increase in blood volume you're experiencing. Iron helps your body form hemoglobin, the protein that carries oxygen to the blood. You need this oxygen to get to your placenta to help your baby develop.

Aside from your prenatal vitamin, you find iron in animal foods like beef, poultry (higher in dark meat), pork, fish, and egg yolks, although you can also get iron in seeds, beans, lentils, dark-green leafy vegetables, dried fruit (like prunes, raisins, and apricots), and whole grains. Manufacturers often add iron into other grains such as rice and cereals as well. In packaged food products, you can find the amount of iron per serving listed on the food label, but be aware that the percentage listed is based on the average 18 mg daily requirement and you now need 27 mg.

Iron, especially the form found in vegetable sources, is often not absorbed in high quantities by your body. To help improve absorption, eat foods that are high in vitamin C along with your iron-rich foods. For example, include oranges, tomatoes, cantaloupe, strawberries, kiwi, peppers, or broccoli in the same meal as your iron-rich foods. The vitamin C in these foods helps your body absorb more iron. Cooking iron-rich foods in an iron skillet may also help boost your iron intake because some of the iron actually gets into the foods.

Your doctor will probably check your iron levels periodically throughout your pregnancy to make sure they're within the normal range. One symptom of iron deficiency is fatigue, but you may have a hard time figuring out whether you're tired because you're iron deficient (called *anemic*) or because you're just plain exhausted from pregnancy! A blood test is the only way to know for sure. If you find out that you're iron deficient, your doctor may recommend that you take a higher dose of supplemental iron. Iron supplements can cause nausea, loss of appetite, and constipation, though, so if you're suffering, talk to your doctor about taking a lower dose and focus on getting as much iron as possible from food.

Calcium

REMEMBER

Calcium helps with blood pressure control, but it's best known for its role in bone health — both maintaining yours and building your baby's. If you don't get enough calcium in your diet (1,000 mg), your body will take it from your bones, leaving you at higher risk of osteoporosis. The good news is that your body actually absorbs calcium better when you're pregnant.

Most prenatal vitamins contain only about 250 mg of calcium, so plan to supplement that amount by eating dairy foods (like milk, cheese, and yogurt) daily. You can also find calcium-fortified soymilk, orange juice, breads, cereals, and nutrition bars. Some vegetables and fruits, like dark-green leafy vegetables, broccoli, okra, and figs, also contain calcium. For packaged foods, calcium has to appear on food labels, so you can easily find out how much calcium the food you're eating contains. Fortunately, the daily recommendation is the same for pregnant and nonpregnant people, so looking at the percent on food labels is a good way to see whether you're getting enough calcium.

Choline

REMEMBER

Although you may not have heard of it, choline is pretty important to your little one. Preliminary evidence suggests that it works along with folate to ensure the proper development of the neural tube and central nervous system. In addition, choline plays a key role in developing the *hippocampus,* which is the memory center of the brain. So if you want your child to remember Mother's Day, get plenty of choline — 450 mg of it.

Choline isn't difficult to get in your diet, but purposely include some of the best food sources daily so you get your fill. Eggs are the best source of choline, with 125 mg; just make sure you eat the yolk because all the choline is in the yolk, not in the white part. You also find choline in meats such as beef, poultry, pork, and fish. If you're looking for vegetarian sources, try wheat germ, cauliflower, broccoli, potatoes, and nuts (especially pistachios). Check the label of your prenatal vitamin to see if it includes choline; most prenatal vitamins have it, but some may not.

Omega-3 fatty acids

REMEMBER

Omega-3 fatty acids have been shown to help reduce the risk of preterm births, preeclampsia, and hypertension in pregnancy. Two specific omega-3 fatty acids found mainly in fish and seafood are essential during pregnancy:

>> **Docosahexaenoic acid (DHA):** Most research emphasizes getting plenty of DHA in pregnancy because the brain is made up primarily of DHA. Aim to get a minimum of 300 mg of DHA a day while pregnant.

>> **Eicosapentaenoic acid (EPA):** EPA is essential to building every structural cell in the body. Aim to get a minimum of 220 mg per day (which is actually the same amount you need when you're not pregnant).

The key to getting plenty of omega-3s in pregnancy is focusing on the best sources of omega-3s while avoiding the sources with higher mercury contents. How do you know which sources are best? Take a look at Table 2-2. It shows a list of high-omega-3 fish that are also low in mercury (and, thus, safe to eat during pregnancy).

TABLE 2-2   **Low-Mercury Sources of DHA and EPA Omega-3s**

Fish	DHA + EPA Content
Atlantic salmon, farmed, 3 ounces cooked	1,835 mg
Coho salmon, farmed, 3 ounces cooked	1,087 mg
Anchovies, 2 ounces canned	924 mg
Sardines, 3 ounces canned	835 mg
Crab, 3 ounces cooked	335 mg
Flounder, 3 ounces cooked	255 mg
Clams, 3 ounces cooked	241 mg
Light tuna, 3 ounces canned	230 mg
Scallops, 3 ounces cooked	80 mg
Shrimp, 3 ounces cooked	80 mg
Catfish, 3 ounces cooked	77 mg

Source: USDA nutrient database (www.nal.usda.gov)

If you're not a fan of fish, look for sources of algae because the algae the fish eat produce their high omega-3 content. But before you start scraping the sides of your fish tank, look for food products on store shelves that boast high DHA contents. Most of these products are fortified with algal oil and contain between 30 and 50 mg of DHA per serving.

TIP

A great nonfish source of omega-3s is a DHA-enhanced egg. Eggland's Best farms feed their hens sea kelp, which results in each egg having about 57 mg of DHA per large egg. Regular eggs have 29 mg on average.

If you can't fathom eating a ton of fish or omega-3-fortified food, consider taking an omega-3 supplement. Your prenatal vitamin may already have some omega-3s in it, so look at the label for DHA and EPA. Aim to get a minimum of 300 mg of DHA but ideally more like a total of 1,000 mg of DHA and EPA combined. If your prenatal vitamin doesn't have enough omega-3s, consider a fish-oil supplement. Just be sure to read the label carefully to see how many pills you need to take to get to the 1,000 mg amount.

Fish oil supplements can cause a nasty case of fish burps. If you don't think you can handle tasting fish for a while after taking a supplement, look for a supplement that's made from high-quality, highly purified fish oil, like Nordic Naturals. Alternatively, choose one that's enteric coated, like Vital Remedy MD's Vital-Oils1000 or a store-shelf brand like Nature Made's Ultra Omega-3 Minis, which give you 1,000 mg of combined DHA and EPA in three small pills that are easier to swallow. If you're a vegan, look for Ascenta brand NutraVege, which has 400 mg of DHA in 2 teaspoons.

The rest of the essential pregnancy nutrients

The preceding five sections describe specific nutrients that have a direct relationship to various key areas of your baby's development, but they're not the only nutrients worth knowing about. The following list highlights four additional nutrients that are important for keeping you and your baby properly nourished:

>> **Vitamin D:** Vitamin D helps build bones and protect the immune system of both you and your baby. Low levels of vitamin D have been linked to increased risk of cesarean (C-section) delivery, preeclampsia, and gestational diabetes for pregnant moms and to weak bones, seizures, respiratory infections, and brain disorders in babies. Vitamin D is difficult to get in the diet, so make sure your prenatal vitamin contains at least 600 international units (IU). If you want to do even better by you and your baby, try to get at least 1,000 IU

of vitamin D per day. (You can take an extra vitamin D supplement to reach this amount.)

REMEMBER

The American Academy of Pediatrics recommends that every pregnant woman get her vitamin D level checked and aim for a blood level above 32 nanograms/milliliter (ng/mL). It takes about 1,000 IU of vitamin D to raise blood levels 10 ng/mL. Many researchers now recommend that all pregnant and nursing women take 5,000 IU of vitamin D daily, but check with your doctor for his or her recommendation.

>> **Vitamin A:** This nutrient is necessary in pregnancy because of its key role in building healthy cells and developing vision in your baby. Do your best to get 2,566 IU (770 mcg) of vitamin A per day.

WARNING

Getting enough vitamin A isn't typically a problem. The concern is consuming too much of this particular nutrient. Some studies have connected high levels of vitamin A to birth defects. Getting too much vitamin A in your diet is pretty hard to do unless you eat liver several times per week (liver is really high in vitamin A), but getting too much from supplements is much easier. Check all the supplements you're taking and make sure that you're not getting more than 10,000 IU total of preformed vitamin A daily. Also make sure your supplement uses beta carotene as its source of vitamin A rather than the potentially problematic form called retinol.

RESEARCHING THE LINK BETWEEN MOM'S NUTRITION AND BABY'S DEVELOPMENT

A recent study found that a mother's nutrition while pregnant can actually alter the function of her child's DNA, predisposing the child to conditions and diseases such as obesity, diabetes, and heart disease. Eating a poor diet during the times that are most critical in the development of your baby may even cause certain organs not to function correctly and may lead to complications in your baby. For example, one study on baboons (hey, they're not so different from humans!) found that poor nutrition during fetal and early life damaged the pancreas and predisposed the offspring to type 2 diabetes later on in life.

Another study looked at survivors of the Dutch Famine in the 1940s. The women who were pregnant during the famine had children who were more likely to develop a preference for fatty foods and to be less active. They also had increased risk of type 2 diabetes, obesity, hypertension, and cardiovascular disease. Although a famine probably isn't on the horizon in your life, this study is a great example of the impact a lack of nutrition during pregnancy can have on your child's lifelong health.

>> **Zinc:** This mineral is essential for keeping your immune system strong and for cell growth in your baby. During your pregnancy, aim to get a minimum of 11 mg of zinc per day; it's okay to get more than that. Good sources of zinc include animal proteins as well as fortified grains, sunflower seeds, wheat germ, tofu, and peanuts. You may also be able to meet your daily zinc requirement just by taking your prenatal vitamin; check the label to be sure.

>> **Iodine:** In pregnancy, iodine helps with brain development and hormone production in your baby, so be sure to get 220 mcg of it daily. You can find iodine in iodized salt, a common staple in many people's homes, as well as in fish (especially saltwater fish), dairy foods, and some vegetables, like potatoes and beans. Some prenatal vitamins contain iodine, but some don't, so don't rely on your vitamin to get your iodine.

Discovering the Numerous Benefits of Fiber

Fiber offers your body several health benefits. Probably the most well-known benefit is its broom-like quality. That is, fiber keeps things moving through your digestive tract, cleaning out the colon. Fiber is the part of complex carbohydrates that literally doesn't get digested. Because your body can't digest it, fiber creates bulk in the stool, leaving you with a softer stool that passes with regularity.

Fiber also keeps you feeling fuller longer and keeps your blood sugar under control while your body tries to digest it. In addition, fiber can help you control your blood pressure, decrease your risk of preeclampsia, and reduce your cholesterol levels. The following sections tell you everything you need to know about how much fiber to get during pregnancy and where to go to get it.

Knowing how much fiber you need

During pregnancy, you need to get 28 g of fiber per day (that's 3 g more than the recommended pre-pregnancy amount). Pregnant women need more fiber in their diets to combat their increased risk of constipation, which is a common occurrence for many expectant mothers due to hormonal changes in the body. (For additional constipation-prevention tips, turn to Book 1, Chapter 4.)

TIP

Eating fiber can leave you feeling a bit gassy. To avoid this experience, increase your fiber intake slowly. Eat a bit more fiber every day for several weeks to get up to the full 28 g per day. Doing so allows your digestive tract to get used to the added fiber.

Filling up on fiber-rich foods

The only place you find fiber is in plant foods. So look to whole grains, beans, fruits, vegetables, nuts, and seeds to get your fill of fiber. Table 2-3 provides you with a list of common plant foods along with their fiber content. (For any foods with a range of fiber contents, just check the label on the food you're about to eat to find out exactly how much fiber it contains.)

TABLE 2-3 **Common High-Fiber Foods**

Food	Fiber Content
High-fiber cereals (like All-Bran, Fiber One, Kashi, Raisin Bran, and Shredded Wheat)	6–14 g
Beans (like black, kidney, garbanzo, pinto, lima, and baked beans), ½ cup cooked	5–9 g
Lentils, ½ cup cooked	8 g
Blackberries, 1 cup raw	8 g
Pear, medium with skin	5 g
Apple, medium with skin	4 g
Russet potato, medium with skin	4 g
Whole-wheat bread, pasta, and brown rice, serving size	2–4 g
Popcorn, 3 cups popped	3.5 g
Banana, medium	3 g
Strawberries, 1 cup raw	3 g
Broccoli, ½ cup cooked	2.5 g
Spinach, ½ cup cooked	2 g
Oatmeal, ½ cup cooked	2 g
Flaxseed, 1 tablespoon ground	2 g
Wheat germ, 2 tablespoons	2 g
Hummus, 2 tablespoons	1.5 g

TIP

Fiber is listed as *Dietary Fiber* on the Nutrition Facts panel on food labels (under the *Total Carbohydrate* line). Looking for this entry is the best way to find the exact amount of fiber in a packaged food.

Sneaking more fiber into your day

Look for opportunities throughout the day to add more fiber to your diet. Start with a high-fiber cereal or a piece of whole-grain toast and be amazed at how easily you can get your required 28 g every day. Here are some additional creative ways of adding fiber to your diet:

» Use whole-wheat flour in place of part or all of the white flour in recipes.

» Leave the skin on fruits and vegetables (if it's edible!).

» Sneak more vegetables into foods by shredding and pureeing them and adding them to casseroles, sauces, and soups.

» Use fresh or frozen fruits and vegetables to make smoothies.

» Add canned beans to salads, soups, and pasta dishes — basically anywhere and everywhere you can think to add them. (Just remember to drain and rinse the beans to cut back on sodium and potentially reduce gas.)

» Use snacks like popcorn, fresh fruit, raw veggies, canned beans, and high-fiber cereal or crackers as midday fiber opportunities.

Realizing Why Proper Hydration Matters

Whether you're pregnant or not, fluid is critical. You could survive for a long time on your body's stores of nutrients, but without fluid, you may not even last a week. Fluid transports nutrients to your cells and transports waste material away from them, keeps your body at the proper temperature (something that's especially important when you're pregnant), and moves fiber through your digestive system. Read on to find out how much fluid you need to stay *hydrated* (having proper fluid balance in your cells) and where to get it.

How much fluid do I need?

REMEMBER

You need 102 ounces (that's 3 liters or 12.7 cups) of fluid per day throughout your pregnancy. Why so much? Well, blood is about 83 percent water, and your blood volume increases when you're pregnant. Also, what do you think your baby is floating around in? You guessed it — fluid! Without that extra fluid, your baby wouldn't have the proper cushioning he needs to protect his delicate, developing body.

TIP

To determine whether you're properly hydrated, look at the color of your urine. You don't need to examine it for hours; just taking a quick peek to see whether your urine is barely yellow can leave you feeling assured that you're hydrated. If it's bright yellow or dark in color, reach for a beverage after you wash your hands. If you're having trouble with vomiting during your pregnancy, you may have a hard time staying hydrated. Check with your doctor about monitoring and improving your hydration.

Where should my fluid come from?

Water should be your primary source for hydration (it's calorie-free and easily available), but the 102-ounce recommendation also includes the water you get from food and other fluids. Food (including fruits, vegetables, rice, pasta, and even bread) typically contributes about 20 ounces of your fluid for the day. The remaining 90-plus ounces comes from everything you drink.

Coffee, tea, soft drinks, sparkling water, juice, and milk all earn you hydration points. Because you're not drinking alcohol and you're limiting your caffeine (see Book 1, Chapter 4 for details), you won't be getting any major diuretic effects from those beverages. Decaffeinated beverages hydrate essentially the same as water.

Note: Tap water is generally safe in the United States, so don't feel like you have to drink bottled water throughout your pregnancy. If you're concerned about the safety of your tap water, use a reverse osmosis filter to be sure it's as safe as you can make it.

What if I can't stay hydrated?

TIP

If staying hydrated isn't easy for you, employ some of these tips to help you hit your 102-ounce fluid goal:

>> Create a fluid checklist for yourself and mark off your progress throughout the day.

>> Carry a water bottle with you at all times. You'll be more inclined to drink up if you have water sitting in front of you.

>> Set a timer to remind yourself to drink on average about 8 to 12 ounces every one to two hours.

>> Add cucumber or fresh orange slices (or pineapple, berries, lemon slices, or lime slices) to keep your water interesting.

>> Drink a tall glass of liquid at every meal.

>> Fill up on liquid-containing foods, like soup, gelatin, fruits, and veggies.

>> Drink water or sports drinks before, during, and after you exercise.

>> Drink more fluid on hot days or if you're traveling by plane.

>> Add more fluid to your daily diet if you've been sick with a fever, diarrhea, or vomiting.

REMEMBER

Don't wait for thirst to tell you to drink. When you feel thirsty, you're likely already at least slightly dehydrated.

Living a Vegetarian Lifestyle While Pregnant

If you're a vegetarian, you can continue to live your lifestyle and have a healthy baby. Although it's probably not the best idea to become a vegetarian right before or during your pregnancy, if you've been one for some time, you've likely mastered the skills you need to plan properly nutritious meals.

The term *vegetarian* means different things to different people. For example, if you're a *lacto-ovo* vegetarian (meaning you eat dairy and eggs), you likely won't have any problem meeting your nutrient requirements as long as you're eating the iron-rich foods listed in the upcoming bulleted list. If you're *vegan* (meaning you don't eat any dairy or eggs), you'll likely have to take dietary supplements to ensure you're getting the proper nutrients.

REMEMBER

Regardless of what being vegetarian means to you, make sure you're getting enough calories and gaining the proper amount of weight as your pregnancy progresses. As a vegetarian, focus on eating beans, soy, nuts, and seeds to get plenty of protein, and if you avoid dairy, choose calcium-fortified milk replacements like soy-based milk, yogurt, and cheese.

REMEMBER

Vegetarian diets generally tend to be lower than traditional meat-containing diets in a few key nutrients that are essential during pregnancy. The following list breaks down these essential nutrients and explains how you can get more of them in your diet (to figure out the amount you need of each nutrient, see the earlier section "Getting the Nutrients You Need"):

>> **Iron:** Choose fortified grains, dark leafy greens, dried fruit, tofu, prunes, beans, and blackstrap molasses. Or consider taking an iron supplement.

>> **Vitamin B12:** Because only animal products like dairy and eggs contain this vitamin, vegans need to get their vitamin B12 from supplements or fortified foods.

>> **Protein:** Incorporate a protein-rich food, like dairy, eggs, beans, nuts, seeds, or soy foods, into every meal.

>> **DHA:** If you avoid fish, getting enough of this omega-3 can be a challenge. Look for algal-oil-fortified foods or choose eggs that have been laid by hens that eat special feed high in DHA. You can also look for an algae-based supplement (see the earlier section "Omega-3 fatty acids" for details).

>> **Calcium:** If you eat your three servings of dairy per day, you'll likely meet your calcium needs. If you don't, look for fortified foods or supplements.

>> **Zinc:** You find zinc in wheat germ, beans, nuts, seeds, milk, and fortified foods.

>> **Vitamin D:** You find a small amount in fortified milk, seafood, and some mushrooms, but you probably still need to consider taking a vitamin D supplement to make sure you're getting enough of this important nutrient.

For more detailed information on good pregnancy nutrition for vegetarians, check out the latest edition of *Living Vegetarian For Dummies* by Suzanne Havala Hobbs (Wiley).

Sticking to Good Nutrition When Faced with Unique Circumstances

Every woman brings with her a unique set of genetics and lifestyle habits that guides how her pregnancy will progress. Various nutrition–related medical complications may creep up on you. For example, if you find out you have gestational diabetes, your best bet is to seek the counsel of a registered dietitian to guide you in exactly how many and what kind of carbohydrates to eat. If you're faced with preeclampsia or high blood pressure, you'll have to watch your sodium intake very carefully. If you develop anemia, you'll need to focus on getting plenty of iron–rich foods and making sure your body absorbs as much of it as possible.

Gestational diabetes

Gestational diabetes, a type of diabetes that can develop in the second half of pregnancy, affects how your body uses *glucose* (blood sugar). Scientists aren't sure why some pregnant women develop gestational diabetes and others don't, because pregnancy itself affects certain hormones that impact how insulin clears glucose out of the blood and gets it into cells. As your pregnancy progresses and your baby grows, the placenta produces hormones that block insulin, which may cause higher-than-normal glucose levels in the blood. Some women develop gestational diabetes in response to insulin's not working as efficiently during pregnancy.

The universal treatment for gestational diabetes — whether you have a mild case or a severe one that requires daily insulin injections — is a diet that moderates your carbohydrate intake. As explained earlier in this chapter, carbohydrates are found mostly in grains, fruits, vegetables, and sweet foods. Although you shouldn't start following a diet that's very low in carbohydrates, you do need to use caution with portion sizes of carb-containing foods. Also try to avoid sugary foods, specifically liquid sources of sugar like regular soft drinks and even fruit juices, and limit portions of desserts, candy, and processed starches, like white bread, white rice, and many low-fiber cereals and crackers.

REMEMBER

Fill up on foods that are high in fiber and protein to prevent spikes in your blood sugar.

Regular exercise is another part of the standard gestational diabetes treatment plan. Exercise can increase your body's sensitivity to insulin, meaning that your body doesn't need to produce as much of it to clear out the excess glucose. Check with your doctor for any limitations you may need to incorporate into your exercise routine.

Polycystic ovary syndrome

Polycystic ovary syndrome (PCOS) is a common hormonal disorder that results in irregular menstruation, cysts on the ovaries, and overproduction of *androgens* (male hormones). PCOS is a leading cause of infertility, in part because many women with PCOS are overweight or obese. If you have PCOS and you're reading this, then congratulations on overcoming this pregnancy hurdle!

WARNING

The big pregnancy complication for many women with PCOS is that PCOS can lead to insulin resistance, which results in high blood sugar and diabetes. If you have PCOS, alert your doctor as soon in your pregnancy as possible so you can be screened earlier for gestational diabetes (see the preceding section for details on this condition). Follow your doctor's instructions on medications and lifestyle modifications, such as a carb-controlled diet and increased exercise, that are necessary to keep your blood sugar under control.

Depending on your pre-pregnancy weight, you may also be advised to adjust the desired amount of weight gain during your pregnancy (to find out the average weight gain numbers, refer to Book 3, Chapter 1). Also consider visiting a registered dietitian (RD) who specializes in pregnancy and PCOS to create an individualized nutrition plan for you.

High blood pressure and preeclampsia

Even if you didn't have high blood pressure (also called *hypertension*) before you were pregnant, you may develop it while you're pregnant, particularly in the second or third trimester. This is especially true if you have a family history of high blood pressure or you're overweight prior to getting pregnant. Your doctor measures your blood pressure at every prenatal visit. Because you likely won't feel any symptoms if you have high blood pressure, it's extremely important that you attend all your prenatal appointments.

Whether you have high blood pressure or preeclampsia, the primary nutrition recommendation is the same: Limit your intake of sodium to less than 2,300 mg per day. (Your doctor may want you to lower your intake to 1,500 mg if your case is more severe, so be sure to check with him or her to find out how much you need to modify your diet.) Chances are most of your daily sodium comes from processed and prepared foods, including soups, sauces (such as soy, BBQ, and tomato), condiments (think pickles and olives), cheese, processed meats (such as ham, pepperoni, and sausage), and restaurant food. Try to avoid these major sodium sources and read labels to see how much sodium is in the foods you're consuming.

TIP

Here are some additional diet-related ways to keep high blood pressure at bay:

>> **Take in more potassium.** Potassium helps you maintain proper fluid balance in your body and has been shown to help with blood pressure control. Every fruit and vegetable has at least a little bit of potassium, but bananas, potatoes, and legumes (beans) have the most. Aim to consume at least five servings of fruits and vegetables every day to get your daily 4,700 mg.

>> **Embrace dairy products.** Calcium has been shown to help keep blood pressure in check, so drink your milk and eat your yogurt (these foods are also good sources of potassium) or take a calcium supplement to get your 1,000 mg per day.

>> **Avoid caffeine.** Caffeine can raise blood pressure, so avoid it if you have blood pressure issues.

>> **Consider taking an omega-3 supplement.** Omega-3 fatty acids (DHA and EPA) have been found to help reduce blood pressure, so eat fatty fish such as salmon or take a fish-oil-based omega-3 supplement. Find out more about omega-3s in the earlier section "Omega-3 fatty acids."

Along with adjusting your diet, you can make two other important lifestyle changes to help control your blood pressure: exercise and stress management. Check with your doctor to find out if you need to incorporate any limitations into your exercise routine and then head over to Book 4 for tips on adding exercise to your day. Controlling stress isn't easy, especially when you're preparing to bring a new life into the world, but getting plenty of rest and relaxation can help you keep it under control.

Anemia

Anemia, or abnormally low levels of red blood cells, is fairly common in pregnancy because of the increased blood volume and the high demand for iron (the mineral that helps make red blood cells, which carry oxygen from the lungs to all parts of the body). To account for the increase in blood volume, pregnant women need to consume about 27 mg of iron per day.

The best way to treat anemia is to consume more iron-containing foods; refer to the earlier section "Iron" for information on this key nutrient and foods that contain a lot of it. Another way to get your daily dose of iron is to take a supplement. Your prenatal vitamin has some iron, but your doctor may recommend that you take even more iron in supplement form if your blood levels are too low. *Note:* Iron in supplements has been known to constipate some people, so eat high-fiber foods and drink plenty of water to prevent that unpleasant side effect.

Food allergies

TIP

If you're allergic to milk or wheat and worried about whether your allergy is causing you to miss out on important nutrients, never fear. To ensure you're eating a diet that's filled with all the nutrients you and your baby need, just make the simple food substitutions recommended in this list of the eight most common food allergies:

>> **Milk:** Milk is rich in calcium and vitamin D, among other nutrients. Choose fortified soymilk in place of regular milk, and look for dairy-free cheeses to get your calcium. If soymilk isn't your thing, take a calcium supplement (500 to 1,000 mg). Also take a vitamin D supplement because it's difficult to get through food.

>> **Eggs:** Eggs are high in choline, so if you can't have eggs, incorporate beef, poultry, wheat germ, cauliflower, broccoli, and soy lecithin into your diet to make sure you're still getting enough choline (refer to the earlier section "Choline" for information on this important nutrient).

>> **Peanuts:** Peanuts have monounsaturated fat, protein, fiber, folate, and other B vitamins. To get these same nutrients, you can eat tree nuts (if you're not allergic to them), beans (garbanzo beans, navy beans, kidney beans, black beans, and so on), or lentils.

>> **Tree nuts:** These nuts include walnuts, almonds, cashews, and pecans. They're full of protein, fiber, unsaturated fats, vitamin E, folate, and B vitamins. To get these nutrients if you're allergic to tree nuts, simply include some vegetable oils, avocados, and whole grains in your diet.

>> **Fish:** Fish, such as salmon, tuna, and cod, is an excellent source of protein and the best place to get the omega-3 fatty acids DHA and EPA. If you're allergic to all fish, turn to other meats and meat alternatives for protein. To get your omega-3 fatty acids, your best bet is to take a fish-free DHA/EPA omega-3 supplement, like Ascenta NutraVege or Spectrum's Vegetarian DHA supplement.

>> **Shellfish:** Shellfish, such as shrimp, lobster, and crab, is a lean protein that offers various vitamins and minerals, including selenium, vitamins D and B12, and zinc. You can get protein and many of these nutrients from other lean meats (lean beef, white-meat skinless poultry, or lean pork) or meat alternatives (soy foods and legumes), and you can take a vitamin D supplement and get selenium from chicken, eggs, nuts, and seeds. You can get your omega-3 fatty acids (DHA and EPA) from a shellfish-free supplement (check the label to make sure it's shellfish-free).

>> **Soy:** Soy is a good source of protein and nutrients such as folate and other B vitamins, potassium, and iron. If you can't have soy, eat meat, eggs, or dairy to make sure you still get these nutrients.

>> **Wheat:** Wheat foods contain complex carbohydrates, folate, iron, B vitamins, and more. Look for wheat-free foods that provide similar nutrients, like rice, potatoes, and quinoa.

Chapter 3
Knowing What Foods to Avoid

When talking about pregnancy nutrition, it's as important to focus on what you shouldn't eat as it is to talk about what you should. This chapter gives you a rundown of what foods (and substances) to avoid throughout your pregnancy to keep you and your baby safe. It also helps you reduce your chances of developing foodborne infections (you're at an increased risk for them now that you have a bun in the oven), discusses food-related toxins, and explains why you should be selective about sweeteners and seafood.

Foods and Beverages That Aren't Safe during Pregnancy

If you look no further in this chapter than this section, you'll still have a solid understanding of the foods and beverages that are of the most concern during pregnancy. Table 3-1 spotlights the foods and beverages that are dangerous when consumed while pregnant. Table 3-2 lists the foods that you don't have to completely avoid but that you do need to be cautious about when eating.

TABLE 3-1　　**Foods and Beverages to Avoid during Pregnancy**

Don't Eat/Drink This	Why Avoid It?
Agave nectar	Can cause uterine contractions
Alcohol	Passes to the fetus; increases your risk of miscarriage or stillbirth; can result in fetal alcohol syndrome and brain damage if consumed in excessive amounts
Commercially prepared meat salads (ham, chicken, tuna salad)	Can be contaminated with *Listeria* bacteria
High-mercury fish (shark, swordfish, king mackerel, tilefish, golden/white snapper)	Can have high levels of mercury
Raw eggs (like those found in cookie dough)	Can be contaminated with *Salmonella* bacteria
Raw honey	Can be contaminated with bacteria that causes botulism (a serious paralytic illness)
Raw shellfish (oysters, clams)	Can be contaminated with *Vibrio* bacteria
Raw sprouts (alfalfa, mung bean, clover)	Can be contaminated with *E. coli* or *Salmonella* bacteria
Raw or undercooked fish (sushi made with raw fish)	Can be contaminated with various bacteria or parasites
Raw or undercooked meat (pork, poultry, beef)	Can be contaminated with *E. coli* bacteria
Soft cheeses from unpasteurized milk (Brie, feta, Camembert, blue cheese, queso blanco, queso fresco)	Can be contaminated with *E. coli* or *Listeria* bacteria
Unpasteurized (or fresh-squeezed) cider or juice (like orange, cranberry, and other drinkable juices)	Can be contaminated with *E. coli* bacteria
Unpasteurized (raw) milk	Can be contaminated with various bacteria

Adapted from www.foodsafety.gov/risk/pregnant/chklist_pregnancy.html

TABLE 3-2　　**Foods and Beverages to Be Cautious of during Pregnancy**

Use Caution with This	Why Use Caution?	Alternative Strategy
Albacore (or white) tuna	Can have moderately high levels of mercury	Limit intake to 6 ounces per week; choose light tuna instead.
Caffeine	Crosses the placenta and can increase the baby's heart rate; is linked to slowing fetal growth	Limit caffeine to 200 mg maximum or choose decaf beverages instead.
Deli meats (turkey, ham, roast beef), cold cuts (bologna), hot dogs	Can be contaminated with *Listeria* bacteria	Always cook these meats until they're steaming hot or 165 degrees or higher (even if the package says *precooked*).

Use Caution with This	Why Use Caution?	Alternative Strategy
Homemade ice cream, custard, eggnog, mousse, meringue, and Caesar dressing	May contain raw eggs, which can be contaminated with *Salmonella* bacteria	Avoid eating it if you don't know whether raw eggs were used, or use pasteurized eggs if you're making it yourself.
Liver (beef and chicken)	Contains high levels of vitamin A, which can be toxic, especially in the first trimester	Limit intake and enjoy other meats in place of liver.
Meat spreads or pâté	Can be contaminated with *Listeria* bacteria	Use canned versions.
Saccharin	Passes to the fetus and may remain in the fetal tissue; may increase cancer risk in offspring	Use the safer sweeteners listed in the section "Being Selective with Sweeteners" later in this chapter, or use small amounts of real sugar.
Smoked seafood	Can be contaminated with various bacteria or parasites	Cook all smoked seafood until it reaches a temperature of 165 degrees or higher.
Stuffing and gravy	Can be contaminated with various bacteria	Cook stuffing until it reaches a temperature of 165 degrees or higher; reheat gravy to a boil.
Undercooked eggs	Can be contaminated with *Salmonella* bacteria	Cook eggs until both the yellow and white parts are firm.

Adapted from www.foodsafety.gov/risk/pregnant/chklist_pregnancy.html

A Warning on Herbals

WARNING

Even though herbal supplements may appear to be "natural," they don't undergo the same safety testing that food products and over-the-counter and prescription medications go through. For that reason, you should avoid herbal products in food and supplements during pregnancy — a feat that's easier said than done these days, because herbals are found not only in supplements but also in many foods. Read labels carefully and watch out for these common herbal products in particular:

>> Agave

>> Aloe

>> Black cohosh

>> Ephedra

>> Ginkgo biloba

>> Ginseng

>> Goldenseal

>> Saw palmetto

>> Willow bark

>> Yohimbe

Focusing on Foodborne Illnesses

Throughout your pregnancy, you and your growing little one are at high risk for getting sick thanks to immune system issues. Your immune system is weaker because your body is so busy growing another person, and your baby's immune system is still developing and not even close to operating at full strength. Consequently, fending off the pesky, disease-causing bugs found on door handles, in the air, and in your food is much more difficult when you're pregnant.

WARNING

Foodborne illnesses, which occur when you eat something that contains a type of bacteria, parasite, or virus that makes you sick, can cause miscarriage or premature delivery in serious cases. In really severe cases, exposure to these harmful organisms can cause death. The best-case scenario for you is a little bit of dehydration and fatigue, but your baby can suffer a variety of problems.

The following sections fill you in on five pesky "bugs" — living organisms that are too small to see but can bring you to your knees — that pregnant women are particularly susceptible to. You can find out how to protect yourself from contracting a foodborne illness from these little buggers.

Campylobacter

Campylobacter jejuni bacteria are one of the major causes of diarrheal foodborne illness in the United States. These bacteria grow in raw or undercooked poultry, other meats, and seafood as well as in unpasteurized milk and untreated water. In fact, some studies have found *Campylobacter* in up to 100 percent of the poultry tested in retail stores.

WARNING

Symptoms occur two to five days after infection and include diarrhea, fever, muscle aches, vomiting, and nausea. In pregnant women, infection of *Campylobacter* can be transmitted to the placenta and can cause miscarriage, stillbirth, or preterm delivery.

The good news is that most modern water-treatment systems easily destroy *Campylobacter*, so the water you drink from your tap is completely safe. To prevent *Campylobacter* infection from spreading in your home, cook meats to proper temperatures and don't cross-contaminate cutting boards and knives.

E. coli

E. coli bacteria have many strains, and all animals, including humans, have *E. coli* in their intestines. One specific strain — *E. coli* O157:H7 — contains toxins that damage the lining of the intestines, causing hemorrhagic colitis, an acute disease. *E. coli* contamination typically happens when people don't properly wash their hands after using the restroom, when raw meats aren't properly handled, or when fruits and vegetables aren't properly washed. Manure (animal feces) is often used as a natural fertilizer, especially for organic produce, so it's no surprise that *E. coli* outbreaks often happen because of contaminated produce.

E. coli contamination typically affects the digestive tract the most; symptoms include diarrhea and bloody diarrhea. The biggest risk of *E. coli* infection during pregnancy is dehydration, which can cause miscarriage or premature labor in severe cases. *E. coli* bacteria are also the most common cause of urinary tract infections in pregnant women.

REMEMBER

To prevent *E. coli* contamination, follow these simple steps:

» Cook all meats well to their proper temperatures (see Table 3-3).

» Drink juices and milk only if they're pasteurized.

» Wash all fruits and vegetables well, whether they're organic or conventionally grown.

» Wash all cutting boards and knives between uses with different foods.

TABLE 3-3   ## Minimum Meat Temperatures

Meat	Minimum Temperature
Precooked ham	140 degrees
Fish	145 degrees
Pork roasts and chops*	145 degrees
Beef steak or roasts*	145 degrees

(continued)

TABLE 3-3 *(continued)*

Meat	Minimum Temperature
Casseroles containing meat or eggs	160 degrees
Ground beef, lamb, and pork	160 degrees
Ground poultry	165 degrees
Chicken breasts	165 degrees
Whole poultry	165 degrees
Leftovers containing meat or eggs	165 degrees

*The U.S. Department of Agriculture (USDA) recommends a three-minute "rest time" for these meats. In other words, allow the meat to sit (or rest) for three minutes before you carve or consume it.

Listeria

Listeria is a type of bacteria that can grow even below the "safety zone" of temperatures (less than 40 degrees), where most other bacteria can't. It can grow in unpasteurized milk and cheese, refrigerated ready-to-eat meats (like cold cuts and deli meat), poultry, and seafood. Fruits and vegetables that haven't been properly washed can also be contaminated, especially if manure was used as a fertilizer.

WARNING

Listeria causes an infection known as *listeriosis.* Symptoms occur a few days to several weeks after infection and can include fever, chills, muscle aches, diarrhea, headache, stiff neck, and confusion. Pregnant women are 20 times more likely to get listeriosis than other healthy adults. In fact, about one-third of listeriosis cases in the United States involve pregnant women. Listeriosis is especially dangerous in the first trimester because it can cause miscarriage, but it also poses a risk to the baby after birth. It can cause mental retardation, paralysis, seizures, and developmental problems in the brain, heart, and kidneys.

REMEMBER

Here are some steps you can take to reduce your risk of contracting listeriosis:

>> **Heat deli meats, cold cuts, hot dogs, and smoked seafood to steaming hot if you choose to eat them.** Even when these meats are fresh and cold out of the refrigerator, they can have high levels of listeria.

>> **Check the labels on soft cheeses like Brie, Camembert, feta, blue cheese, Gorgonzola, and queso blanco or fresco to make sure the ingredient list includes *pasteurized* milk.** If it doesn't, don't buy the cheese!

>> **Avoid refrigerated pâtés or meat spreads.** Eat them only if they're canned and shelf stable (meaning they're safe to shelve without refrigeration).

>> **Wash fruits and vegetables prior to eating them.** Simply rub your produce well while holding it under running water.

Salmonella

Salmonella bacteria is carried by animals and is found in raw meats. It also exists in soil, so it can contaminate fresh fruits and vegetables. *Salmonellosis* is one of the most common foodborne illnesses in the world. In pregnant women, it can pass to the fetus and cause miscarriage or developmental delays in the baby. Symptoms for Mom include fever, nausea, vomiting, diarrhea, and stomach cramps, but a woman can be infected without experiencing any symptoms.

WARNING

Raw sprouts, like alfalfa and broccoli sprouts, are one of the most common produce items to carry *Salmonella*. Because sprouts are so difficult to wash properly, you should completely avoid them while pregnant. Eggs are another major source of *Salmonella* contamination. Eat pasteurized eggs, and cook your eggs thoroughly until both the whites and yolks are firm. If you're eating a dish that contains eggs, make sure it's cooked well.

Other ways to prevent *Salmonella* poisoning include washing all fruits and vegetables thoroughly and cooking meats to their proper temperatures (refer back to Table 3-3).

Toxoplasma

Toxoplasma gondii is a parasite found in undercooked or raw meats that causes an illness called *toxoplasmosis.* It lives in the soil, so unwashed fruits and vegetables can also be contaminated. This parasite is the main reason water can make you sick in some countries; fortunately, the water supply in the United States is treated and safe.

WARNING

Pregnant women are at a 20 to 50 percent higher risk of developing the toxoplasmosis infection. Symptoms include swollen glands, muscle pain, a stiff neck, and fever, but not all pregnant women experience symptoms. Even if you don't experience signs of toxoplasmosis infection, your baby could be infected. Infection in babies can cause mental retardation, blindness, and hearing loss.

REMEMBER

Heating meats to their proper temperatures before eating them is key to preventing toxoplasmosis because heat destroys the infection-causing parasite. Make sure you separate raw meat in the grocery cart and your refrigerator, and use a separate cutting board and clean knife when preparing meat at home. Also wash all fruits and vegetables before eating them.

WARNING

Cat feces can also carry *Toxoplasma* (especially if your cat is a mouse hunter outside), so if you can, ask someone else to change out the cat litter, or use disposable gloves and give your hands a thorough wash if you're doing it yourself. Also be sure to wash your hands after handling your cat, especially before preparing meals, and keep your cat off all food preparation and eating surfaces in your home. Keep your cat's risk low by feeding him dry or canned food, not raw meat scraps.

Because *Toxoplasma* exists in the soil, use gardening gloves while digging in the soil outside and wash your hands thoroughly before touching your mouth or your food.

Tackling Food-Related Toxins

The microorganisms that cause foodborne illnesses aren't the only things that can harm you and your baby. Toxins can also be found in foods as well as in the containers that house them. This section reveals three toxins that are of particular concern during pregnancy and explains how you can reduce your (and your baby's) exposure to them.

Mercury

Mercury is a metal that exists naturally in the environment, but industrial pollution produces high levels that enter the air and water supply in large amounts. Humans typically come into contact with mercury by eating fish. Mercury builds up in your bloodstream and passes to your baby, and although it does eventually leave your body naturally, it can take more than a year to do so. For that reason, limiting your exposure to high-mercury fish is vital, ideally even before you become pregnant (for a list of the most popular high-mercury fish, refer back to Table 3-1).

Nearly all fish have some mercury because they feed on mercury-containing organisms. But some fish have decidedly lower mercury levels than others. Head to the later section "Hitting the Seafood Counter" for a list of safe and unsafe fish to eat during pregnancy.

WARNING

Symptoms of mercury poisoning can include itching; burning skin; sensitivity in hands, feet, and mouth; lack of coordination; impairment of peripheral vision; muscle weakness; and speech impairment. However, you may not notice any symptoms at all from mercury poisoning. But even if you don't have any symptoms, your baby will. Mercury can affect your baby's developing nervous system, and the effects can carry on through childhood. To play it safe and still satisfy your seafood craving, eat no more than 12 ounces of low-mercury fish each week throughout the course of your pregnancy.

Pesticides

Very little evidence connects pesticides to significant risk to unborn babies. However, large amounts of pesticides can lead to low-birth-weight babies, premature labor, or miscarriage.

TIP

One surefire way to reduce your exposure to pesticide residue on the produce you're eating is to go organic when it comes to the following fruits and vegetables, which tend to have the most pesticide residue: apples, bell peppers, blueberries, celery, cherries, grapes (imported), kale and collard greens, nectarines, peaches, potatoes, spinach, and strawberries. If you don't go organic with your fruits and vegetables, be sure to wash all dishes, cutting boards, and utensils that may have been exposed to any pesticide residue before using them again.

Plastics

Plastics contain several potentially harmful chemicals. Leading the pack are bisphenol A (BPA), which makes plastic clear and strong, and phthalates, which make plastic more flexible. Unfortunately, many foods come in packages made from these materials. Here's what you need to know about these chemicals and how they relate to your pregnancy:

>> BPA has been linked to miscarriage and negative effects on the brain and prostate gland in fetuses and children.

>> Phthalates have been connected to birth defects, specifically in male genitals, and after-birth exposure to these harmful chemicals can still have negative effects on the reproductive systems of baby boys.

TIP

Heating plastics can leach some of the BPA and phthalates from the containers into the food you consume; to reduce your (and your baby's) exposure to toxins found in plastics, follow these steps:

>> Heat only those plastics that are made specifically for cooking. Avoid any plastics that have the number 7 or the letters *PC* (which stand for polycarbonate) in a triangle on the container.

>> Don't microwave food in plastic containers. Transfer your food to a ceramic or glass container before warming it up.

>> Wash plastics by hand to prevent exposing them to high heat in the dishwasher.

Being Selective with Sweeteners

If you've ever looked at the ingredient list for a box of cookies, a can of soda, or even a loaf of bread or jar of peanut butter, you're probably well aware that sugar isn't the only sweetener out there. Many foods and beverages contain *nonnutritive sweeteners*, which sweeten food without contributing significant calories. (Nonnutritive sweeteners are also commonly referred to as *artificial sweeteners*, although not all of them are artificial.) Other foods are made with *nutritive sweeteners*, which do contribute calories.

REMEMBER

It's important to note that in order to be in the food supply in the United States, a food ingredient or food additive must go through an approval process with the U.S. Food and Drug Administration (FDA). The agency is responsible for reviewing safety studies to ensure that every food ingredient and food additive is safe to eat. The safety data reviewed must include safety for everyone — children, adults, the elderly, and pregnant and lactating women. The FDA uses panels of scientists to rigorously review all data available on that particular food ingredient in an objective and independent fashion.

That being said, you may still have some concerns about whether a particular sweetener is safe to consume during pregnancy. This section gives you the information you need to make your own decisions regarding whether to include the following sweeteners in your diet.

WARNING

Even if you never pick up a blue or pink packet of sweetener, you may be consuming nonnutritive sweeteners without realizing it, depending on the foods and beverages you're eating and drinking. If you prefer to avoid everything artificial (including artificial colors and flavors) throughout your pregnancy, you need to diligently read ingredient lists on food labels.

Acesulfame K

Acesulfame K (brand name Sunett and commonly called Ace-K) is a nonnutritive sweetener that's used quite frequently in food products, often in combination with other nonnutritive sweeteners. You can find acesulfame K listed among the ingredients of more than 4,000 foods, including soft drinks, ice cream, chewing gum, baked goods, breakfast cereals, and canned fruits. Although you may also find packets of acesulfame K, it's not as popular as the other nonnutritive sweeteners in packet form.

REMEMBER

The FDA has found acesulfame K to be safe for use in pregnancy in moderation. What's moderation? The acceptable daily intake (ADI) is set at an equivalent of 2 gallons of an acesulfame-K containing beverage every day.

Agave nectar

Agave nectar is a natural, nutritive sweetener that comes from the tequila plant. You find agave as a sweetener option in natural food stores and in some coffee and tea houses.

WARNING

Just because something is natural doesn't mean it's safe. In terms of pregnancy safety, agave is surrounded by controversy. For instance, some people link it to cramping or increased risk of miscarriage. Agave contains a large number of *saponins,* which are naturally occurring substances that can cause uterine contractions. For this reason, you may want to avoid agave while pregnant. After all, it's better to be safe than sorry.

Aspartame

Aspartame (brand names Equal and Nutrasweet) is one of the most widely known nonnutritive sweeteners. You find it in the blue tabletop sweetener packets as well as in a wide variety of soft drinks, chewing gum, yogurt, and many reduced-sugar items. The FDA has approved the use of aspartame for pregnant women, but many experts still recommend using caution with how much you consume. In fact, the ADI for aspartame is set at about 97 packets or 20 cans of diet soda each day. As long as you're not downing can after can of diet soda, you'll be fine adding a couple of blue packets to your foods or beverages and eating a few aspartame-containing foods per day.

WARNING

Aspartame breaks down to phenylalanine, so if you have phenylketonuria (PKU), steer clear of this sweetener.

High-fructose corn syrup

High-fructose corn syrup (HFCS) is an inexpensive nutritive sweetener that many manufacturers use to sweeten their foods. In recent years, HFCS has drawn a lot of blame for the ever-increasing number of diabetes and obesity cases in the United States. However, scientific studies don't support this theory. HFCS is no worse for you than table sugar; however, it does contain calories without nutritional value.

HFCS is simply syrup made from cornstarch mixed with fructose, another type of sugar found naturally in fruit. HFCS is actually very similar in composition to table sugar. You can find HFCS in a wide variety of products, including soft drinks, yogurts, candy, cookies, crackers, and condiments. Studies have determined that HFCS is safe to consume when you're pregnant, but remember that it does have calories. (To be exact, it has 16 calories per teaspoon — the same as table sugar.)

Honey

Honey contains trace amounts of minerals, as well as dormant *Clostridium botulinum* bacteria, which can cause a severe paralytic illness known as *botulism*. The honey you find on store shelves has been pasteurized to eliminate the toxins created by the bacteria, but you may find raw honey at farmers' markets.

WARNING

Avoid eating raw, unpasteurized honey while pregnant. And don't feed children under age 1 any type of honey because they don't have mature enough immune systems to break down and destroy the bacteria.

If you want to eat pasteurized honey while pregnant, remember that it does contain calories (21 per teaspoon), so be careful how much you use as you sweeten your tea.

Saccharin

The pink sweetener packets you see on many restaurant tables contain another well-known nonnutritive sweetener called *saccharin* (brand name Sweet'N Low). Saccharin isn't used in as many food products as other nonnutritive sweeteners, which is nice because the safety of saccharin during pregnancy is questionable. To date, no studies prove that saccharin is harmful in pregnant humans, but some animal studies have shown increased cancer risk in offspring when mothers consume the sweetener during gestation.

WARNING

For many years, saccharin was on the National Institute of Health's list of possible cancer-causing agents because of some older studies. However, more recent studies haven't confirmed the cancer findings, so the institute removed saccharin from the list in the 1990s. Even so, because saccharin crosses the placenta and may remain in fetal tissue, many health professionals recommend that you don't use it during pregnancy.

Stevia

Stevia (brand names Truvia and PureVia) is the new kid on the block when it comes to nonnutritive sweeteners. You find it in the green tabletop packets as well as in many foods, including yogurts, soft drinks, juices, and ice cream. Stevia is a natural sweetener that comes from the stevia plant. This plant contains several sweet components, one of which is called *rebiana*. On food labels, you may see rebiana (rather than stevia) in the ingredient list. The ADI for rebiana is 29 packets or 64 ounces of rebiana-sweetened beverage every day.

Sucralose

Sucralose is one of the newer nonnutritive sweeteners out there, and it goes by the brand name Splenda. You find it in the yellow tabletop sweetener packets as well as in soft drinks, yogurts, ice creams, and other reduced-sugar items. The FDA has approved the use of sucralose in pregnancy, but as with aspartame, you should use moderation with the amount you consume. The ADI for sucralose is equivalent to about 28 packets of sucralose each day, so definitely stick with less than that amount.

TECHNICAL STUFF

Even though sucralose claims to be "made from sugar," it has been chemically altered not to be absorbed by the body, so it belongs in the classification of artificial sweeteners.

Hitting the Seafood Counter

Fish should definitely be on your weekly shopping list. After all, eating fish and seafood is especially good for your health during pregnancy (and while nursing). Fish contains protein and iron, two nutrients you need while pregnant (see Book 3, Chapter 2 for why these nutrients are so important). Plus, eating fish has been linked to reduced risk of cardiovascular disease and reduced risk of dying from any cause in adults. The benefits you get from eating fish come mainly from the omega-3 fatty acids that are so prevalent in many fish and seafood. These same omega-3s, especially DHA and EPA, are part of the building blocks of the brain, which is why pregnant women and young children should get plenty of DHA and EPA.

REMEMBER

All these benefits sound great, but what about the bad things you've heard about fish, like mercury, polychlorinated biphenyls (PCBs), and dioxin? Although these contaminants are important to be aware of, many experts believe that the benefits of eating fish outweigh the potential risks. Just to be safe, though, the Environmental Protection Agency (EPA) and the FDA have come up with a recommendation that pregnant women eat no more than 12 ounces of seafood per week.

You can minimize any potential seafood-related risks even more by choosing the right kinds of fish to include in your max of 12 weekly ounces. The following sections outline the fish to watch out for as well as the safest fish to eat.

Knowing which fish to be cautious of

The main concern with fish is mercury. Mercury occurs naturally in the environment and is present in trace amounts in almost all fish, but most of the mercury comes from industrial pollution that gets into the water. Bacteria in polluted water change the mercury into a form called *methylmercury,* which can be toxic. Fish consume the methylmercury by eating the organisms that live in and absorb the water.

WARNING

Methylmercury passes from your blood to your baby and can have a negative effect on his developing nervous system. Fish that are highest in methylmercury are the larger, predatory fish because they spend their days eating smaller fish, who've eaten even smaller fish, who've eaten teeny-tiny fish, who've eaten the organisms that absorbed methylmercury. Avoid the following high-mercury fish while pregnant and nursing, and don't feed them to small children:

>> King mackerel

>> Shark

>> Swordfish

>> Tilefish (also known as golden bass)

Although fish that contain moderate amounts of mercury are safe for most people to consume, pregnant women and women who are nursing should avoid the following moderate-mercury fish:

>> Ahi tuna

>> Chilean sea bass

>> Grouper

>> Mahi mahi

>> Marlin

>> Orange roughy

>> Spanish mackerel

Aim to eat the lower-mercury fish listed in the next section rather than their moderate- or high-mercury counterparts.

TIP

If you're worried about eating fish because of *PCBs* and *dioxins* (chemical contaminants found in the environment), keep in mind that the levels found in fish are similar to those found in beef, chicken, and pork. In fact, only 9 percent of the PCBs and dioxins in the U.S. food supply come from fish and seafood; the other 90 percent come from other foods. If you eat fish caught in local waters, check the local fish advisories to see whether they warn about contaminated waters.

Discovering which fish are best

The EPA and FDA recommend that pregnant or nursing women choose fish and seafood that are low in mercury to get the recommended limit of 12 ounces per week. Choose from these low-mercury options:

>> Anchovies

>> Catfish

>> Cod

>> Light tuna (*not* albacore, or "white," tuna, which is safe to consume only in 6-ounce amounts per week as part of your overall fish allowance)

>> Pollock

>> Salmon (*not* smoked salmon or fresh salmon jerky, which may contain harmful bacteria)

>> Sardines

>> Shrimp, crab, clams, and scallops

>> Tilapia

TIP

Not sure what 12 ounces of fish looks like? A 3-ounce portion is the standard recommended portion size. For 12 ounces, you could have four servings of one of the following 3-ounce portions: six large shrimp, six large scallops, a tuna salad sandwich, or a 3-ounce fillet that fits in the palm of your hand.

4

Staying Fit While Pregnant

Contents at a Glance

Chapter 1

Recognizing the Benefits of a Fit Pregnancy

Congratulations on your pregnancy! With a healthy lifestyle and good advice from your healthcare provider, you're going to deliver a healthy, happy baby in a few months.

One of the most significant benefits of a fit pregnancy is that you gain less fat than nonexercisers do during their pregnancies. And for the weight you do gain (keeping in mind that weight gain during pregnancy is healthy and absolutely necessary), if you're a fit woman, you'll have an easier time shedding your weight after you deliver.

REMEMBER

If you're tempted to think of these 40 weeks as a time to throw caution to the wind and eat whatever you want, you'll probably gain far more weight than you need to and will have a difficult time getting back to your pre-pregnancy size. To stay fit during your pregnancy, you have to approach your pregnancy with a different mindset: not throwing caution to the wind but using common sense in every decision. You do so by incorporating healthy eating habits and burning additional calories as you work out. (Book 3, Chapters 1 and 2 cover how many extra calories you need during your pregnancy, how many *more* calories you can eat without gaining more weight than your doctor recommends, and your nutritional needs to support you and your baby during your pregnancy.)

Besides helping you manage your weight, a fit pregnancy brings other incredible benefits, from making your pregnancy more comfortable to improving your mood to helping your body get back to normal after you deliver. Even your baby benefits from your workouts. This chapter is chock-full of the benefits of a fit pregnancy that you and your baby can enjoy.

REMEMBER

Much of the current research on the benefits of fitness during pregnancy comes from fitness pregnancy guru James F. Clapp III, MD, who has been researching the effects of exercise on women and their babies since the 1970s. His research and writing has shown the world how beneficial fitness during pregnancy is to moms and babies alike. His groundbreaking book, *Exercising Through Your Pregnancy* (Addicus Books), coauthored by Catherine Cram, MS, was updated in 2012.

What Does "Fit Pregnancy" Mean?

In a nutshell, a *fit pregnancy* means that during the nine months between the time you conceive and the time you go into labor, you're doing the following:

>> **You're setting yourself up for an easier labor and delivery.** This is what you've been waiting to hear, isn't it? Women who exercise during pregnancy deliver their babies about five days earlier, spend less time in labor, experience fewer complications during labor and delivery, have fewer inductions and cesarean deliveries, and need fewer drugs to relieve pain than women who don't exercise.

>> **You're establishing cardiovascular fitness.** Getting fit while you're pregnant means that your heart and lungs (your *cardiovascular system*) get stronger, healthier, and more efficient. This means that not only will you be a mother, but you'll also likely live to be a great-great-grandmother!

>> **You're developing strength.** You tone your arms, chest, abdomen, butt, hips, and legs. You may never look like a bodybuilder (and probably don't want to), but you can make yourself strong. This strength comes in handy with all the bending and lifting you'll be doing in a few months.

>> **You're improving your flexibility.** By stretching after your workout and on your days off, you'll become far more flexible, which means you'll experience fewer injuries and be far less limited in what your body can do throughout the rest of your life.

>> **You're balancing exercise with proper nutrition.** Exercise and nutrition go hand in hand; the food you eat fuels your body (doing so either efficiently or inefficiently), and the exercise you do changes the amount of food you need to eat to maintain your weight. This is why you see articles about food in workout magazines and articles about workouts in health-food magazines. The two are inseparably linked. Book 3 tells you what you need to know about nutrition during pregnancy.

Being fit during pregnancy doesn't mean training for a triathlon or getting certified as a fitness instructor (although if those ideas become future goals of yours, that's terrific). And you don't have to start eating macrobiotic food or anything like that. Instead, a fit pregnancy is about normal people taking seriously the advice of physicians and researchers to get in shape and stay that way.

Coping with the Changes Your Body Is Experiencing

Your body undergoes dramatic changes during pregnancy, and these physical changes can make women downright uncomfortable for much of the 40-week duration. These changes range from how your heart and lungs operate to how you process the food you eat to how your muscles and joints change (Book 1, Chapter 4 covers these changes). One of the best ways to alleviate the discomfort of many of the changes your body is experiencing is to exercise. That's right: If you exercise during pregnancy, you'll spend nine months being far more comfortable than you'd be if you didn't exercise.

Easing back pain and soreness

As your abdomen increases in size and you gain the weight required to have a healthy baby, you'll likely see a shift in your posture (either a greater curve in the low back or a hunched-over appearance in the shoulders). You may also experience some low-back pain as the curvature of your lower spine changes with the added weight of your baby and body fluids.

WEATHERING GESTATIONAL DIABETES

Gestational diabetes, a form of diabetes that appears during pregnancy and may increase your risk of developing type 2 diabetes later in life, often leads to delivering a very large baby and increasing the risk of complications during labor and delivery. But here's the good news: Research shows that pregnant women experiencing gestational diabetes who exercise just three times per week lower their blood sugar.

During pregnancy, your growing baby changes your center of gravity, and muscles in your legs, hips, butt, back, and shoulders either lengthen or shorten because of this shift. Without exercise, these muscle changes can lead to poor posture, which in turn leads to back pain, stiffness, and soreness.

Exercising during pregnancy, however, helps get those muscles back into balance and improves your posture. And many types of exercise specifically strengthen your back and abdominal muscles, helping you get rid of low-back pain.

Fine-tuning your circulatory system

Exercising during pregnancy increases the volume of blood your heart pumps with each beat, increasing the amount of oxygen and nutrients delivered to your baby. This increase in cardiovascular fitness also provides a safety margin for you and your baby by enabling your cardiovascular system to pump out adequate blood flow during times of physical stress.

The increased cardiovascular functioning helps you weather the physical challenges of pregnancy better and with less fatigue.

Helping you sleep better and giving you more energy

During pregnancy, many women tend not to sleep well at night and experience extreme fatigue during the day. Exercise, however, can lick these problems, making you sleep more soundly at night and feel refreshed throughout the day. It's true! If you lie awake at night or sleep fitfully, set up a regular fitness routine; you'll find yourself dozing faster and more soundly as your body recovers from the paces you're putting it through.

REMEMBER

Essentially, exercise creates a system in which you're very alert throughout most of the day and then you crash at night, sleeping like a log. As long as you exercise in the morning, afternoon, or early evening, you should feel sleepy at your bedtime. However, because exercise makes you alert, if you work out three or fewer hours before your bedtime, you'll throw off your body clock and be alert at night and dead tired throughout the next day.

Developing muscle tone and flexibility

Exercise at any point in your life builds muscle tone, and if you stretch regularly, you'll also improve your flexibility.

If you currently watch your flabby arms wiggle when you brush your teeth, tend to hide your legs under sweat pants, and could barely touch your toes even when you weren't pregnant, exercise can change your life. Imagine being able to lift heavy objects without help and without hurting your back, wear sleeveless shirts and short shorts with pride, and snake yourself under couches and dressers to retrieve lost toys. A whole new world is waiting for you if you just add exercise to your daily routine.

The best news, though, is that you're not only improving your appearance but also getting your body ready for some difficult tasks ahead: labor, delivery, and motherhood.

GETTING INTO A GREAT MOOD

Have you heard of distance runners getting high on endorphins? That's not an illegal substance they're taking; rather, *endorphins* are natural, pain-relieving chemicals that the brain releases during physical activity, not just during distance runs. Get on the exercise bandwagon, and you, too, can experience a daily dose of free, safe, mood-enhancing drugs sent throughout your body by your brain. You'll feel relaxed and calm instead of tense and stressed.

Exercise also helps you work through whatever's bothering you. Many women find that by using their 20- to 60-minute workouts to sort out the problems of the day, they tend to be less upset over minor frustrations.

Controlling weight gain

During pregnancy, you need to gain weight regularly so that your baby grows properly and is well-nourished. (Book 3, Chapter 1 tells you how much weight most women gain and in which areas of the body.) Exercising while pregnant helps you gain a healthy amount of weight that tends to come off fairly easily after you deliver.

A study by Dr. Clapp showed that women who regularly exercised to the end of their pregnancies gained nearly 8 pounds less than nonexercising pregnant women, yet they were still well within the normal weight gain limits for a healthy pregnancy.

Preparing Your Body for Labor and Delivery

Anyone who tells you that childbirth is a breeze isn't being very honest with you. Childbirth is hard, and you don't want to approach it without being physically ready. One of the best ways to get yourself ready is by exercising during your pregnancy.

Having a less complicated delivery

Several research studies have shown that women who exercise have fewer complications during delivery, including instances of fetal intervention because of abnormal fetal heart rates, *forceps deliveries* (in which a large tong-like tool helps the baby come out), and *cesarean deliveries* (in which the baby is surgically removed from the uterus). Women who exercise during pregnancy also tend to need fewer drugs for pain relief.

Spending less time in labor

According to a study by Dr. Clapp, labor is significantly shorter (by about one-third) for women who exercise regularly during pregnancy than for a control group made up of physically active women who didn't continue exercising during pregnancy.

Also, babies of women who exercise regularly throughout pregnancy are born about five days earlier than those of women who don't exercise, making pregnancy that much shorter (and five days is a really big deal when you're in your third trimester).

Passing the Benefits to Your Baby

You're not the only one who benefits from your fit pregnancy — your baby gets in on the action, too! Women who exercise during pregnancy see the following benefits in their babies.

A better-functioning placenta

Okay, so your baby may not thank you for producing a better-functioning placenta the way he would thank you for, say, a car when he turns 16, but a better-functioning placenta is actually better for your baby than any hot rod will ever be!

The *placenta* is an organ that develops inside your uterus during your pregnancy. Throughout your pregnancy, the placenta transports nutrients, oxygen, and waste products between your baby's and your blood supply via his umbilical cord. The better the blood flow to and from the placenta, the healthier the baby. A study by Dr. Clapp showed that regular exercise during pregnancy leads to a placenta that grows about 30 percent faster in mid-pregnancy and has about 15 percent more blood vessels and surface area at the end of pregnancy. This effect on the placenta may have an added benefit of providing a safety margin for the fetus in times of stress-caused decreases in uterine blood flow.

A leaner child

Dr. Clapp discovered that when women exercise regularly (three to five times per week) during pregnancy, their babies are born with less fat. And though babies of exercisers are leaner, they're not born with low birth weight; in fact, they're well within normal limits — the same size range as babies born to mothers who didn't exercise, in terms of weight, limb lengths, and head and chest circumferences. They're just leaner.

And this leanness continues. Dr. Clapp's studies showed that by age 5, children of women who exercised while pregnant are generally still leaner than children born to women who didn't exercise during pregnancy. What a great way to help your baby start life as a healthy person!

Bouncing Back after Your Baby Is Born

Studies show that women who exercise during pregnancy have a much easier time returning to their pre-pregnancy weight and size than women who don't exercise while pregnant. In addition, having a fit pregnancy also gets you up and around faster after you deliver and helps you not crumple while carrying your ever-growing baby in your arms.

Recovering quickly

Babies don't give you much time to recover from your pregnancy. They have needs, and they want those needs met *now!* In order to do a bang-up job as a new mother, you need to be up and out of bed as quickly as possible, and exercising through your pregnancy is just the way to do that. Not only do women who exercise throughout pregnancy have shorter labors and deliveries, but they also get back to their lives faster than women who haven't exercised.

Getting back to your pre-pregnancy weight

Exercising during pregnancy helps you keep the amount of weight you gain at a healthy level. Research also shows that women who become or stay fit during pregnancy have less weight to lose after they deliver, and those women find that the weight they do gain comes off more easily and quickly than it does for their nonexercising counterparts. And given that an inability to lose weight is one of the top two complaints of new mothers (the other is lack of sleep), this is welcome news.

Carrying your baby

Have you ever lifted a 10-pound sack of potatoes off the display at the supermarket and barely been able to carry it over to your cart? Your baby's going to weigh almost as much as that sack of potatoes at birth and will quickly exceed that weight as he grows. Exercising now gives you time to strengthen your arms, back, hips, and legs so you can lug Junior around with ease.

Chapter 2

Designing a Safe Prenatal Fitness Program

Think of this chapter as the fine print — all the information that you need to know but that exuberant friends, trainers, and fitness book authors may have glossed over. This chapter helps you get your healthcare provider on board with your prenatal fitness goals so you don't ever put your baby at risk. It also tells you how to continuously monitor — and modify — your and your baby's responses to your exercise routine. You discover some key signals that indicate you should call or visit your physician immediately. Safety may not be the most exciting topic you'll ever read about, but this chapter is jam-packed with tips and advice.

Consulting Your Healthcare Provider

Here's the bottom line on your healthcare provider's role in your pregnancy fitness goals: Always consult with him or her before starting an exercise program. Discuss your goals and the type of activity you plan to do, making sure it's safe for you to get started.

REMEMBER

Your number-one goal for your pregnancy is to deliver a healthy child — that has to take precedence over your fitness goals. If your healthcare provider feels that your exercise routine will put your baby at risk, don't push it. In nine months, you can pick up your fitness regimen and work out wholeheartedly, knowing that you have a healthy baby at home.

The American Congress of Obstetricians and Gynecologists (ACOG) has devised guidelines for exercising during pregnancy and after delivery, and that advice serves as the basis for this and every other book on fit pregnancy. Go to www.acog. org for info on ordering these guidelines. In addition, ACOG issued a set of *contra-indications* (medical conditions and complications) and put them into two categories:

>> **Relative contraindications:** These conditions *may* indicate that something's amiss and may mean that you shouldn't start or continue your exercise program. We cover these contraindications in the later section "Knowing How Much May Be Too Much." That section also includes some potential warning signs that may indicate a problem is developing and that you should stop exercising and check with your healthcare provider.

WARNING

Keep the relative contraindications in mind whenever you exercise, and if you ever experience any of them, stop exercising and call your healthcare provider right away. Together, you can decide whether continuing to exercise is appropriate for you.

>> **Absolute contraindications:** These contraindications are listed in the last section of this chapter, "Understanding Conditions That Make Exercise Off-Limits." If you began your pregnancy with any of these conditions or if they develop during your pregnancy, your healthcare provider will very likely tell you that exercise isn't an option during your pregnancy. And if you are cleared to exercise but begin to develop any of the absolute contraindications, call or visit your healthcare provider as soon as possible.

Developing an Exercise Plan

Exercise has four main components: intensity, duration, frequency, and type. By putting these components together, you build strength, cardiovascular fitness, and flexibility without injuring yourself or being uncomfortable. All four pieces of the exercise puzzle fit together, though, so you need to think of each as you and your healthcare provider develop a workout plan.

REMEMBER

As Book 1, Chapter 4 points out, when you're pregnant, your body goes through a number of changes, some that are so subtle you may not be aware of them. These changes are important to keep in mind as you develop and engage in your pregnancy exercise program:

>> **Shifts in your center of gravity:** As your uterus pushes your abdomen up and out, your center of gravity may also change, and you may find that you can't balance as well as you used to, which can result in falling down. This is why, as your pregnancy progresses, many healthcare providers urge you to stay away from activities that require excellent balance.

>> **Joint instability:** During pregnancy, your body releases a hormone called *relaxin,* causing your joints to loosen slightly and allowing the joint in front of the pelvis to widen so that your baby's head can pass through that region during birth. Be cautious with activities that require quick movements or a lot of balance.

>> **How much heat you generate:** Throughout your pregnancy, you're like a little furnace, generating far more heat — and therefore raising your body temperature faster — than you did before you were pregnant. Both you and your baby can suffer if you overheat, so take extra care during these 40 weeks to stay away from situations that can raise your body temperature too high, like exercising outdoors in high heat or in a hot, unvented gym.

Intensity

The *intensity* of your workout is the effort you put forth as you exercise — hard, moderate, or easy. With some sports, you measure your intensity in miles per hour, revolutions per minute, per-lap time when swimming, and so on, so that you know empirically whether you're working harder or easier than the day before. In other sports, you can't measure intensity directly.

TIP

Regardless of what the speedometer is telling you, the important measure of intensity is how hard you *think* you're working out, based on how you feel (for example, saying, "Whew, that workout was hard" versus "Today's workout felt easy"). A specific tool, called the Borg Rating of Perceived Exertion (RPE) Scale, lets you assign a number to your response. The scale ranges from 6 (no effort at all) to 20 (maximum effort), with 13 being somewhat hard.

You want to feel challenged and slightly winded while exercising, so keep your workouts in the 12 to 14 range or at a level that feels moderate to somewhat hard (you can talk while exercising without feeling exceedingly short of breath).

REMEMBER

A rating of 12 on the RPE Scale won't always correlate with the same mile-per-hour rate throughout your pregnancy. One day, you may give a 12 rating when you're walking at a pace of 16 minutes per mile. On another day, later in your pregnancy or as a result of not sleeping well, you may give the same 12 rating when walking at a pace of 20 minutes per mile. Even though you're walking more slowly, you may feel that the two efforts are equally hard. And that's what's important — how the workout feels to you, not what the clock or speedometer says.

Duration

Duration refers to the amount of time you spend exercising each day. When you're exercising at a 12 to 14 rating on the RPE Scale (see the preceding section) and you don't feel any discomfort or fatigue, you can begin to gradually increase the duration of each workout from 15 or 20 minutes up to 30 minutes or more.

Duration and intensity are super-glued together: You may be able to exercise without discomfort or fatigue for 45 minutes at a level of 12 on the RPE Scale but for only 30 minutes when you're exerting yourself at a level of 14. If, during a workout, you have trouble exercising for a longer duration, scale back your intensity from a 14 to a 12. If you still experience fatigue or discomfort at 12, reduce the duration by 5 or 10 minutes.

Frequency

Frequency refers to how often you work out — that is, how many days per week. Most experts agree that exercising for three to six days per week at a duration of 30 to 60 minutes per workout keeps you in good shape. How many days per week you can comfortably exercise depends on the following:

>> **How fit you are right now:** The fitter you are, the more days per week you can work out without experiencing discomfort or fatigue.

>> **How your pregnancy is progressing:** Is your baby growing normally? Are you gaining weight normally? Do you feel good? If you answer no to any of those three questions, cut back on the number of days you're working out each week.

>> **The intensity and duration of your workouts:** If you're working out at a 14 on the RPE Scale for 45 to 60 minutes, you may find that three or four days per week is a more comfortable frequency than five or six days per week.

TIP

You need one day off per week while you're pregnant, even if you're convinced that you can work out seven days per week. You can, however, stretch your muscles seven days per week. And if one of your days is only a strength-training day, seven days is okay. But doing cardiovascular workouts all seven days will cause you to experience too much fatigue. Enjoy that day and the extra time you have as a result of not working out, and you'll be better prepared for the days that you do work out.

Type

The *type* of exercise refers to what activity you choose as your workout. Book 4, Chapter 3 helps you pin down the activities that tend to work best during pregnancy, and if you're new to exercise, Book 4, Chapter 4 asks you some questions that may help you decide what sort of exercise routine you're looking for. Ultimately, you want to choose activities that meet the following criteria:

>> You enjoy the activity.

>> The activity doesn't put your baby at risk (see Book 4, Chapter 3).

>> You can still do the activity as your center of gravity changes throughout your pregnancy.

>> The activity makes sense as one to do during pregnancy. If you're doing an activity that you can't easily modify, or if your RPE Scale rating is more than 14 and modifying the duration and frequency doesn't lower the intensity, consider changing to a different type of activity.

Monitoring Your Body

The key to safeguarding your and your baby's health is to monitor your body while you're working out and throughout the rest of your day. This is the time to notice details about your body and to keep tabs on how you feel. Along with your health-care provider, you need to closely monitor telltale signs:

>> Whether your baby is growing normally

>> Whether you're gaining weight normally

>> Overall, whether you feel good (you have energy and would tell others that you feel "good") or bad (you're tired all the time, seem to be getting sick pretty often, and so on)

If your baby is growing as scheduled, you're also gaining weight normally, and you feel great, you can continue your workout routine. If any of the preceding three signs are negative, you need to modify your routine until you're feeling good, gaining weight, and helping your baby gain weight again.

In addition, try to stay aware of other body signs, including pain or discomfort, your weight after a workout, the amount you're sleeping, and the color of your urine. Here are specific tips on what to watch and measure:

>> **Hot bod:** When you're pregnant, you produce more heat, so you need to closely monitor whether you're overheating. You can avoid overheating by working out indoors (in an air-conditioned area) during times of high heat and humidity and by staying well-hydrated all day long. If you become lightheaded, feel faint or nauseated, sweat more than usual, or feel uncomfortably hot, stop exercising, hydrate, and rest until you feel better. Avoid hot yoga classes (Bikram) and hot tubs or saunas, as these activities don't allow your body to effectively regulate heat.

>> **Finger on the pulse:** Although your heart rate is no longer considered an adequate measure of how intense your workout is, checking your heart rate is an effective way to determine how rested you are and how your body is handling pregnancy overall. Check your heart rate every morning, before you get out of bed (but not directly after your alarm goes off, when your heart may be racing). Take your pulse for one full minute. Keep a daily record of your pulse, and if you find that one morning it's significantly higher (for example, you go from 70 beats per minute to 90), your body may be fatigued, you may be getting sick, or you may be training too much. Whenever your morning resting pulse is elevated, consider taking that day off from your workout routine.

WARNING

>> **No pain:** Although you may feel some initial soreness when you begin an exercise program or increase the duration or intensity of your workouts, you shouldn't feel pain as a result of exercising. The later section "Knowing How Much May Be Too Much" explains some common types of pain that may indicate you're overdoing your exercise program, but the general rule is this: If exercise hurts, stop your workouts and call your healthcare provider.

>> **Talk time:** Pregnancy isn't the time to exercise to or past the point of exhaustion. You should always be able to carry on a conversation while exercising; if you can't, you need to reduce the intensity or duration of your workout.

>> **Toilet test:** If you aren't getting enough fluids, you can get dehydrated, which is bad for you and your baby. The color of your urine is an excellent indicator of whether you're drinking enough fluids. After you urinate, take a peek at the color of the water in the bowl: If your urine is light yellow or nearly clear, you're drinking just the right amount. If the color is orange, dark yellow, or a medium yellow, you need to drink more fluids, and you may want to curtail your exercise routine until the color lightens.

>> **Too tired:** You're bound to feel a little tired as you're exercising, but how do you feel the rest of the day? Do you feel overly tired, fatigued, or downright exhausted? If so, pull back — take a day or more off, reduce the total time you're exercising each week, and/or reduce the intensity of the workout.

REMEMBER

When monitoring your health throughout your fit pregnancy, keep in mind that if your exercise routine feels good to you, you're probably doing everything right. If the routine feels too intense or your body's not responding well after you finish exercising for the day, you need to reduce the intensity and/or duration of your workouts or take a short-term break from exercising. Whenever something just doesn't feel right, contact your healthcare provider for advice.

Modifying, Modifying, Modifying Your Routine

During pregnancy, whenever something isn't quite right, you need to modify your exercise routine to keep it safe and effective. Your baby's health is your most important priority right now, and if modifying your exercise regimen ensures a safe, healthy baby, that's the only healthy course of action to take. No matter how much you want to continue your current routine, you shouldn't do anything that compromises your baby's health.

You may need to modify your routine monthly, weekly, or even daily according to your body's response to both your pregnancy and your exercise routine. Pregnant women generally make certain modifications throughout each trimester, as the following sections discuss.

First trimester (weeks 1–13)

During the first trimester, you want to continue whatever physical activities you've been doing. If you're new to exercise (see Book 4, Chapter 4), get into exercise very gently. Either way, consider the following potential modifications and tips during this trimester:

>> If your breasts are sore, you experience morning sickness (or nausea/vomiting any time of day), or you're experiencing extreme fatigue, cut back on your routine or forgo exercise until you feel better.

>> After 12 weeks, you can modify supine exercises by using a wedge or pillows to raise your upper body off the floor.

>> If you were exercising before you got pregnant, you can probably wear your sports bras throughout much of the first trimester. You may find, however, that at the end of this trimester, you need a larger size. If you haven't yet invested in a good sports bra, go to a sporting goods store, running store, or fitness store and try on several until you find one that's comfortable. Don't buy too many: You'll quickly outgrow them, and because sports bras are made of fast-drying material, you can quickly wash one or two out, as needed, and wear them over and over.

Second trimester (weeks 14–26)

During the second trimester, you may feel better than at any other time during your pregnancy. Continue to monitor your body's reaction to exercise, and if you feel good enough to do so, consider increasing the duration or intensity of your workouts. Also keep the following potential modifications and other tips in mind:

>> Sometime during this trimester, you want to shop for a new sports bra, because your existing one is probably getting too tight.

>> If you feel unbalanced during these weeks, consider discontinuing any activity that can throw you off balance, like gymnastics, tennis, downhill skiing, skating, horseback riding, trail biking, and hiking in the woods over rutty trails. Replace with swimming, water aerobics, or a stationary bike, which doesn't require excellent balance.

>> Because your baby is growing and becoming more vulnerable if you fall or are hit in the abdomen, your healthcare provider may ask you to stop ball sports (soccer, basketball, racquetball, and so on), contact sports, and outdoor biking. (Note that because of your expanding abdomen, you may find a recumbent bike more comfortable than a traditional stationary bike.)

>> If you're doing step aerobics, make sure that your step is no higher than 4 inches off the ground, unless you feel absolutely stable and balanced with a higher step.

>> If you're rowing, you may find that this super-intense sport is too fatiguing for the rest of your pregnancy. Pay careful attention to how you're feeling and how well you and your baby are gaining weight.

>> If you're weightlifting, don't overwork your thigh muscles, because machines that work the thighs also tend to place stress on the ligaments around the pelvis and cause discomfort.

>> After the fourth month, avoid lying on your back for long periods, or you run the risk of feeling faint from the pressure your uterus puts on the *vena cava*

(the large vein that sends blood from your lower body to your heart). If you feel faint while on your back, roll over on your side to reestablish blood flow.

» If you're doing yoga, remember to modify poses for comfort and avoid any moves that cause pain. After the first trimester, use a wedge or pillows to raise the upper body when doing supine exercises.

» Many healthcare providers recommend that you stop competing in sports events during the second trimester, although this depends on your sport and how you're feeling. If you're in your second trimester and want to continue participating in a competitive sport, ask your healthcare provider for advice.

» Be careful not to overstretch or make sudden moves during this trimester (and the next and for about five months after you deliver). While you're pregnant, a hormone called *relaxin* gets you ready for childbirth by relaxing all your ligaments and joints. Use extra care to make sure you don't overstress your joints with fast and ballistic movements.

Third trimester (weeks 27–40)

In the third trimester, depending on how you feel, you may need to switch to low-impact activities, such as walking, swimming, and indoor cycling. In fact, some women are so fatigued and have so much difficulty moving around that they aren't able to exercise at all during the third trimester, but if you can, keep it up: Studies show that women who exercise during the third trimester achieve the greatest benefits from that exercise: reduced fat gain, shorter and less complicated labor and delivery, and shorter recovery after delivery from exercise.

As you go through your third trimester, keep the following potential modifications and tips in mind:

» As with the second trimester, avoid overstretching. And if you haven't already discontinued outdoor cycling, now is definitely the time to begin cycling indoors.

» In addition to needing a new sports bra, you may need a support belt or belly brace.

» If you've been running, you may decide to stop that activity and walk instead. If you're doing aerobics, avoid jumps in the last trimester. If you've been cycling indoors on a traditional indoor bike and didn't switch to a recumbent bike in the second trimester, you may need to do so now.

Knowing How Much May Be Too Much

WARNING

Following is a list of symptoms that *may* mean something's wrong. Only your healthcare provider can determine whether exercise is causing these symptoms and whether the symptoms are anything to worry about. If you experience any of the following, however, stop exercising and call your healthcare provider immediately:

>> **Contractions:** Contractions are a positive sign only if you're within a week or two of your due date. Otherwise, contractions may indicate premature labor.

>> **Dizziness:** This can be a sign of *anemia* (a low red blood cell count that results in weakness and fatigue) or other conditions.

>> **Shortness of breath not during exercise:** Shortness of breath is normal during exercise but may signal a problem if you experience it when you're not working out.

>> **Headache:** Although many pregnant women report an increase in headaches during their pregnancies (often brought on by fatigue and stress), if you experience a severe headache or a less severe one that doesn't seem to go away, contact your healthcare provider. Headaches can be an early sign of *preeclampsia* (pregnancy-induced high blood pressure).

>> **Increased swelling in your legs:** This can be a sign of preeclampsia, which is characterized by high blood pressure and fluid retention in the extremities. It can also indicate *deep-vein thrombosis,* a blood clot that develops in a vein.

>> **Muscle weakness:** Muscle weakness can take a couple of different forms: total-body weakness (in which you feel weak all over) or specific muscle weakness (such as weakness in your right arm or the left side of your body).

>> **Vaginal bleeding and/or leaking of amniotic fluid:** Leaking blood or other fluids can be the result of several complications, including *placenta previa* (in which the placenta blocks all or part of the cervix), *placenta abruption* (separation of the placenta from the uterus before delivering your baby), premature labor, and miscarriage.

>> **Not feeling your baby moving:** Your baby will probably be calm during exercise, but you should start to feel several movements again within 20 to 30 minutes after you stop. If your baby's normal movements have diminished or stopped, your baby may be experiencing problems. (Keep in mind that fetal movement isn't expected until around 20 weeks.)

TIP

Review this list with your healthcare provider, and ask him or her about any other symptoms you should watch for, based on your own medical history and circumstances.

REMEMBER

If you're asked to reduce or completely cut out exercise as a result of one or more of these symptoms, keep in mind that this period of rest may be temporary. Ask your healthcare provider to reevaluate your condition at each prenatal visit and see whether you and your baby are now in a safe condition and can return to some level of exercise.

In addition, the following physical conditions may mean that you won't be able to successfully work out while pregnant. If you've experienced any of the following contraindications, take extra time with your healthcare provider to ensure that exercising during pregnancy is right for you:

>> Irregular beating of your heart that hasn't been explained

>> *Intrauterine growth retardation* (IUGR), which means that your baby isn't measuring up to what's normal for her gestational age

>> A history of a sedentary (nonactive) lifestyle

>> Orthopedic (bone, muscle, joint, ligament) limitations that exercise may worsen

>> A history of heavy smoking

>> Being extremely overweight or underweight

>> Severe anemia

>> Chronic bronchitis

>> Type 1 diabetes that isn't well controlled

>> Hypertension (high blood pressure) that isn't well controlled

>> Hyperthyroidism (overactive thyroid) that isn't well controlled

>> Seizure disorder that isn't well controlled

Understanding Conditions That Make Exercise Off-Limits

REMEMBER

A few medical conditions usually — although not always — make exercising during pregnancy an unwise choice. Your healthcare provider is the only one who can verify which conditions make pregnancy workouts off-limits for you, and many physicians ask their patients not to exercise during pregnancy if they're diagnosed with or have a history of any of the following:

>> Carrying multiple babies who may be delivered early

>> Heart disease that restricts activity

>> Incompetent cervix (the cervix dilates prematurely)

>> Lung disease that restricts activity

>> Persistent vaginal bleeding in the second or third trimester

>> Placenta previa after 26 weeks

>> Pregnancy-induced hypertension (high blood pressure along with edema and increased protein in the urine)

>> Premature labor during this pregnancy

>> Ruptured amniotic membranes

A WORD ABOUT UNDERGARMENTS

Although undergarments aren't visible, they're extremely important for your overall comfort. If you're wearing an uncomfortable sports bra, the most comfortable T-shirt or pair of shorts in the world isn't going to overcome the discomfort you feel because of that bra. So make the first layer you put on your most important.

The principal element to look for in your undergarments is comfortable support, not fashion. After all, no one's going to see these articles of clothing except you. Also keep the following in mind as you shop:

- **Size:** Don't buy anything that feels too tight or too short. You're always better off with slightly loose clothing than gear that's too tight.

- **Chafing points:** While standing in front of the dressing room mirror, move around to see where underwear or a sports bra may rub (*chafe*) your skin. You don't want your skin to be raw after you work out.

- **Fabric:** The most comfortable fitness clothes have at least a percentage of poly-ester, sometimes under brand names like CoolMax and DriFit. The rest is usually cotton or *Lycra,* a fabric that makes clothing stretch and give a little.

Chapter 3

Knowing Which Activities Are Best (And Which to Avoid)

I f you've mentioned to friends and family that you want to start or continue exercising throughout your pregnancy, you've probably already heard a laundry list of activities you shouldn't do. Although some of that information may be accurate, some may also be old wives' tales. This chapter helps you understand which sports and other activities are well-suited to pregnancy and which you want to avoid.

WARNING

Before beginning any exercise program, talk to your healthcare provider about your plans to make sure that the activities you plan to do are safe for you and your baby.

Discovering the Best Ways to Stay Fit While Pregnant

Staying fit during pregnancy has never been easier or more fun! Whether you decide to keep your workout indoors or enjoy nature; join a gym or pool or work out at home; take a class or exercise on your own; go with basic clothing and equipment or outfit yourself with the latest and greatest stuff — and whether you're new to working out or you're an old pro — you can stay fit throughout your pregnancy in a way that fits your lifestyle and interests.

This section introduces you to the activities that women often find most comfortable and effective during pregnancy.

TIP

If you've never exercised before, check out Book 4, Chapter 4, which helps you get started. That chapter also helps you think about your own interests and personality when choosing an activity.

Gym balls, resistance bands, and low-weight bars or hand weights

An excellent way to increase strength and flexibility is to work out with the following:

>> **Gym ball:** You've probably seen these in advertisements or in fitness magazines — they're large balls that you sit on, lie on, or lean against in order to do a variety of exercises. Some are perfectly round, which means that part of the exercise you're doing comes from keeping yourself from rolling off (thereby making the workouts even more challenging); others sit on a flat base, which many pregnant women prefer. As your abdomen grows and your center of gravity changes, staying on a rolling object can seem less and less possible!

>> **Resistance bands:** Resistance bands are like extraordinarily large rubber bands, although they usually have special plastic or rubber handles that help you control them. When you pull up or out on your resistance bands, they resist your pull the way a heavy weight does. Doing workouts with resistance bands can make a variety of muscles much stronger.

>> **Weight bars or hand weights:** Using weights — either individual ones that you hold in your hands or a long, weighted bar that you hold over your head or behind your neck — can quickly improve your strength and muscle tone.

REMEMBER

If you combine workouts that improve strength and/or flexibility with workouts that challenge your heart and lungs (*aerobic* workouts), you turn your body into a finely tuned machine.

Fitness walking and running

Fitness walking is an excellent exercise for beginning and experienced exercisers alike, because you can control the intensity, duration, and frequency of your workout — walking faster, longer, and more often as you become fitter.

Running is another great way to get and stay fit but is usually reserved for women who were running before getting pregnant and who continue to progress normally in their pregnancies. Why? Running is a whole-body activity that can be very physically demanding — more so than you may be up for during your pregnancy. However, if you think running will be the best activity for you during your pregnancy and you haven't been running up 'til now, talk to your healthcare provider about whether running makes sense for you. Keep in mind that you may need to modify your running pace and distance as your pregnancy progresses.

Swimming and water aerobics

Except for the discomfort you may feel wearing a swimsuit while you're pregnant, you won't find a better pregnancy workout than swimming or water aerobics.

TIP

In order to swim or do water aerobics, you need access to a pool, not a lake, a river, or the ocean, which could introduce infection into your vagina. Check with your local high school or YMCA to see whether a community pool is available in your area that offers convenient times for open swimming or offers water aerobics classes, especially ones designed for pregnant women.

DANCING THROUGH THE TULIPS

Not every activity that's healthy has to be considered a sport. Dancing, for example, can be an excellent way to become or stay fit during your pregnancy and after you deliver. Just find a comfortable surface (like carpeting or an exercise mat) in a private place (unless you want the neighbors to be your audience) and then tune in to your favorite playlist.

Gardening is another way to get fit that may not seem like exercise. If you're pulling weeds, hoeing, raking, or shoveling, you're getting an excellent workout. Just be careful when lifting and bending so you don't injure your growing and changing body.

Low-impact aerobics, Zumba, yoga, and Pilates

Low-impact aerobics (which is similar to high-impact aerobics but without jumps, kicks, deep bends, step-ups, and so on) and Zumba are popular ways to work out while pregnant, and you can probably find classes in your area. Call your local community health agency, high school, gym, and dance studio to see what they offer; ask, especially, whether they offer prenatal classes so you can work out with other pregnant women. If you can't find a class in your area, you can set up your own workout area in your home and follow an aerobics DVD.

REMEMBER

If you're used to doing high-impact or step aerobics, your pregnancy continues to progress normally, you aren't experiencing any discomfort (as discussed in Book 4, Chapter 2), and your healthcare provider doesn't object, you can continue with higher-impact aerobics throughout your pregnancy. You may be able to modify your routine by reducing the height of the step and the height of your kicks.

Yoga, on the other hand, is a gentle way to work out that strengthens and sculpts your body, and many yoga studios offer special classes for pregnant women. A few yoga poses may not work well for you during pregnancy, but for the most part, yoga and pregnancy go well together. Yoga is also a terrific way to calm your mind, so if you start to feel stressed, give it a try. If you can't find a class in your area, set up a yoga studio in your own home with a mat and a good DVD.

WARNING

As always, avoid exercise environments that are hot, such as those found in hot yoga (Bikram) classes. Your body won't be able to regulate heat loss effectively, and that can be dangerous to your baby.

Pilates is another low-intensity exercise to try. As in yoga, the movements are slow and gentle, but they tend to be a little more rigorous than yoga. Pilates equipment is rather expensive, so look for a class in your area and talk to the instructor about accommodations during your pregnancy.

Cycling

Because cycling is a seated activity that actively works your heart and a variety of important muscles (legs, butt, back, and so on), it's very popular among pregnant women. You can cycle indoors (on a stationary bike) or out. Whether you can cycle outdoors depends on your experience, how well you're able to balance as your pregnancy progresses, and whether the temperature is moderate (without excessive heat or humidity). Avoid high-traffic routes to avoid being exposed to excessive amounts of exhaust. Check with your healthcare provider to get additional feedback and advice.

TIP

Cycling indoors doesn't have to be a boring experience, especially if you can ride while watching Netflix or Hulu. Riding indoors while lifting light hand weights also works your upper body, creating an incredible total-body workout.

Indoor machines

If you have access to indoor exercise machines, either at home or in a gym, you have an excellent way to exercise indoors, away from the cold, rain, and heat. Whether you choose to use a treadmill, weight machine, elliptical, or rowing machine, you're going to get an excellent workout in the comfort of your home or a gym.

Cross-training

Cross-training is combining two or more types of exercises into one workout; it can also mean working out with one type of exercise on one day and another type of exercise on another day. Cross-training is an effective way to work a variety of muscles and ease the boredom that may come from one particular type of workout.

Considering Additional Activities, Depending on Your Background

Traditional wisdom has been that pregnant women should avoid the following activities because of the risk of falling or getting hit, potentially harming the baby. Chances are, however, that if you're already doing these activities, you're pretty darned good at them and don't have much risk of falling or otherwise injuring yourself or your baby. If you're already participating in these activities, keep in mind that you need to modify your workout for comfort and safety as your pregnancy progresses, and always make sure your healthcare provider is on board with your exercise regimen. As long as you and your baby are doing well, you may be able to continue with your pre-pregnancy exercise activities throughout your pregnancy. Remember that your healthcare provider must be aware of exactly what type of exercise you plan on doing, especially if it includes one of the following activities:

>> **CrossFit or boot camps:** Do these only if you're already experienced and plan to scale back the intensity as your pregnancy progresses.

>> **Cross-country skiing:** Avoid hills and difficult trails.

REMEMBER

Contact sports (such as soccer, volleyball, basketball, and hockey): Contact sports are almost always off-limits to pregnant women because of the risk of falls and other injuries. Be sure that your healthcare provider understands exactly what sort of contact sport you have in mind.

>> **Downhill skiing:** Continue downhill skiing only if you're an expert skier.

REMEMBER

Keep in mind that you can't control those skiing around you, and falls are common. Also, most ski places are located at high elevations, and that can cause issues related to reduced oxygen availability — dangerous for mother and baby.

>> **Figure skating:** Steer clear of jumps and backward skating.

>> **Horseback riding:** Avoid any jumps or risky riding.

>> **Mountain biking:** Stay on flat, stable surfaces.

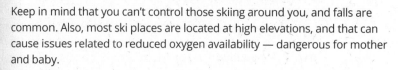

UNDERSTANDING THE LIMITATIONS OF ALTITUDE

Some pregnancy fitness experts advise you not to train at altitude during your pregnancy unless you already live in an area of high altitude. Research has confirmed that women who've been training at sea level before pregnancy struggle to train at high altitudes throughout their pregnancies. (Heck, anyone who's been training at sea level — pregnant or not — struggles to train at high altitude!)

If you live at a low elevation, talk to your healthcare provider before exercising at a high elevation to find out whether it's a good idea for you. If you're cleared to train at altitude, keep a close eye out for the following signs of altitude sickness:

- Lightheadedness

- Nausea

- Dizziness

- Extreme fatigue

- Racing pulse

If you experience any of these symptoms, stop exercising. If the symptoms continue (or even begin to occur) when you're training at a lower elevation, contact your healthcare provider.

See Book 4, Chapter 2 for more safety precautions that you need to consider. If you have any concerns about doing any activity, avoid it — pregnancy is only 40 weeks of your life, and your chosen sport can wait that long.

If you're new to exercise, don't take up any of the activities listed in this section. They all require either a high fitness level or a superb sense of balance (or both) and aren't for the uninitiated. Instead, choose from the activities listed earlier in "Discovering the Best Ways to Stay Fit While Pregnant."

REMEMBER

Before taking part in these activities, talk with your healthcare provider. Your skill level, as well as other factors, may determine whether these activities are safe. Always use common sense and err on the side of caution.

Steering Clear of Certain Activities

Two activities are absolutely, positively off-limits to you during your pregnancy, which means that no matter how much you want to continue or try them, you just can't without risking your baby's health. Plan a water vacation next year and try the two activities in this section at that time.

Scuba diving

Scuba diving — deep-sea diving with breathing gear strapped to your back — is absolutely out of the question at any time during your pregnancy. The intense underwater pressure (pressure that you don't necessarily feel because of the equipment you're using) is harmful to your baby.

TIP

If you're a die-hard scuba diver, ask your healthcare provider whether you can snorkel during your pregnancy. Snorkeling is done in shallow waters, so your baby doesn't have to withstand the deep-sea water pressure.

Waterskiing

Waterskiing presents two challenges that make it off-limits:

>> If you fall while skiing — and many people do — the force of the impact on your abdomen is incredibly high, putting your baby at great risk. In addition, during a fall, a jet of water can enter your vagina at a high force, possibly causing damage.

>> You risk infection from contaminated lake or river water entering your vagina. For this same reason, don't swim in a lake, river, or ocean while you're pregnant.

Finding Activities Even When You're on Bed Rest

If a symptom or condition keeps you from exercising — or if your doctor or midwife sees a change in your baby's health during your pregnancy — you may get a directive from your healthcare provider to spend weeks (or even months) in bed, with little time standing or walking. For an active woman, bed rest may feel like the kiss of death, and you may be concerned that all your fitness gains in the first two trimesters will be wasted during a period of bed rest. However, bed rest doesn't have to mean that you completely stop exercising your muscles and stretching. With the thumbs-up from your healthcare provider, the exercises and stretches in this section can help you maintain some of your strength and flexibility.

REMEMBER

Don't do any of the exercises listed here if you haven't first shared them with your healthcare provider and received the go-ahead. The purpose of bed rest is to help you and your baby get back to a more normal pregnancy, so unless your doctor or midwife tells you that these bed-rest exercises are acceptable, don't put yourself or your baby at risk. If you're doing these exercises while on bed rest, your healthcare provider must carefully supervise you. Stop any exercises if you experience warning signs or symptoms, and consult with your healthcare provider immediately.

TIP

If you're feeling down in the dumps and could use some support from women who can feel your pain, or if you just want more information about bed rest and high-risk pregnancies, visit www.sidelines.org.

Stretching

Gently stretching several times a day improves your circulation and minimizes muscle tightness and discomfort. Do the following stretches up to three times per day for one or two sets of 10 to 12 repetitions (reps), starting off with less than that (one or two sets of 5 to 10 reps once or twice per day) and building up:

>> Make circular motions with your ankles, wrists, neck, and shoulders (like giant shrugs) and with your arms outstretched to your sides. Be gentle. Start with small circles and gradually increase the diameter without going beyond what feels comfortable.

» Bring your chin to your chest, hold for 3 seconds, and then lift your chin back up. Also do the same stretch to each side of your neck, bending your neck so that your ear nearly meets your shoulder.

» Extend your arms in front of you, bend your elbows, and extend your arms out again.

» Lift each arm all the way up and down.

» Lying on your side or back, stretch your arms as far above your head as you can and push your heels downward (away from your head) as far as you can to get a whole-body stretch.

Strengthening muscles

Strength training is not only possible while you're on bed rest, but it's also a great way to keep from losing muscle mass during this time of inactivity. You want to do the following exercises in one or two sets of 10 to 12 reps, two or three days per week. Keep some light weights (1 to 3 pounds) or cans of vegetables or soup near your bed so that they're ready when you are. Avoid lifting anything that requires a lot of effort; you should be able to do 10 to 12 reps without straining.

Bicep curls

This exercise works the *biceps*, the muscles on the inside of your arms, above your elbows. The biceps are the muscles you notice the most when you're wearing a tank top — fit celebrities often have biceps you'd kill for.

1. **Sit up with your hands by your sides.**

2. **Hold weights in your hands with your palms facing up.**

3. **Take a breath and then exhale as you slowly lift your hands to your chest.**

   Keep your elbows as stationary as possible.

4. **Inhale as you slowly lower your hands to your starting position.**

5. **Repeat.**

Shoulder raise

This exercise strengthens the muscles around your armpits and shoulders.

1. **Straighten your arms by your sides, holding light weights.**

   You may need to rise up a bit in your bed.

2. **Take a breath, and then exhale as you slowly raise your arms to shoulder level (or as high as you can go).**

3. **Inhale as you slowly lower your arms to your starting position.**

4. **Repeat.**

   Modify this exercise by raising the weights with your arms straight out in front of you.

Chest press

The chest press works your chest and the muscles around your armpits.

1. **Lie on your back with several pillows propping you up so that you're in a semi-reclining position, and grip a light weight in each hand.**

2. **Put your hands on your chest, facing outward.**

   Make sure the backs of your hands are sitting against your chest.

3. **Take a breath, and then exhale as you slowly press the weights out and away from your chest until your arms are straight.**

4. **Inhale as you slowly lower your hands to your starting position.**

5. **Repeat.**

Triceps extension

This exercise works the *triceps*, the muscles on the outside of your arms, above the elbows.

1. **Hold a light weight in your right hand.**

2. **Lift your arm above your head so that your bent elbow is next to your ear and your hand is near the back of your shoulder.**

   If you're in a sitting position, lean forward before lifting your arm.

3. **Take a breath and exhale as you slowly straighten your elbow so that your hand is above your head and your arm is straight.**

4. **Inhale as you slowly lower your arm to your starting position.**

5. **Repeat.**

6. **Follow the same steps for the left arm.**

Abdominal press

This exercise helps you maintain abdominal strength during bed rest and also helps get your tummy back into shape after you deliver.

1. Sit or lie on your side.

2. Take a deep breath and exhale, slowly pulling your belly button toward your spine.

3. Hold the position for 3 seconds (count elephant-1, elephant-2, elephant-3).

4. Inhale and slowly release for a count of 3.

5. Repeat, working up to 10 to 12 reps.

Tummy leg slides

This exercise tightens your tummy and works your leg muscles.

1. Sit comfortably with pillows supporting your back and with your knees bent and your feet resting on the bed.

2. Take a deep breath, and as you exhale, tighten your tummy. Keep your tummy tightened as you slide one leg out (knee straight) and then slide your leg back in (knee bent).

   Use a count of 3 to slide out and then in. Exhale as you slide your leg out and inhale as you slide in.

3. Repeat.

4. Follow these same steps for the other leg.

Exercising your pelvic floor muscles

Kegel exercises (exercises for your pelvic floor muscles) are essential for pregnant women. You can perform these simple exercises while on bed rest, getting the go-ahead from your healthcare provider in advance, of course.

Doing pelvic floor exercises with control strengthens the pelvic floor muscles and, at the same time, gets you used to what it feels like to contract and relax your pelvic floor, which comes in handy at pushing time during delivery. These exercises are simple to perform after you get the hang of which muscles to contract.

One way to locate your pelvic floor muscles is to notice the muscles that contract when you stop your flow of urine. Use the urine stop-and-start test when sitting on a toilet to figure out how to locate and isolate the pelvic-floor muscle group. After you've figured out how to contract your pelvic floor muscles, use the following exercise to strengthen them.

To do the pelvic floor exercise:

1. **Slowly contract your pelvic floor muscles throughout a count of 5.**

2. **Hold for 5 seconds and then release for a count of 5.**

As you do Kegel exercises, keep these suggestions in mind:

» Start with 10 to 20 slow repetitions (reps), twice a day, and build up to 25 or more reps, twice a day. If your pelvic floor muscles fatigue quickly, do fewer reps each time, but do the exercises more than twice a day.

» Remember that no one can tell you're doing these exercises, so you can do them anywhere. In fact, try to use certain activities (for example, driving to work, brushing your teeth, or taking a shower) as your cue to do your exercises.

» Contract your pelvic floor muscles each time you lift, laugh, sneeze, or cough to provide support.

Don't fatigue your muscles to the point of being unable to perform any more pelvic floor contractions. If you're unable to hold for 5 seconds, alternate slow contractions and holds with the *quick-contraction technique:* Contract your pelvic floor muscles by quickly squeezing and releasing, repeating for 20 or more reps. Keep in mind, however, that the longer you hold each contraction, the more effectively you build pelvic floor strength, so your ultimate goal is to build your reps and contraction hold times from 5 seconds to 10 seconds or more.

The muscles of the pelvic floor provide support for the pelvic organs. Keeping these muscles strong helps prevent conditions such as incontinence and prolapsed organs.

Chapter 4

Getting Up and Moving

Never exercised before? No problem! Just because you may have hated gym class and didn't play sports when you were in school doesn't mean you're doomed to be fitness-challenged during your pregnancy. This chapter helps you find a fitness routine that fits your interests, lifestyle, and goals.

If you've been an athlete — competitive or not — you probably find yourself in a quandary: Can you maintain your current level of fitness and activity while simultaneously doing everything in your power to protect your growing baby? The good news for you is that although your workouts need to change somewhat during your pregnancy (information you'll find in this chapter), you can continue to be active and maintain much of your fitness. And after you deliver a healthy baby, you can gradually ease back into your old routine and regain any lost fitness in just a few months — head to Book 4, Chapter 5 for that info.

For the Novice Exerciser

Your options for working out are nearly endless, which means that you can find fun ways to work out. The key is to choose an activity — or activities (who says you have to choose only one?) — that suits your personality and gives you a great workout.

Homing in on your favorite activities

Liking the activity you're doing helps you stick to a workout routine. The problem is, if you've never exercised, you may not know what activities you do and don't enjoy. Here are some questions and advice that can help you narrow down your list of potential workout activities:

>> **Do you like being outdoors?** If so, walking is your best bet, and fitness walking is a great workout. If you aren't ready to walk briskly for 15 minutes, try a combination fitness walk/leisurely walk, in which you walk powerfully until you feel fatigued and then begin walking slowly until you're ready to speed up again. Just be sure to avoid exercising outdoors when heat and humidity increase the possibility of heat exhaustion or heat stroke.

>> **Do you dislike being outside in extreme weather?** Swimming, Zumba, yoga, indoor cycling, and any number of indoor exercises (stair-stepping, elliptical training, or rowing on indoor fitness machines) keep you out of the cold. If you opt for stair-stepping, be sure you're using a step machine (such as a StairMaster) rather than participating in a high-intensity step-aerobics or CrossFit class, which may be too intense during pregnancy if you've never exercised before.

>> **Did you like riding a bike as a kid?** Chances are you'll still like cycling now. Choose low-traffic areas that don't make you breathe exhaust, which can be bad for you and your baby. Remember, though, that pregnancy plays with your balance. If you're not an adept cyclist, stick to indoor cycling on a stationary or recumbent bike.

>> **Did you like swimming as a child?** People who love water tend to always love it, so take up swimming or water aerobics. Swimming, considered one of the safest activities in which you can participate, is also a whole-body workout that tones your arms and legs.

>> **Do you want to work out with others or alone?** If you want to be around people, consider joining a gym or enrolling in a prenatal yoga class, low-impact aerobics class, or water-aerobics class. If you prefer to work out alone, you can do nearly any activity; just be sure to keep your phone with you at all times.

>> **Are you looking for an activity that will calm you?** Yoga, swimming, and walking are activities that give you quiet time to meditate. Yoga and Pilates are excellent ways to move and breathe slowly and gently while still strengthening muscles, so they're recommended during pregnancy. Some yoga and Pilates routines, however, don't elevate your heart rate enough to strengthen the heart muscle, improve your breathing, and burn calories. Consider alternating yoga or Pilates one day with another activity the next.

WARNING

Remember that pregnant women should avoid hot exercise environments, so hot yoga (Bikram) or any classroom that isn't cool and well-ventilated is not recommended.

REMEMBER

To get the benefit of exercise, you want to keep moving at a brisk pace for a minimum of 15 minutes, which means that activities that don't elevate your heart rate, that allow for plenty of rest, and that offer options to ride or sit instead of walk aren't going to get you very fit. A *workout* during pregnancy is any activity that takes your Rating of Perceived Exertion (RPE) to 12 to 14, which is considered "moderate" to "somewhat hard." (See Book 4, Chapter 2 for the lowdown.)

You've heard it before: Check with your healthcare provider before beginning any exercise activity. Also check out Book 4, Chapter 2 for more safety precautions.

Exercise basics: Warming up, cooling down, stretching, and hydrating

Every workout routine — no matter what activity you decide to pursue — must include four important elements: warming up, cooling down, stretching, and *hydrating* yourself (drinking fluids). This section gives you a brief overview of these exercise basics.

>> **Warming up:** Every time you exercise, you want to ease into your workout, starting off gradually and giving your body time to warm up. This means that you ease into your workout, starting out more slowly than you intend to go during the bulk of your workout. The amount of time you take to warm up depends on how fast your body adjusts to physical activity, but for most people, five or ten minutes is plenty.

REMEMBER

Many people like to stretch *before* exercising, but this introduces the possibility of getting injured. Stretching can be as challenging to your body as the rest of your workout routine, so if you stretch *cold* muscles (muscles that have been resting), you're essentially working out without a warm-up. Instead of trying to warm up with a stretch, do your stretches after you finish your workout.

» **Cooling down as you finish:** As you near the end of your workout routine, gradually downshift to your warm-up pace again. This helps ease your body from the intensity of your workout and avoids stopping suddenly, which can cause muscles to tear.

Never end your workout with a big, ferocious finish and then stop — your muscles just can't downshift quickly enough, and a quick stop can also make you feel lightheaded or dizzy.

If you work out for 15 minutes, the majority of your workout is spent warming up and cooling down. As you increase the length of each workout, keep your warm-up and cool-down periods the same, thus increasing the amount of time that you maintain your workout pace.

» **Stretching afterward:** Right after you finish your workout — and before you sit down, take a shower, or relax in any other way — you need to stretch. Stretching today keeps you from getting sore tomorrow.

» **Drinking plenty of fluids:** After you stretch, take time to hydrate your body. Drink at least 16 ounces (2 cups) and up to 32 ounces (4 cups) of fluids within 30 minutes of completing your workout, and drink a total of 64 ounces (8 cups) throughout the day.

DEBUNKING "NO PAIN, NO GAIN"

The idea that you can't make fitness gains without feeling pain is still popular, but it's a bunch of malarkey. To be at your fittest, you need to exercise regularly and with effort, but you shouldn't feel pain with any regularity.

Of course, during the first week to ten days that you work out — and anytime you start exercising again after taking time off — you will feel soreness. Soreness is different from pain.

Pain comes from overdoing your activity — that is, exercising for too long or with too much vigor before you're ready to do so. *Soreness,* on the other hand, comes from working muscles you haven't worked before (or haven't worked for a long time), so chances are good (like, 100 percent) that you'll experience soreness.

Soreness makes every muscle you use during exercise feel like a giant bruise, and it feels awful for the first day or two after you begin exercising. But the main difference between soreness and pain is that soreness begins to fade after four to seven days (although it may not disappear completely for a few weeks), and as long as you continue exercising regularly, it won't come back.

Avoiding injuries

In general, injuries are caused by the following situations, so avoid them in your own training:

» **Doing too much, too soon:** Getting fit takes time, and you need to build up the length and intensity of your workouts very, very gradually. From week to week, never increase the average duration of your workouts more than 5 minutes: The first week, your average may be 15 minutes per workout; the second week, the average should be no more than 20 minutes; the third week, 25 minutes; and so on. And increasing even less than that is perfectly acceptable.

» **Not stretching after a workout:** Without stretching, your muscles, ligaments, and tendons tighten up, becoming more prone to tears and sprains.

» **Wearing worn-out shoes:** Replace your athletic shoes about every six months, even if they don't look worn out. If you don't replace your shoes twice per year (or more often), you risk joint pain in your knees, ankles, and hips; shin pain; foot pain and/or bruises; and so on.

» **Working out on hard surfaces:** Concrete is the hardest surface on which you can exercise, and all that pounding can add up to the wear and tear on your back, joints, and muscles and lead to an injury. Instead, work out on asphalt (blacktop) roads or bike trails (asphalt is softer than concrete), dirt roads or trails (as long as the footing is even enough not to throw you off balance), an exercise mat or pad placed over a hard surface, or even a rug or carpet in your living room.

» **Not getting enough sleep:** Your body needs eight hours of sleep to recover from the stress of being pregnant each day, plus a little more to account for exercise.

Setting up your first fitness routine

To set up an effective fitness routine, you need to establish a convenient time to work out, set up a workout plan that includes some variation (so you don't get bored), keep track of your workouts, and stay motivated. The following sections get you started.

TIP

Developing a fitness routine isn't easy, mainly because you've never had to include exercise in your day-to-day routine before. You can pick up a new habit, though, by doing an activity for just 21 days. This means that if you exercise today and stick to it for the next 21 days, in only three weeks, exercise will be a daily part of your life.

Carving time out of your day

To allow time to work out and stretch, allot 30 to 60 minutes each day that you exercise. Most women work out at one of three times throughout the day: morning (before work or other commitments), midday (lunchtime), and late afternoon or early evening (after work but more than three hours before bedtime).

REMEMBER

Any of these times can work, depending on your schedule and your preferences. A fourth option — exercising a few hours after dinner — isn't a good idea, because you increase your heart rate too close to your bedtime. Exercising less than two or three hours before your bedtime can interrupt your sleep and lead to increased fatigue the next day. You can also get your 30 to 60 minutes in multiple, shorter sessions throughout the day. Research shows that this provides benefits equivalent to one session of the same cumulative length.

Creating a workout plan

Although a one-size-fits-all workout plan doesn't exist, Tables 4-1 through 4-3 give you an idea of what a beginner's exercise routine may look like. Modify these tables to match your own goals and the number of weeks you're into your pregnancy, and always determine whether and how much you'll work out by how you feel and what your baby is telling you.

These tables list the number of minutes to work out. If your form of exercise involves stopping and starting (such as with weightlifting or with exercise balls and resistance bands), don't count the minutes in between each type of exercise in your total minutes. And keep in mind that the minutes in these tables include time to warm up and cool down. Also, the term *CT* in these tables means "cross-train" — that is, switching from your normal activity to a very different one.

TABLE 4-1   **Four-Days-Per-Week Workout Plan**

Week	Monday	Tuesday	Wednesday	Thursday	Friday	Saturday	Sunday
1 (60 min)	15	Off	15	Off	15	Off	15
2 (66 min)	15CT	Off	18	Off	18	Off	15
3 (70 min)	15CT	Off	20	Off	15	Off	20
4 (75 min)	15CT	Off	20	Off	20	Off	20CT
5 (80 min)	15	Off	25	Off	15CT	Off	25
6 (85 min)	20CT	Off	20	Off	25	Off	20

TABLE 4-2   Five-Days-Per-Week Workout Plan

Week	Monday	Tuesday	Wednesday	Thursday	Friday	Saturday	Sunday
1 (75 min)	15	Off	15	15CT	Off	15	15CT
2 (81 min)	15	Off	18	15CT	Off	18	15CT
3 (88 min)	20	Off	20	15CT	Off	18	15CT
4 (96 min)	20	Off	23	15CT	Off	18	20CT
5 (105 min)	25	Off	25	15CT	Off	20	20CT
6 (115 min)	25	Off	30	20CT	Off	20	20CT

TABLE 4-3   Six-Days-Per-Week Workout Plan

Week	Monday	Tuesday	Wednesday	Thursday	Friday	Saturday	Sunday
1 (90 min)	15	15CT	Off	15	15CT	15	15CT
2 (96 min)	18	15CT	Off	18	15CT	15	15CT
3 (103 min)	20	15CT	Off	20	15CT	18	15CT
4 (111 min)	20	18CT	Off	20	15CT	20	18CT
5 (120 min)	20	20CT	Off	25	15CT	20	20CT
6 (130 min)	25	20CT	Off	25	18CT	22	20CT

REMEMBER

Wondering why each week increases? Because even though 15 to 20 minutes of activity is enough to raise your heart rate and expend calories, more is better, up to a point. Research varies, but for nonpregnant women, working out between 30 and 60 minutes per day, four to seven days per week, is generally considered the ticket to excellent overall health and fitness. During your pregnancy, however, especially if you've never exercised before, 20 to 30 minutes per day, four to six days per week, is terrific; as you become more fit, try to continue to increase your duration and frequency to six to seven days for 40 minutes or more of exercise.

Keeping track of your workouts

To track your workouts, download an app or use a paper calendar (remember those?) that has spaces for each day. Make note of what workout you did and for how long. You may also want to note how you felt ("tired," "sore," "full of energy," and so on) and what may have contributed to that feeling ("got a great night of sleep," "bad morning sickness," and so on). This information can help you monitor your progress. And whenever you feel a workout slump coming on, you can look back at your fitness progress for a strong dose of motivation.

For Fitness Buffs and Competitive Athletes

If you love to exercise or are a fierce competitor, you may think that nothing will change during the next 40 weeks: You'll just keep exercising the way you have been, deliver your baby, and not skip a beat.

It's a fine dream, but a dream nonetheless. *A lot* is going to change over the next nine months:

>> Morning sickness (or any-time-of-day sickness) may interrupt your usual workout schedule.

>> You'll be far more fatigued than you've ever been, so a seven-days-per-week workout schedule may no longer be possible.

>> Your balance will be off, making you susceptible to falls and injuries and putting some forms of outdoor exercise off-limits.

>> Your weight gain (which is absolutely necessary to deliver a healthy baby) makes getting around more difficult than usual.

>> The increasing size of your breasts and abdomen and the tenderness of your breasts may keep you from being physically capable of doing your pre-pregnancy exercises.

>> You may experience a host of minor illnesses or other complaints that make you less able to start or finish a workout. These problems run the gamut, including (in alphabetical order) backaches, breathlessness, gassiness, headaches, heartburn, hemorrhoids, rashes, swelling and fluid retention, and urinary incontinence and increased urination. And that's just in the first trimester!

>> Your body isn't going to recover nearly as fast as it has been able to, so you'll be able to do fewer hard workouts and will need more easy or rest days between harder efforts.

None of this means, however, that you can't continue to be highly active. It just means you need to make a few modifications.

TIP

If you're an elite athlete and hope to continue training at a high level during your pregnancy, consider being monitored by a physician or taking part in a supervised prenatal training program to minimize the risk of danger to you and your baby.

Modifying your workouts to accommodate your pregnancy

Whether you need to modify your workouts depends on how you and your baby are faring during your pregnancy:

>> Is the baby growing normally?

>> Are you gaining weight normally?

>> Do you feel good?

If you can answer "yes" to the preceding questions and your healthcare provider doesn't have any objections to your continuing your pre–pregnancy workouts, you don't need to modify your routine. If any of your answers change, however, that's when you need to modify.

REMEMBER

If all the physical stresses placed on your body during pregnancy sound terribly unfair, given how fit your body was before you became pregnant, remember that, in just nine short months, you'll have a healthy baby as your reward. Until then, give yourself time to come to terms with the fact that your workouts will indeed change.

The following tells you how you may decide to modify your current routine:

>> **Intensity:** In order to keep yourself healthy, you'll likely need to decrease the intensity of your workouts. If you can measure your workout intensity, expect your pace to slow down as you progress through your pregnancy. If you participate in a sport in which you can't measure intensity directly, pay careful attention to how your body feels during and after each workout. If you find yourself increasingly fatigued, are sore in muscles that have been long developed, or can't seem to work out as long as you used to, reduce the intensity of your workouts.

>> **Duration:** If you want to continue the duration of each workout and you feel great, do so. If you aren't feeling as good as you and your healthcare provider would like, consider reducing the duration. If, for example, you want to continue running 7-minute miles, you may find that you're comfortable running for 30 or 40 minutes per workout instead of 60.

If you don't want to reduce the duration, you can reduce the intensity. For example, you may be able to run 60 minutes at 9-minute miles (reducing the intensity) and keep up the same duration (the 60 minutes of exercise). You can also alternate higher-intensity, lower-duration days with lower-intensity, higher-duration days.

>> **Frequency:** Even elite athletes tend to have trouble working out seven days per week while pregnant.

REMEMBER

If staying in good shape isn't enough for you — that is, if you're planning to stay in the finely tuned, ready-for-competition shape that you were in before you became pregnant — you may need to rethink your ambitions. Trying to stay in top shape during the 40 weeks of pregnancy may mean making your workout routine a higher priority than your baby's health, a concept that may have tragic consequences. Your goal during pregnancy should be to avoid losing so much ground that you can't quickly get yourself back into shape after you deliver your healthy baby. But you're not going to run a marathon or play in a tournament a week after labor — you may, however, be able to perform at a high level four to six months after childbirth.

>> **Competition:** The most notable change in exercise for a pregnant athlete is that your healthcare provider will likely advise you to stop competing by the second trimester (weeks 15 to 27). Although your doctor or midwife may recommend that you stop competing earlier or later than that, the fact remains that pregnancy will very likely set limits on your competition for at least a few months. Use common sense about this, thinking about what — if any — competitive gains you'll make by continuing your racing schedule; listen carefully to your healthcare provider's advice.

TIP

Many athletes have made successful returns to competition after delivering healthy babies, and some even find that time off from competition renews their interest in it and makes them more successful.

Finding alternate activities

If, after you reduce the intensity, duration, and/or frequency of your workouts, your body still isn't managing your exercise routine well and you're feeling fatigued or you and your baby aren't as healthy as you should be, talk to your healthcare provider about whether you can try a less-intense activity than the primary activity you've been doing. Table 4-4 gives you some ideas, but your healthcare provider may have others.

TIP

To quickly resume your training regimen after you deliver your baby, you want to work similar muscles with your alternate activity as you do with your primary activity. For example, cycling, speed-skating, and cross-country skiing all use similar muscle groups, but they use very different muscles from running, which is similar to walking and aerobics. So if you're a speed-skater looking for an alternate activity, you want to choose cycling over walking.

TABLE 4-4   **Alternate Activities**

If You Find That You Can No Longer . . .	Try . . .
Do CrossFit or boot camp	Reducing the intensity of your workouts, using lighter weights, and substituting out some of your higher-impact movements
Weight train with heavy weights, including doing squats, bench presses, and incline bench presses	Lifting lighter weights with more reps; avoid deep-knee bends and pushing weights over your head when lying on your back or in an inclined position
Mountain bike	Indoor cycling on a stationary bike
Perform gymnastics moves	Walking, doing low-impact aerobics, using resistance bands, and/or weightlifting
Play soccer, basketball, or hockey	Weightlifting and the following: walking, using a stair-stepping machine, or using an elliptical trainer
Row	Weightlifting, swimming, and walking
Run or hike	Walking or doing low-impact aerobics
Ski (downhill or outdoor cross-country) or skate	Indoor cycling or using a cross-country ski machine

REMEMBER
Even if you seem to be physically handling your workouts and don't want to reduce their intensity, duration, or frequency or change activities altogether, your healthcare provider may still ask you to change sports until after you deliver. This is especially true if you participate in very demanding activities like rowing and running, ball sports or contact sports that can result in blunt trauma to your baby (but may be considered okay), or activities that can result in a hard, serious fall that can hurt your baby. See Book 4, Chapter 2 for additional information on sports that you may be asked to give up as your pregnancy progresses.

Easing back into your routine after delivery

As a fitness buff or competitive athlete, you may long for the day when you feel fit again, attack your workouts with vigor, and maybe even compete in your sport. Returning to your old routine will happen, but it takes time and patience. This section gives you a few tips.

TIP
Take as much time as you need to get back to your old routine. Because you've likely reduced the intensity, duration, or frequency of your workouts, you'll need some time to build back up again. Most women need to take a minimum of two weeks off from exercise after the birth of a baby. This time allows you to recover from the stress of labor and delivery and allows your body to heal. In order to

determine whether you're ready to get back into your exercise routine, ask yourself the following questions:

>> Have you recovered from labor and delivery, and do you feel ready to start exercising again?

>> Is your baby feeding well, and is she on a feeding schedule that allows for a long enough break for you to exercise?

>> Has your healthcare provider given you the go-ahead to start exercising?

>> If you had a cesarean section or episiotomy, is your incision healed, and are you able to move around comfortably and without pain?

If you feel ready to get started, start back slowly — and reduce or discontinue exercise if you experience any increase in vaginal bleeding or have pain or discomfort.

Although every woman and every pregnancy is unique, consider the following tips for a safe return to your old fitness routine:

>> **Start your first post-delivery workouts as though you've never worked out before.** See the earlier section "For the Novice Exerciser" for some beginner's guides to working out, and follow whichever one allows you to work out without feeling any pain or significant discomfort. You may experience some muscle soreness and fatigue, but you shouldn't feel any sharp pains.

>> **Increase your weekly minutes no more than 10 percent per week for the first couple of months, no matter how antsy you feel about getting back into great shape.** This may mean that your return to your pre-pregnancy fitness level takes from four to six months. As you become stronger, you can start to increase your duration and intensity beyond 10 percent, but always use your body's response as a guide.

REMEMBER

If you end up having a cesarean delivery, returning to your old exercise routine may take a couple of months longer than it would if you'd delivered vaginally. This timeline doesn't hold for all women, given that people heal at different rates, but it's a general timeline to consider if you're trying to set goals for the year after you deliver.

>> **Be cautious when stretching or doing any quick, stop-and-start movements for three to five months after delivery.** The hormone relaxin has made your ligaments and joints much less stable than they were before you were pregnant, so use care and avoid quick and jerky movements.

>> **Start with one moderately high-intensity workout every one or two weeks and gradually increase to a maximum of two high-intensity days per week.** The demands of breastfeeding and new motherhood are hard

enough on your body to consider doing more than two hard workouts per week at this stage.

» **Take one or two easy days (of lower intensity) after each hard workout.** Follow a hard–easy–medium–easy–hard–easy or hard–easy–easy–hard–easy–easy workout schedule.

» **If you're nursing, keep up your caloric intake so you produce enough milk.** You may need as many as 500 more calories per day than you did before you became pregnant and started nursing. Make sure you're eating enough calories for the amount of exercise you're doing and hydrate well.

» **Don't try to lose weight too quickly, especially if you're breastfeeding.** By eating right and gradually increasing the intensity, duration, and frequency of your workouts, you'll naturally lose the weight in a relatively short time frame without dieting.

WARNING

Continue to monitor your urine color, body weight, temperature, and overall physical well-being as your body returns to its pre-pregnancy state. Exercise only after you're released to do so by your healthcare provider, and call him or her if your body isn't adjusting well to working out.

Chapter 5

Recovering from the Labor Marathon and Getting Up and at 'Em

Wheeew! You made it through that marathon called labor and delivery (see Book 2, Chapters 4 and 5), and you now hold in your arms a beautiful baby. Thanks to all the stretching and exercising you did throughout your pregnancy, your body was in good shape for this event, and you can expect it to heal more quickly than if you hadn't stayed fit and active. However, right after you deliver your baby, you need to allow some time for your body to recover.

This chapter focuses on the first days and weeks after you deliver your baby, a time when you need to be especially gentle with yourself, and shows you how to keep from injuring yourself as you lift and carry your baby, who will gain weight rapidly in the coming weeks.

All that bending, lifting, and carrying is definitely exercise, but sometime in the days and weeks after you deliver and as you begin to develop a daily routine with your new bundle of joy, you may begin to miss your old workout routine. You may not miss the discomfort and the sweat, but certainly you'll miss the extra energy and natural high that come from exercising and the wonderful sense of accomplishment that you get when you complete a workout. The question is, when should you return to physical activity — and at what level? And if you take several weeks off, how do you start up again? This chapter dishes the dirt.

Resting Up First

The first few days after you deliver your baby is not the time to be thinking about your workout routine. After all, you've just been through the mother of all workouts — labor and delivery — and now's the time to rest. But you may have trouble getting the rest you need while meeting your baby's many needs during this time. Here are some tips for getting rest with a new baby in the house:

>> **Always nap when your baby naps.** For the first few weeks of your baby's life, don't try to use your baby's nap times to catch up on housework, check email, exercise, or do anything else except sleep.

>> **Take as much time away from work as you can afford.** Even if you're the very definition of a workaholic and can't imagine being away from your work for more than a few hours, you have to let it go for a few weeks, for your own health and the health of your baby. You desperately need sleep right now, and trying to sneak in a few hours of work each day takes away potential nap times.

>> **Get someone to help you with housework.** Don't let housework interfere with your rest time — whether your partner does your share of the chores, you enlist a family member or friend to help with laundry and cleaning, or you hire outside help, get as much help as you need so you can take care of yourself and your baby.

>> **Arrange to do an activity you fully enjoy at least once or twice per week.** Whether you quietly read a book, binge-watch Netflix for a few hours, take a bubble bath, go shopping, or do whatever else interests you, spend some time pampering yourself. Take advantage of the time your partner is bonding with your baby, take up friends and family on offers to babysit, or hire a babysitter who's experienced with infants for a few hours. Spending time by yourself doing activities you love makes you better able to relax and actively participate in your child's care.

>> **Limit visits from well-meaning friends and family.** Establish set hours during which friends and family can visit, times when you and your baby are awake.

>> **Continue taking your prenatal vitamins, eat well, and drink plenty of fluids.** If you aren't getting the proper nutrients and drinking enough fluids, you may become malnourished and/or dehydrated — both add to fatigue. Research shows that including plenty of protein (in lean meats, lean dairy products, beans, nuts, and so on) and vitamin C (most notably in citrus fruits and many green vegetables) in your diet helps your body recover quickly. (Book 3, Chapter 1 offers some post-pregnancy nutrition advice.) Also drink eight to ten glasses of water and other fluids every day.

>> **Take care when getting out of bed or getting up from lying down, especially if you had a cesarean delivery.** Rising straight up from lying on your back puts tremendous stress on your low back and abdomen, especially when your muscles are weak from the physical changes of pregnancy. Getting up that way also stresses any incisions and stitches you may have. A better way to get off your back and onto your feet is to roll over to one side and push yourself up slowly with your arms into a sitting position; then drop your legs down in front of you and use your arms to help press up your body as you stand.

Caring for Baby without Stressing Your Body

Just as you have to master proper lifting technique when you go to work for UPS or FedEx and carry those heavy boxes around, as a new mother, you need to be trained in your new job of hoisting and carrying your baby. The fact is, new mothers who are instructed in proper lifting techniques suffer fewer back injuries and other aches and pains, so this section gives you the lowdown on how to stand properly when lifting any object (not just your baby), how to lift your baby from various positions, and how to carry her without straining yourself.

Standing up straight

Before lifting and carrying your baby, practice good posture. When you're standing correctly, your lower back isn't curved in, and your shoulders aren't hunched. Instead, your shoulders are back, your pelvis is tucked under your hips, and your chest is pressed slightly forward.

When you think of good posture, envision your body functioning in a way that allows for balanced, relaxed movement. When your body is balanced with all parts working together normally, your muscles don't have to work overtime to maintain balance. The most relaxed way to stand is with

>> Your eyes level and focused forward

>> Your shoulders relaxed and slightly rotated down and back

>> Your pelvis in a neutral position and not tilted forward or back, and your weight balanced over the center of your foot (to find the neutral position of your pelvis, tilt it forward and back several times until you find a comfortable spot in the middle)

TIP

If you drew a line from your head to your feet while standing with proper posture, the line would run straight down, in between your ears, shoulders, hips, knees, and ankles. When your posture is poor, your neck may lean forward, you may hunch your shoulders and hump your upper back, and your low back may sway. All these awkward positions can lead to headaches, neck and back stiffness and pain, and weakness and discomfort in your hands and legs.

Lifting your baby from the floor or a stroller (and putting her down)

To pick your baby up off the floor or out of a stroller, do the following:

1. **Kneel down with one knee on the floor and the other foot planted flat on the floor.**

   You can also squat, keeping both feet flat and both knees deeply bent.

2. **Move in as close as possible to your baby (or to the stroller) so you don't have to reach out very far, as shown in Figure 5-1.**

3. **Bring your baby close to your body *before* you lift.**

4. **Breathe in, and then exhale, contracting your tummy. Take another breath and exhale as you lift.**

   This breath supports your low back.

5. **Lift your baby, holding her tight and using your leg muscles, not your back, to gradually rise to a standing position, as shown in Figure 5-2.**

TIP

To lift a baby from a baby carrier, whether on the floor or on a car seat, follow the same steps as those just outlined: Kneel or squat in front of the carrier, position the handle up and out of your way, and slide your baby out. Keep your baby straight while you pull her toward you to release her from the carrier. Reverse these steps to put your baby into a carrier.

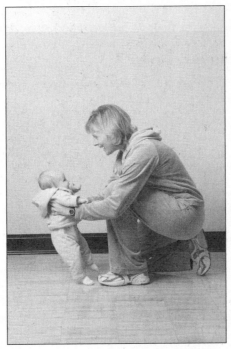

FIGURE 5-1:
Bending down
to pick up
your baby.

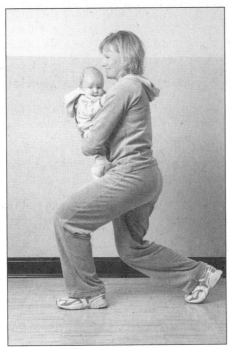

FIGURE 5-2:
Gradually rising
to a standing
position.

Recovering from the
Labor Marathon and
Getting Up and at 'Em

To put your baby down (on the floor or into a stroller), reverse the process:

1. **Hold your baby close to your body.**

2. **Squat or kneel (see the preceding list for proper form), and then set your baby on the floor or into the stroller.**

   Avoid hunching your back and/or lifting or setting your baby down while bending from your hips — doing so puts too much stress on your low back. Do all your lifting and lowering with your legs, keeping your back fairly straight and your abdominal muscles contracted.

Lifting your baby from a changing table or crib

To lift your baby from a changing table or crib, do the following:

1. **Stand as close as possible to the edge of the changing table or side of the crib, with one foot forward and one foot back. Slightly bend both of your knees.**

   Be sure that the table or crib is at the proper height for you. The top of the table should be at about waist height. If the crib has a drop-down side, be sure to drop it down before putting your baby in the crib or getting him out.

TIP

   If you're a shorter woman and have trouble reaching into the crib, don't buy a crib that doesn't have drop-down sides. Test drive a few models before you buy by reaching down into them in the showroom.

2. **Slide your baby toward you by pulling his bottom blanket until he is at the edge of the crib.**

3. **Prepare to lift your baby by reaching one hand around and under his back and the other hand around and under his neck.**

4. **Sit your baby up and slide him toward you so that he's as close to you as possible, as shown in Figure 5-3a.**

5. **Before you lift, breathe in, tightening your lower abs, and exhale as you lift.**

   This abdominal contraction supports your low back — use it anytime you're lifting.

6. **Lift your baby up into your arms, shifting your weight to your back leg and keeping your back straight as you lift. Refer to Figure 5-3b.**

   Never twist and lift your baby or twist and set him down — doing so puts tremendous stress on your low back.

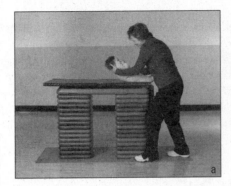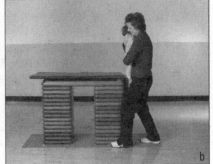

FIGURE 5-3:
Lifting your baby from a changing table.

Photograph by John Urban

REMEMBER

To set your baby down into a crib, reverse this process, setting your baby down into the crib as close to the side as possible, without twisting your back as you set him down and while bending your knees slightly.

EXERCISE AND BREAST MILK PRODUCTION

Studies show that exercise doesn't interfere with your ability to produce breast milk. The *La Leche League* is an organization of women who help other new mothers successfully breastfeed. The league is famous for its breastfeeding guidelines, which help you monitor whether your baby is getting enough breast milk. The following is a sampling of the League's guidelines that let you know you're breastfeeding successfully:

- Your baby nurses 8 to 12 times per day, whenever she is hungry and until she is satisfied.

- Beginning her fourth day, your baby wets five to eight diapers per day and has two to five bowel movements per day.

- Beginning her fourth day, your baby gains 4 to 7 ounces of weight per week.

- You can hear your baby swallowing as she breastfeeds.

- Your baby is growing normally.

If your baby doesn't feed this often, wet this number of diapers, gain this amount of weight, or appear to be growing normally, contact your healthcare provider immediately. And visit the league's site at `www.lalecheleague.org` for breastfeeding information and local contacts in your area. Book 5 covers breastfeeding in detail.

When lifting your baby from a crib that doesn't have a collapsible side (which means that you have to reach down in to lift your baby), always first slide the baby near the side of the crib closest to you. (To slide your baby closer to you, always place him on a blanket, which you can slide toward you when you're lifting him up.) Prepare to lift him by placing your hands under his back and neck. Then, keeping your back straight and bending your knees, breathe in, tighten your lower abs, and exhale as you hold and lift your baby, letting your legs do as much of the lifting work as possible.

Carrying your baby

As you probably already know, you're going to be carrying your baby a lot, and you're not always going to want or be able to carry her in the same way. Following are a few ways to carry your baby safely and comfortably.

The football carry

Carrying your baby like a football (see Figure 5-4), in the crook of your arm and resting on your forearm and wrist, is convenient when she's still a newborn. You may feel pressure on your wrists, however, so alternate arms frequently. As she grows, however, this method becomes too difficult.

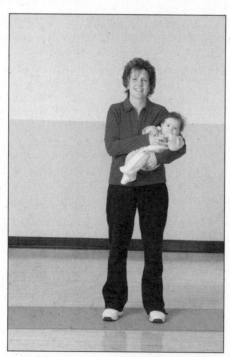

FIGURE 5-4: The football carry.

Photograph by John Urban

The hip carry

When you're preparing a meal, doing laundry, talking on the phone, or negotiating any other task that takes up one hand, use the hip carry, shown in Figure 5-5. Without thrusting out your hip, simply straddle your baby over one hipbone, alternating hips from time to time.

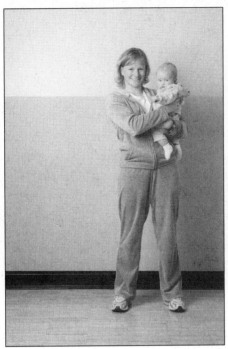

FIGURE 5-5:
The hip carry.

Photograph by John Urban

The front carry

When you need to carry your baby for long periods and don't need your hands for any other activity, use the front carry (see Figure 5-6). Keep your baby tight to your body as you walk. As your baby becomes too heavy for you to lift even in a front carry, put her in a stroller or other carrying device. Try to keep your shoulder blades pulled back to avoid slouching.

The hands-free carry

If you use a *baby backpack* (in which your baby sits in a sling attached to your back), a *baby front pack* (same idea, but your baby sits on your front side), or a *baby sling* (a device that goes over one shoulder and under the opposite armpit so that your baby can lie down in front of you), be sure to set your baby in the pack or sling on a table, and then strap the pack or sling to your body. If the back or sling has a waist strap, use it to keep some of the weight off your back. Keep the pack securely fastened to your body to avoid having the weight pull away from you and cause added muscle strain.

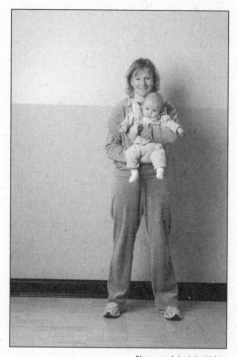

Photograph by John Urban

FIGURE 5-6:
The front carry.

TIP

If you're having a lot of discomfort from a backpack or front pack, head back to the store where you purchased it and have them help you fit it properly to your body.

Pushing your baby in a stroller

When taking your baby with you on a walk, keep a straight back as you push and use your legs and buttock muscles to do the work. Make sure that the handle height of the stroller fits you well so you don't have to bend forward or raise your hands into an uncomfortable position to push. If the handgrips are too hard, purchase some foam and tape it securely to the grips to add cushioning.

TIP

If you plan to fitness walk or run with your baby in a stroller, invest in a *running stroller*, which is made specifically for those activities. The wheels on a running stroller move easily through rough terrain, and the stroller is easy to propel. Running strollers cost more than standard strollers, but you won't regret your decision to buy one. Talk with other moms who walk or run with a stroller to find out which brands work well and hold up to consistent use.

Deciding When to Exercise and What Activities to Do

You'll likely have one of these reactions to exercise after delivering a baby:

>> **You see exercise as an utter impossibility.** If you fall into this category, start with stretches and keep in mind that a ten-minute walk is far better than no walk at all; any exercise tends to ease constipation and hemorrhoids (which many moms are all-too-familiar with right after delivery).

   Gradually build up your walks or other exercises to your pre-delivery routine, following the guidelines in Book 4, Chapter 4, and even consider exercising more than you did when you were pregnant. You'll speed weight loss and quickly get your body back to its pre-pregnancy shape.

>> **You can't wait to get back to exercising so you can lose your pregnancy weight gain.** If this describes you, good for you! Remember, though, that you do need time to heal from labor and delivery, so don't rush resuming your exercise routine. If, shortly after delivery, you work out too intensely or for too long, you run a high risk of injuring yourself, which means you'll have to go even longer without exercise. Instead, take several weeks or months to build back up to your pre-delivery exercise routine, and then continue to increase your duration and frequency as much as your schedule allows.

REMEMBER

To get back to your exercise routine after delivering your baby, make sure you fit all the following guidelines:

>> Your healthcare provider has given you the go-ahead to get started.

>> Any incisions or tears have healed.

>> You feel ready to get back to exercise.

>> Your postpartum recovery is progressing normally, and you're healthy.

>> You feel good after exercise, you don't experience any increase in vaginal bleeding, and you don't feel any other physical discomfort.

REMEMBER

If you've had a cesarean delivery, don't forget that it's major surgery. You must give yourself time to recover. This means avoiding excess exertion (including going up and down stairs and lifting your baby from the floor or over your head), limiting your activities (you'll need to wait at least until your six-week checkup before working out again), and taking good care of your incision. Keep an eye on the wound and call your healthcare provider if the area becomes increasingly red, feels warm, or starts to drain fluid and also if you run a fever.

Returning to Your Pre-Pregnancy Weight and Strengthening Your Abs

The good news about your post-pregnancy weight is that you'll lose about 12 pounds shortly after delivering your baby. However, you gained more than 12 pounds during your pregnancy, which means you have some work to do. Instead of trying in one or two weeks to lose weight that you gained over a period of nine months, give yourself time to lose the weight you need to lose — no more than a half pound per week. With diet and exercise, you can get back to your pre-pregnancy condition. For an entire book full of dieting techniques, tips, and tricks, check out *Dieting For Dummies*, 2nd Edition, by Jane Kirby, RD, and the American Dietetic Association (Wiley).

To firm your abdominal muscles and regain strength, begin gentle abdominal exercises as soon as you feel ready. Traditional sit-ups put too much stress on your abdomen and back, so avoid those for the next few weeks and months. A better way to safely strengthen your abdominal muscles is through a series of exercises developed by physical therapist Shirley Sahrmann. These exercises, which are described in the following sections, are designed to strengthen the muscles below your belly button — the ones that you rely on most for low-back support but that are most weakened during pregnancy. As you do these exercises, progress slowly and be patient with your body. Your abdominal muscles and the skin around your abdomen need time to firm up.

The Sahrmann abdominal exercise series contains five levels of exercises, all developed to progressively strengthen the lower abdominal muscles without putting stress on your low back. The beginning ones appear here, and you can find all five levels of this technique in *How to Raise Children Without Breaking Your Back* by Hollis Herman, MS, PT, OCS and Alex Pirie (Ibis Publications).

REMEMBER

If you've had a cesarean delivery or experienced *diastasis recti,* the separation of the abdominal muscles, check with your healthcare provider before starting any abdominal exercises.

Basic breath

The first exercise, the basic breath, shows you how to isolate and control your abdominal muscles.

1. **Lie on your back with your arms at your sides, your knees bent and together, and your feet resting on the floor.**

2. **Inhale and exhale a few times to get yourself ready.**

    Don't flatten your back or tilt your pelvis; just let the natural curve in your back remain. Breathe in and out slowly and deeply.

3. **Exhale and tighten your tummy muscles, pulling your navel toward your spine.**

    Concentrate on contracting the muscles below your belly button without flattening your back. Put one hand under the small of your back and the other hand on your belly, as shown in Figure 5-7, if that helps you maintain the proper position.

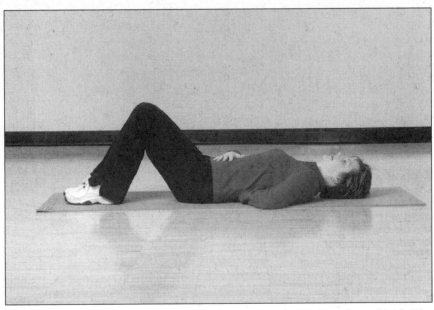

FIGURE 5-7:
The basic breath helps you control your abs.

Photograph by John Urban

4. **Hold the contraction for a count of 5 (keep breathing normally as you hold), and then relax. Repeat 5 to 10 times.**

Leg slides (Sahrmann exercise #1)

When you're able to contract, hold, and relax your abdominal muscles without moving your back or losing the contraction in your tummy, you've mastered the basic breath, which means that you can move on to leg slides, which work the lower abdominal muscles.

1. **Lie on the floor with your knees bent and your arms at your sides. Hold your tummy in by doing the basic breath contraction.**

   Place your right hand on your belly, if needed.

2. **While continuing to breathe and holding the abdominal contraction, keep your right leg bent and slowly slide your left leg forward until it's straight and resting on the floor, as shown in Figure 5-8.**

   Don't flatten your back; keep the natural curve in your spine.

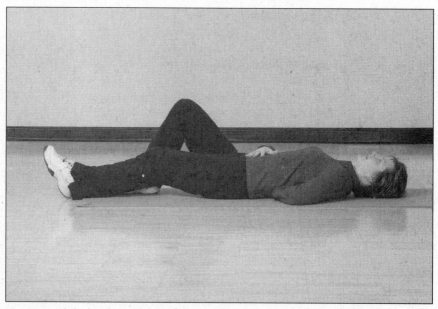

FIGURE 5-8:
The leg slide strengthens your lower abdominal muscles.

Photograph by John Urban

3. **Slide your left leg back to the bent-knee position.**

4. **Relax your tummy and repeat Steps 2 and 3 with your right leg.**

   Start with 5 repetitions on each leg. With time, build up to 20 leg slides on each leg.

Leg raises (Sahrmann exercise #2)

Leg raises are more difficult lower abdominal exercises; do these only after you master 20 repetitions of leg slides. If your back keeps coming up off the floor or your tummy pops up while doing this exercise, go back to doing leg slides until your abdomen strengthens.

1. **Lie on the floor with your knees bent and your arms at your sides. Hold your tummy in by doing the basic breath contraction.**

    Place your right hand on your belly, if needed.

2. **Raise your left knee toward your chest, as shown in Figure 5-9a.**

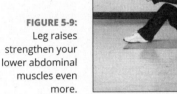

FIGURE 5-9: Leg raises strengthen your lower abdominal muscles even more.

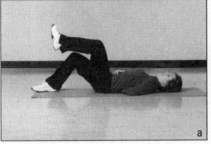
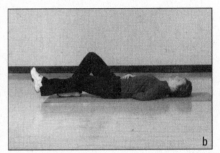

Photograph by John Urban

3. **Slowly straighten and lower your left leg until it's parallel to and about 2 to 3 inches above the floor, as shown in Figure 5-9b.**

    Be sure to keep your left leg just barely off the floor.

4. **Return your left leg to its starting position and relax your tummy. Repeat with your right leg.**

    Start with 5 repetitions on each leg. With time, build up to 20 leg raises on each leg.

5

Feeding Your Baby: Breast, Bottle, or Both?

Contents at a Glance

Chapter 1

Feeding Your Baby: A Primer for Breast and Bottle

One of the first big decisions any new parents make is whether to breast-feed their infant or use formula and bottles. Although the majority of parents these days choose to breastfeed, the decision is by no means an easy one. If you find the decision difficult, take comfort in the fact that both choices are sound and legitimate. This chapter lays out the basic first steps you need, no matter which way you go.

Deciding between Breast and Bottle

Ask almost anyone — your obstetrician, your pediatrician, your friends, total strangers — and they will advise you to breastfeed. In fact, the American Academy of Pediatrics, the World Health Organization, and the Institute of Medicine all recommend exclusive breastfeeding for six months, followed by a combination of breast milk and complementary foods for up to at least 12 months of age. "Exclusive" breastfeeding means no food or drink other than breast milk — including water — unless medically indicated. Back in the 1950s, bottle-feeding became all the rage when scientists developed techniques to pasteurize and store cow's milk in formulas appropriate for infant nutrition. Breastfeeding has regained popularity largely because people and scientific studies have recognized its many medical benefits.

However, the decision of whether to breastfeed isn't simply a medical one. It also involves issues of convenience, aesthetics, body image, maternal bonding, and even conditions surrounding delivery. The decision about how to feed your baby is a personal one that every mother must decide for herself. Figuring out how to breastfeed takes an incredible commitment, so don't feel pressured to do it if your heart isn't in it or if the thought of doing it makes you feel stressed or uncomfortable. If you decide that bottle-feeding is the best decision for you and your baby, don't feel guilty about it.

REMEMBER

You may hear that breastfeeding offers the best opportunity for a mother to bond with her baby, but bottle-feeding can also be a very warm and loving way to interact with your baby — not only for the mother but also for her partner and whoever else may help care for the baby. And although breastfeeding offers certain undeniable benefits, bottle-fed babies are — and remain — perfectly healthy.

This section looks at these two options a bit closer and helps you make a decision that's right for you. Whatever your decision, make it before you deliver so you have adequate time to prepare for the moment when your baby starts feeding. Some women elect to try out breastfeeding for a little while to see how they like it. Some decide from the beginning to use a combination of both breast and bottle (filling the bottle with either formula or breast milk that has been pumped and refrigerated).

Sizing up the advantages of breastfeeding

Breastfeeding gives your baby a tailor-made formula for good nutrition and a whole lot more. The following are some advantages for the baby:

>> Human breast milk can strengthen the baby's immune system and help reduce the risk of allergies, asthma, and sudden infant death syndrome (SIDS). It can also decrease the chances of pneumonia in the baby's first year of life.

>> Babies who are exclusively breast-fed for six months have a decreased number of ear infections (otitis media), fewer gastrointestinal infections, and a lower chance of developing necrotizing enterocolitis (NEC), a serious illness

more commonly seen in premature babies but occasionally seen in term infants.

» When breast-fed babies grow up, they have lower chances of developing inflammatory bowel disease (Crohn's disease or ulcerative colitis), celiac disease (a problem with digesting gluten), diabetes, childhood leukemia, and lymphoma. They also have a lower risk of adolescent and adult obesity.

» Breast-fed babies, when they enter school, have higher intelligence scores and higher ratings by their teachers.

» Mother's milk contains nutrients that are suited to a baby's digestive system. The most commonly used formulas contain proteins from cow's milk that aren't as easily digested, and your baby can't readily use the nutrients it contains.

» Human milk also contains substances that help protect a baby from infections until his own immune system matures. These substances are especially plentiful in the *colostrum* that mothers' breasts secrete during the first few days after the baby is born.

» Babies are more likely to have an allergic reaction to formula than to mother's milk.

Following are some advantages to breastfeeding for the mom:

» Moms who breastfeed have less postpartum blood loss and an increased rate of *involution* (the uterus getting back to its normal, pre-pregnancy size). They also have lower rates of postpartum depression and are less prone to child abuse and neglect.

» If you breastfeed your baby, you have lower risks of adult-onset diabetes, rheumatoid arthritis, hypertension (high blood pressure), hyperlipidemia (high cholesterol), cardiovascular disease, breast cancer, and ovarian cancer later in life.

» Breastfeeding is emotionally rewarding. Many women feel that they develop a special bond with their baby when they breastfeed, and they enjoy the closeness surrounding the whole experience.

» Breastfeeding is convenient. You can't leave home without it. You never have to carry bottles or formula with you.

» Mother's milk is cheaper than formula and bottles.

» You don't have to warm up breast milk; it's always the perfect temperature.

» Breastfeeding provides some degree of birth control (although it's not totally reliable — see the later section "Looking at birth control options").

>> *Lactation* (milk production) causes you to burn extra calories, which may help you lose some of the weight you gained during pregnancy.

>> A breast-fed baby's bowel movements don't have as strong an odor as those of babies who are formula-fed.

>> Breast milk is pretty much organic — no additives, no preservatives.

>> Some studies suggest that women who breastfeed may reduce their lifetime risk of breast cancer.

There are a few situations in which breastfeeding is not recommended:

>> If the infant has a rare genetic disorder called *classical galactosemia*

>> If the mother is HIV-positive (see the next section)

>> If the mother has untreated tuberculosis or brucellosis

>> If the mother is taking certain medications, such as amphetamines, chemo-therapeutic agents, ergotamines, or statins

Patients often ask whether they can breastfeed if they're taking medications for psychiatric problems (psychotropic drugs — some antidepressants fall in this category). The jury is still out on this issue, but most providers feel that medications commonly used today for depression and anxiety are relatively safe and that *not* treating the problem could cause more danger to the baby than any small risk these medications may pose. Ask your doctor about medications you take on a regular basis.

Checking out why some moms choose bottle-feeding

You may decide to choose bottle-feeding for any of the following reasons:

>> You don't want to breastfeed. If your heart isn't in it, it ain't gonna happen. Too much trial and error is involved in making breastfeeding work for someone who's not truly committed to succeeding.

>> You've tried breastfeeding, and your breasts don't produce enough milk to feed your baby (or babies!).

>> Bottle-feeding better fits your lifestyle. Although many working mothers breastfeed, others feel that juggling the requirements of their job with those of breastfeeding is just too difficult.

>> Some women find the whole concept of feeding their baby a "bodily secretion" unpleasant.

>> Bottle-feeding enables others to feed the baby.

>> If you have a chronic infection — HIV, for example — bottle-feeding helps ensure that you don't pass the infection to the baby via breast milk. (Women who carry the hepatitis B virus can breastfeed as long as the baby has received the hepatitis B vaccine. If you are hepatitis C positive, it's generally safe to breastfeed as well, according to the Centers for Disease Control and Prevention.)

>> If you or your baby is very sick after delivery, bottle-feeding may be your only option. A mother or baby who's in the intensive care unit (ICU) because of a complicated delivery often can't initiate breastfeeding.

The mother can use a mechanical pump to empty the milk from her breasts and freeze the milk to feed to the baby up to six months later. Even if the baby can't use the pumped milk at this time, pumping at least keeps the supply of milk flowing. Occasionally, a mother can restart the flow of milk later on, when she or the baby recovers, but this option isn't always possible and often requires the assistance of a lactation specialist.

>> If you've had surgery on your breasts, bottle-feeding may be your best bet; you may not be able to lactate. No medical evidence indicates that lactation has any effect on the progression of breast cancer after it has already been diagnosed, but some women who have had surgery or other treatment for breast cancer are unable to lactate. Also, some evidence suggests that women who have had breast implants produce less milk. However, many of these women produce some milk and can still breastfeed.

Latching onto Breastfeeding

Pregnancy goes a long way toward preparing your body for breastfeeding. The key pregnancy hormones cause the breasts to enlarge and prepare the glands inside the breasts to lactate. But you can prepare yourself for day-to-day nursing by checking out your nipples (if you've never really done this before) to see whether they are flat or inverted. You can certainly breastfeed if you have either of these issues, because your baby latches onto the areola, not onto the nipple, but drawing the nipple out a bit before delivery might help make things easier.

Be aware that stimulating your nipples late in your pregnancy can elicit uterine contractions. When you're near the end of your pregnancy, ask your practitioner before doing this kind of stimulation. One way to get around this problem is to avoid the nipple itself and just rub petroleum jelly, an antibacterial ointment, or baby oil over the areola.

Inverted or flat nipples often correct themselves before the baby is born, but a few techniques during pregnancy can help things along:

>> Use the thumb and forefinger on one hand to push back the skin around the areola. If this doesn't bring out the nipple, gently grasp it with your other thumb and forefinger, pull it outward, and hold it for a few minutes, as shown in Figure 1-1. Do this exercise several times a day.

>> You can also try wearing special plastic breast cups (available at most drugstores) designed to help draw out the nipple over time. This may or may not help, but it won't hurt.

FIGURE 1-1:
One method
of correcting
inverted nipples.

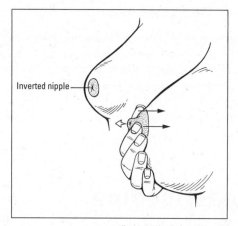

Inverted nipple

Illustration by Kathryn Born, MA

Start one of these preparation techniques for short sessions during the second trimester and then gradually increase the amount of time you work your nipples or wear the cups until your nipples stay out on their own.

Looking at the mechanics of lactation

The flood of estrogen and progesterone that your body experiences during pregnancy causes your breasts to grow — sometimes to an astonishing size. This growth starts early, within three to four weeks of conception, which is why the first sign of pregnancy for many women is breast tenderness. As pregnancy progresses, small amounts of serum-like fluid can leak from the nipples. But serious milk production doesn't start until after the baby is born.

During the first days after delivery, the breasts secrete only a yellowish fluid known as *colostrum*, which doesn't contain much milk but is rich in antibodies and protective cells from the mother's bloodstream. These substances help the newborn fight off infections until her own immune system matures and can take over. Colostrum is gradually replaced by milk.

REMEMBER

Don't be alarmed if your baby doesn't seem to get much milk during the first few days. The colostrum is very beneficial on its own. Your baby probably won't even have much of an appetite until she's three to four days old. And she's likely to need the first few days to practice sucking movements.

When your baby starts sucking on your breasts, it signals your brain to have the breasts produce milk. About three or four days after delivery, milk production sets in. When milk enters the ducts, the breasts become engorged with milk (see Figure 1-2). The engorgement can be so great that your breasts feel rock-hard and sometimes very tender. Don't worry, though. When your baby starts feeding regularly and your milk starts flowing, the engorgement is no longer so intense. The *letdown reflex* (milk entering the ducts) occurs each time your baby feeds. After you've been nursing for a while, you may find that the mere sound of your baby crying or the feel of your baby cuddling next to you can trigger the reflex.

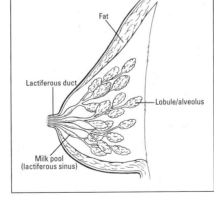

FIGURE 1-2: Your breasts contain a network of milk ducts, which start delivering colostrum during the first days after delivery.

Illustration by Kathryn Born, MA

Checking out breastfeeding positions

You can breastfeed in one of three basic positions, as shown in Figure 1-3. Use whichever position works and is comfortable for you and your baby. Most women alternate among the positions.

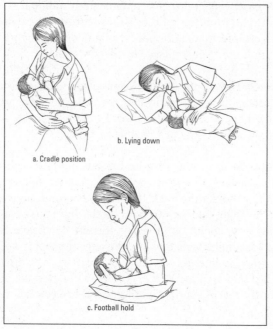

FIGURE 1-3:
The three basic positions for breastfeeding.

a. Cradle position

b. Lying down

c. Football hold

>> **Cradling:** Cradle your baby in your arms with her head next to the bend in your elbow and tilted a bit toward your breast. (See Figure 1-3a.)

>> **Lying down:** Lie on your side in bed with the baby next to you. Support the baby with your lower arm or pillows so that her mouth is next to your lower breast, and use your other arm to guide your baby's mouth to the nipple. This position is best for late-night feedings or after a cesarean delivery when sitting up is still uncomfortable. (See Figure 1-3b.)

One concern about breastfeeding while in bed is that you may fall asleep and unknowingly roll over your baby. You may decide to keep a cradle or crib next to your bed so you can put your baby back to sleep right after you finish feeding, without disrupting your night's sleep too much.

>> **Football hold:** Cradle your baby's head in the palm of your hand and support the body with your forearm. For extra support, you can place a pillow

underneath your arm. Use your free hand to hold your breast close to the baby's mouth. (See Figure 1-3c.)

Getting the baby to latch on

If you choose to breastfeed, you can get started immediately after delivery, wherever you happen to be — the birthing room, the delivery room, or the recovery room. Begin as soon as the nurses have checked your baby's health and your baby has settled down a bit from the delivery. Expect to feel a little awkward at first, and try not to get too frustrated. Many babies don't want to breastfeed immediately. Have patience — you and your baby will eventually get the hang of it.

Babies are born with a suckling reflex, but many of them don't follow it enthusiastically right off the bat. Sometimes babies need some coaxing to latch onto the breast:

1. **Arrange yourself and your baby in one of the basic breastfeeding positions (see the preceding section).**

2. **Gently stroke the baby's lips or cheek with your nipple.**

   This action usually causes the baby to open her mouth. If your baby doesn't seem to want to open her mouth, try expressing (gently pressing out) a little milk — colostrum, really — and rubbing some on the baby's lips.

3. **When the baby's mouth is wide open, bring her head to your breast and gently place her mouth over your entire nipple.**

   This prodding usually causes the baby to start sucking. Make sure that the entire areola is inside the baby's mouth, because if it isn't, she doesn't get enough milk and you get sore nipples. However, don't stuff your breast into your baby's mouth. Rather, bring the mouth to your nipple, and let the infant take in the breast.

WARNING

The tip of the baby's nose should be barely touching the skin around your breast. The only way the baby can breathe while feeding is through her nose, so be careful not to completely cover the baby's nose with your breast. If your breast obstructs the baby's nose, use your free hand to depress your breast in front of her nose to let some air in.

Orchestrating feedings

After your baby latches on, you know that she is sucking when you see regular, rhythmic movements of the cheeks and chin. Several minutes of sucking may go by before your milk letdown occurs. In the beginning, let your baby feed for about

5 minutes on each breast per nursing session. Over the course of the first three or four days, increase the amount of time on each breast to 10 to 15 minutes. Don't get too hung up about timing the feedings, though; your baby will let you know when she's had enough by not sucking and by letting your nipple slip away.

If your baby stops sucking without letting go of your nipple, insert your finger into the corner of her mouth to break the suction. (If you just pull your breast straight out, you'll end up with sore nipples.)

When switching from one breast to the other, stop to burp your baby by laying her over your shoulder or your lap and gently patting her back. Figure 1-4 shows you some of the various burping positions. Burp her again when the feeding is finished.

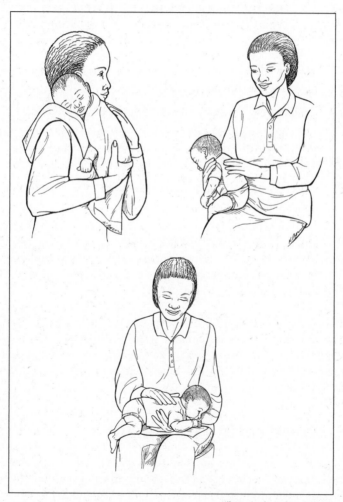

FIGURE 1-4:
There's more than one way to burp a baby. Here are a few of the tried-and-true positions.

Illustration by Kathryn Born, MA

Typically, mothers initially breastfeed about 8 to 12 times a day (averaging 10). This pattern enables your body to produce an optimal amount of milk, and it allows your baby to get the proper amount of nutrition for healthy growth and development. Try to space the feedings fairly evenly throughout the day; of course, your baby has some influence on the schedule, and some babies prefer to cluster feed, nursing very frequently over a several-hour period.

You don't have to wake your baby for a feeding unless your pediatrician specifically advises you to do so. You especially don't have to wake your baby at night; if the baby's willing to sleep through, just count yourself lucky. (However, going through the night without feeding may leave you with overfull, sore, and leaky breasts.) Nor do you have any reason to withhold a feeding if your baby is hungry — even if only an hour or so has passed since the last feeding. Also keep in mind that the number of feedings in a day may be less than average if you supplement breastfeeding with some formula feedings.

You can tell that your baby is getting enough milk if your baby

>> Nurses ten times a day on average

>> Gains weight

>> Has six to eight wet diapers a day

>> Has two to three bowel movements a day

>> Produces urine that's pale yellow (not dark and concentrated)

WARNING

If your baby isn't meeting these criteria or if you have any concern that your baby isn't getting enough milk, call your pediatrician. Some women, no matter how diligent they are, need to supplement breast milk with formula because they just can't produce enough breast milk to totally meet their baby's needs.

Maintaining your diet

During breastfeeding, as during pregnancy, your nutrition is largely a matter of educated common sense. Your breast milk's quality isn't significantly affected by your diet unless your eating habits are truly inadequate. However, if you don't take in enough calories or water, your body has a difficult time producing adequate milk. You may also find that your baby reacts a different way to certain foods — for example, she may be extra gassy. If you pay attention to how your baby responds, you can figure out what foods to avoid.

BREASTFEEDING MULTIPLES

It may seem daunting, but some women with multiples successfully breastfeed. Your body can make enough milk for two or more babies at once, especially if you're persistent and work up your milk production to a high level. Even so, arriving at a system that works for you takes some experimentation. You may breastfeed two babies at once or feed each one separately. The advantage to the first alternative is that you don't spend all your time breastfeeding, but the second method is easier. You don't have to deal with one baby finishing first and needing to be burped while the other one is still sucking. (Holding one baby over your shoulder and keeping another one at your breast can be tricky, no matter how many pillows and props you use.) You may breastfeed one baby, bottle-feed the other, and then alternate at the next feeding. You may breastfeed each baby a little at each feeding and then supplement with the bottle. Or you may breastfeed the babies for most of the day and then supplement with a bottle before bedtime when your milk supply is low.

Women who breastfeed twins need to take in even more calories and fluids. You need about 400 to 600 extra calories per day for each baby you're breastfeeding. (Imagine how much you'd have to consume to breastfeed triplets! About 1,200 to 1,800 extra calories per day!) Also, you need to increase your fluid intake from 8 to 10 glasses per day to about 10 to 12 glasses per day.

If you do decide to try breastfeeding multiples, count on needing help from other family members and friends. Don't be afraid to ask for it.

REMEMBER

Breastfeeding women should take in 400 to 600 more calories a day than they would normally eat. The exact amount varies according to how much you weigh and how much fat you gained during pregnancy. Because lactating does burn fat, breastfeeding helps get rid of some of the extra fat stores you may have. But avoid losing weight too fast, or your milk production will suffer. Also, avoid gaining weight while you're breastfeeding. If you find that you're putting on more pounds, you're most likely taking in too many calories or not exercising enough.

You also need extra vitamins and minerals — especially vitamin D, calcium, and iron. Keep taking your prenatal vitamins or some other balanced supplement while you're nursing. Also, consume extra calcium — either a supplement or extra servings of milk, yogurt, and other dairy products. Omega-3 fatty acids are also important for your developing baby — you should consume about 200 to 300 mg of these every day.

Breast milk is mainly water (87 percent). To produce plenty of breast milk, you must take in at least 72 ounces of fluid per day, which is about nine glasses of water, milk, or juice. Don't go overboard, however, because if you drink too many fluids, your milk production may actually decrease. You also don't want to markedly increase your calorie intake with high-sugar, high-carbohydrate, or high-calorie fluids. A good way to tell whether you're getting the right amount of fluid is to monitor your urine output. If you urinate infrequently or if the color is a deep yellow, you probably aren't getting enough. If you constantly run to the bathroom, you may be drinking too much.

TIP

If you find that your baby is fussy and has a hard time sleeping, you may be consuming too much caffeine. Try cutting back on the coffee or cola until you find the level your baby tolerates.

Looking at birth control options

Although breastfeeding decreases the likelihood of ovulation, it by no means guarantees that you won't become pregnant. For a woman who chooses not to breastfeed, it takes an average of 10 weeks after the birth to resume ovulation — that is, to become fertile again. About 10 percent of women who do breastfeed also begin ovulating again after 10 weeks, and about 50 percent start up again by 25 weeks — about six months — after their babies are born. Clearly, breastfeeding isn't a great form of birth control.

Before you resume intercourse, consider using some effective form of birth control, because chances are you don't want to become pregnant again right away. You can use birth control pills (some are okay with breastfeeding), barrier methods (condoms, a diaphragm, and so on), or long-acting progesterone shots (such as Depo-Provera). One of the newer forms of birth control (Nexplanon) is a tiny reservoir that contains a progesterone-like substance and is placed below the surface of the skin on the inner part of your arm. The reservoir slowly releases the medication and can prevent you from getting pregnant for up to three years. They can even be implanted while you're in the hospital recovering from your delivery, and they don't interfere significantly with breastfeeding. Discuss your options with your practitioner before discharge from the hospital or at your six-week checkup.

Determining which medications are safe

Just about any medication you take gets into your breast milk but usually only in tiny amounts. If you need to take a medication while breastfeeding, try taking the lowest dose possible and, as a rule, take it just after you finish a breastfeeding session. That way, your body breaks down most of the medication by the time you need to breastfeed again. In general, don't deprive yourself of medications that you really need just because you're afraid that some of it may get to the baby and cause harm. Check with your doctor about medications to be sure that they're fine to take while breastfeeding.

The following medications are okay to take while breastfeeding:

>> Acetaminophen (such as Tylenol)

>> Antacids

>> Most antibiotics

>> Most commonly used antidepressants (see the earlier section "Sizing up the advantages of breastfeeding")

>> Antihistamines

>> Aspirin

>> Most asthma medications

>> Decongestants

>> Most high blood pressure medications

>> Ibuprofen (such as Advil or Motrin)

>> Insulin

>> Most seizure medications

>> Most thyroid medications

Handling common problems

One of the greatest misconceptions about breastfeeding is that it comes easily and naturally to everyone. Breastfeeding takes practice. Problems can range from a little nipple soreness to, in rare cases, infections in the milk ducts.

Sore nipples

Many women experience some temporary nipple soreness during the first few days that they breastfeed. For most women, the pain is mild, and it goes away on its own. For some, however, the soreness gets progressively worse and can lead to chapped or cracked nipples and moderate to severe pain. If your breasts are heading in this direction, take action before your suffering gets out of hand. The following list outlines some remedies:

>> Review your technique to make sure that your baby is positioned correctly. If the baby isn't getting the entire nipple and areola in her mouth, the soreness is likely to continue. Try changing the baby's position slightly with each feeding.

>> Increase the number of feedings, and feed for less time at each feeding. This way, your baby won't be as hungry and may not suck as hard.

>> Definitely continue to feed on the sore breast, even if only for a few minutes, to keep the nipple conditioned to nursing. If you let it heal completely, the soreness will start all over when you feed from that nipple again. You may want to feed on the least sore breast first, because that's when your baby's sucking is most vigorous.

>> Express a little breast milk manually before you put the baby to the breast. This action helps initiate the letdown reflex so that the baby doesn't have to suck as long and hard to achieve letdown.

>> Don't use any irritating chemicals or soaps on your nipples.

>> After your baby finishes feeding, don't wipe off your nipples. Let them air-dry for as long as possible. Wiping them with a cloth may cause needless irritation.

>> Exposing the nipples to air helps to toughen the skin, so try to walk around the house with your nipples exposed as much as possible. If you wear a nursing bra, leave the flaps open while you're at home. Your nipples will toughen from the fabric of your clothes rubbing against them.

>> If you're using pads to soak up leakage from your breasts, change them as soon as they get moist, or they may chafe your nipples.

>> Try massaging vitamin E oil or ointment, olive oil, or lanolin into sore nipples and then letting them air dry. Udder Cream and Bag Balm, products developed to treat chapped teats on milk cows (yes, cows), have found new popularity among breastfeeding women. Many drugstores and cosmetics stores now sell these creams.

>> Apply dry (not moist) and warm (not hot) heat to the nipples several times a day. You can use a hot water bottle filled with warm water.

Pain from breast engorgement

When the breasts become engorged with milk, they can hurt. One way to avoid painful engorgement is to begin breastfeeding right after the baby is born. Other strategies include wearing a firm — but not tight — bra and massaging the breasts before feeding. Massaging facilitates letdown and relieves some of the engorgement. You can also try placing warm compresses on your breasts. (Some women feel that ice packs work better — try both and see which works best for you.)

Clogged ducts

Sometimes, some of the milk ducts in the breast become clogged with debris. If this happens, a small, firm, red lump may form inside the breast. The lump may be tender, but it's usually not associated with a fever or excruciating pain. The best way to treat a clogged breast duct is to try to completely empty that breast after each feeding. Start the baby out on that breast, when she's most hungry. If the baby doesn't completely empty the breast, use a breast pump on that side until all the milk is drained. Applying heat to the lump and massaging it manually is helpful. You can also try letting the spray from a warm shower fall on your breast to promote milk release. Most important, keep feeding.

BREASTFEEDING RESOURCES

If you have special problems or if you want more in-depth information about breast-feeding, contact one of the following organizations:

- La Leche League International or La Leche League USA, 1400 N. Meacham Rd., Schaumburg, IL 60173; phone 1-877-4 LA LECHE; website www.llli.org or www.lllusa.org

- American Congress of Obstetricians and Gynecologists, 409 Twelfth St. SW, Washington, D.C. 20024; phone 800-673-8444; website www.acog.org

- American Academy of Pediatrics, 141 Northwest Point Rd., Elk Grove Village, IL 60007; phone 800-433-9016; website www.aap.org

- International Board of Lactation Consultant Examiners; phone 703-560-7330; website www.iblce.org

- International Lactation Consultant Association; phone 919-861-5577; website www.ilca.org

- American College of Nurse-Midwives, 818 Connecticut Ave. NW, Ste. 900, Washington, D.C. 20006; phone 240-485-1800; website www.midwife.org

If the lump persists for more than a few days, becomes very painful, or is associated with a fever, call your doctor to make sure that you're not developing an abscess.

Mastitis (breast infection)

Breast infections (mastitis) occur in about 2 percent of all breastfeeding women. Bacteria from the baby's mouth usually cause the infections, which are most likely to happen two to four weeks after delivery (but can occur earlier or later than that). Infections are more common in women who are breastfeeding for the first time, who have chapped nipples with cracks or fissures, and who don't empty their breasts completely at feedings.

The symptoms of mastitis include a warm, hard, red breast; high fever (usually over 101 degrees Fahrenheit); and malaise (like when you have the flu and your whole body feels achy). The infection in the breast may be diffused, or it may be localized to a particular segment of the breast (known as a *lobule*). If the infection is localized, the redness may appear as a wedge-shaped area over the infected portion of the breast (see Figure 1-5). If these symptoms develop, call your doctor immediately. More than likely, he'll prescribe an antibiotic and may even want you to come into the office for an examination.

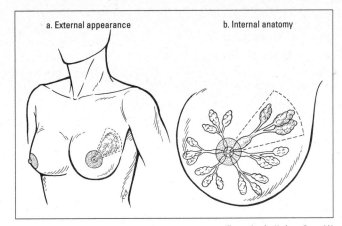

a. External appearance   b. Internal anatomy

FIGURE 1-5: An outer view and an inner view of a wedge-shaped mastitis.

Illustration by Kathryn Born, MA

Continue to breastfeed your baby while you have the infection. It's not harmful to the baby; after all, the bacteria probably came from the baby's mouth. If you stop breastfeeding, the breast will become engorged, making your discomfort even worse. Acetaminophen (such as Tylenol), ibuprofen, or warm compresses may help relieve the pain from mastitis while the antibiotics take effect (usually in about two days). Drink plenty of fluids, and get as much rest as you can to allow your body's natural healing powers to work. Take your medication for the fully prescribed amount of time to help make sure that the infection doesn't recur.

Breast abscess

If mastitis isn't treated aggressively or if a milk duct remains clogged, a breast abscess can develop. In fact, breast abscesses form in as many as 10 percent of all cases of mastitis. Symptoms of a breast abscess are extreme pain, heat and swelling over the area of the abscess, and high fevers (over 101 degrees Fahrenheit). Sometimes doctors can treat abscesses with antibiotics, but often the abscess needs to be drained surgically.

FOR PARTNERS: OFFERING LACTATION SUPPORT

LeBron James makes dunking a basketball look as simple as flushing a toilet, but that doesn't mean you can do it. If your partner chooses to breastfeed, keep in mind that it's not as easy as it looks, especially at first. Issues will arise, and although you can't be the one to solve those issues, your support is a major factor in her success. Be positive and upbeat, listen to your partner when she talks, and thank her profusely for making such a wise decision for both the baby's health and hers.

The most important role for Dad is to stay informed about the process of breastfeeding. Many complications can arise, and the more you know about how to help your partner through those issues, the more likely Mom and baby will be able to work through them.

One of the most common reasons women have for ceasing breastfeeding is that it's uncomfortable or painful. (Breastfeeding *should not hurt* after Mom and baby establish the correct feeding positions.) But sometimes problems do arise — sore nipples, pain from breast engorgement, clogged ducts, and more can frustrate even the most dedicated breastfeeding moms.

Remember that it's the mother's decision to quit breastfeeding if she so chooses; it should never be your suggestion. If lactation issues arise, don't tell her to throw in the towel and go buy some formula, no matter how frustrated or tearful she becomes. Listen to her concerns, help her find resources to correct problems, and ultimately be supportive no matter what she decides.

Whenever your partner decides for any reason to stop breastfeeding, thank her for the time she has invested in doing so and congratulate her on her achievements. You both should be proud of the hard, rewarding work you've done.

WARNING

If you develop a breast abscess, you can continue to breastfeed on the other side, but you should stop feeding on the side of the abscess until the problem subsides. Check with your doctor before resuming feedings on that side.

Bottle-Feeding for Beginners

Suppose you've decided to forgo breastfeeding in favor of formula. Or you've been breastfeeding for a while, and you want to switch. This section goes over what you need to know to get your baby started on bottles.

Stopping milk production

If you decide to formula-feed, you need to stop the process of milk production in your breasts. Milk production is triggered by warmth and breast stimulation. To stop the production of milk, create the opposite environment. Here are some suggestions:

» Make the change gradually, dropping one feeding every day or two.

» Wear a tight-fitting bra, preferably one without underwire that can compress the delicate tissues. Sports bras often work well. Wear the bra 24/7 except when showering.

» Apply ice packs to your breasts when they become engorged (usually around the third or fourth day after your baby is born).

» Keep ice packs inside your bra, or use small packages of frozen vegetables, like peas or corn, which you can easily fold to fit within a bra. (We don't recommend going out in public this way, though.)

» Place cold cabbage leaves inside your bra. Cabbage works chemically to reduce the production of milk.

» Let cold water run over your breasts during a shower. Pat nipples dry instead of rubbing, which can irritate the tissue.

TIP

If you're going to breastfeed for a short period of time (6 to 12 weeks), consider giving your baby one bottle of formula per day while nursing to help make the transition easier.

Engorged breasts can be very uncomfortable. If you're in a great deal of discomfort, you may want to ask your doctor about pain medication. Fortunately, the engorgement usually lasts only 36 to 48 hours and seldom requires medical help.

Choosing the best bottles and nipples

TIP

You won't have any trouble finding a wide choice of bottles and nipples. Some babies definitely demonstrate a preference for one type of bottle or nipple over another. You may have to experiment to discover what tools work best for you and your baby. Four-ounce bottles are good for the first few weeks or months. Later, when your baby drinks more, you can switch to the 8-ounce bottles. Make sure that the bottles you use don't contain the potentially harmful chemical BPA. If you buy new bottles, this shouldn't be a problem, but older bottles may not be BPA-free.

Here is some information on bottles:

>> Some bottles are actually plastic holders in which you insert little transparent plastic bags that hold the milk or formula. The advantage of this type is that you can throw away the empty milk bag, and you don't have to worry about sterilizing the plastic container. Also, because the plastic bag is designed to collapse, less air gets into the bag and into the baby's stomach.

>> Some bottles are angled, which also helps to allow less air to be taken in by the baby, leading to less gas.

>> Nipples come in a wide variety. Newborn nipples have a smaller hole, and the size of the hole increases with the age of the baby (nipples generally come in newborn, 3- and 6-month sizes, and then larger ones for older babies). Orthodontic nipples are designed to mimic nature's design. Some nipples are made out of latex; others, of silicone. Silicone nipples are clear, have less of an odor, and are firmer. Your baby may demonstrate a strong preference for one type over another or may not notice much of a difference.

Feeding your baby from a bottle

Your mother, grandmother, or any number of well-intentioned friends may tell you to sterilize bottles by boiling them in water, but most pediatricians think that this step is unnecessary. After all, a mother who breastfeeds doesn't have to boil her nipples!

Many parents choose to warm their baby's bottle, but heating it isn't necessary. If you choose to, though, you can warm a bottle in different ways. Many parents purchase bottle warmers especially designed for this task. But if you don't want to take up kitchen counter space with another appliance, you can place bottles in a container filled with hot water.

WARNING

If you use the microwave to heat your baby's bottle, be careful. The breast milk or formula may heat unevenly, and some parts of it may be too hot for the baby. However, if you shake the bottle after warming it, it may be okay. Just make sure you squirt some onto your wrist to check the temperature first. Some formula manufacturers don't recommend microwaving their product, so make sure to read the information on the side of the packaging.

Saving leftover formula or breast milk generally isn't a good idea. However, some pediatricians say that reusing a bottle once is okay, so talk it over with your baby's doctor. In any case, don't leave a bottle filled with milk sitting outside the refrigerator for very long, because warmth encourages the growth of bacteria that can upset your baby's stomach.

Choose your formula with the help of your pediatrician. Call his office prior to delivery and find out what he suggests you use. Many formulas come premixed, but some come in either a powder or concentrated liquid form, both of which require you to add water. The powder and concentrated liquid forms cost less, but they may not be available in as wide of a variety.

All kinds of formulas are available, including organic formulas. The jury is still out as to whether there are clear medical benefits to organic formulas. They may be more costly, and some have extra sugar, so check with your pediatrician about whether organic is the way to go.

WARNING

Some babies develop an allergic reaction to their formula; they may have an upset stomach or develop a skin rash. If your baby becomes allergic, talk with your pediatrician. He may want to switch your baby to a soy-based formula or to a hypoallergenic formula.

WARNING

Pediatricians generally caution against propping up a baby's bottle by laying it on a pillow next to the baby's mouth, because propping implies that the baby is being left unattended. Also, laying a baby flat on her back with the bottle propped creates more potential for choking. Propping a bottle may also promote tooth decay.

The most common position for bottle-feeding your baby is to hold the baby cradled in one arm, close to your body. Put a pillow on your lap, which eases the strain on your arms and neck. Most parents find it easier to always hold the baby in the same arm and in the same direction. For example, if you're right-handed, you may want to hold your baby in your left arm and the bottle in the right. When the baby is a little older and has better control of her head and neck muscles, you may want to lay her in front of you along your legs for a change of pace. This way, you and your baby can make eye contact.

Here are some other tips for parents who are bottle-feeding (whether with formula or breast milk):

>> Don't swaddle the baby too much or keep her too warm during feeding. The baby may get so comfortable that she falls asleep instead of feeding.

>> Change the baby's diaper in the middle of a feeding if she falls asleep. This may help to wake her up so that she can finish the rest of the bottle. However, it's usually not necessary to coerce a baby into finishing a feeding; she knows what she needs and may stop before the bottle's empty because she's full.

>> To check whether your baby is hungry, put the tip of your finger into her mouth to see whether she starts to suck.

>> Keep the bottle tilted in such a way as to completely fill the nipple with the formula or milk, thereby minimizing the amount of air your baby gets.

TIP

Burp your baby at least once midway through a feeding and again at the end of a feeding. Babies often take in air along with the milk or formula they drink, and burping helps them get rid of it. It also makes them more comfortable and able to eat more.

Dealing with Baby's Developing Digestive System

Your baby has a brand-new digestive system, and it requires considerable breaking-in. Long story short: Babies spit up. A lot. Whether they're breast-fed or bottle-fed, newborn babies are likely to vomit as often as two times per day. Try these suggestions for dealing with spitting up:

>> Keep a cloth over your shoulder when burping or holding your baby so you don't have to constantly change, or ruin, your clothes.

>> Keep a small bib on your baby during and after feeding so you don't have to constantly change, or ruin, all the baby's clothes.

>> Burp your baby after each feeding.

>> If you're bottle-feeding, stop partway through the bottle to burp the baby instead of allowing the baby to drink the entire bottle in one shot.

>> Don't play with the baby too much after feeding. Jiggling the baby or moving the baby around a lot can lead to more spitting up.

WARNING

>> If your baby seems to be spitting up large quantities or if the spitting up is very forceful, let your pediatrician know.

Sometimes, spitting up or vomiting several times a day is a sign of something as simple as overfeeding, or it may indicate a condition known as *gastroesophageal reflux*, or *GER*, which is a digestive disorder caused by gastric acid from the stomach flowing into the esophagus. It's common in babies, although it can occur at any age. If your newborn is showing symptoms such as pain when spitting up, irritability, inconsolable crying, gagging, choking, or refusal to eat, you should definitely speak to your pediatrician. In this case, she may have *gastroesophageal reflux disease,* or *GERD,* a more serious disorder.

Your pediatrician diagnoses GERD by conducting a medical history, physical exam, and certain diagnostic tests. These tests may include an upper gastrointestinal series, *endoscopy* (placement of a flexible tube with a light and camera lens into the organs of the upper digestive system), pH testing, and gastric emptying studies.

The need for treatment for reflux depends on your baby's age, overall health, and medical history; the extent of the problem; and your baby's tolerance for specific medications, procedures, and treatments. Sometimes reflux can be improved through feeding changes. Try these suggestions:

>> After feeding, place your baby on her stomach with her upper body elevated at least 30 degrees, or hold her in a sitting position for about 30 minutes.

>> If bottle-feeding, keep the nipple filled with milk or formula so your baby doesn't swallow too much air.

>> Adding a feed thickener, such as rice cereal, may be beneficial for some babies who are about 6 months or older. Check with your pediatrician.

>> Burp your baby frequently during feedings.

IN THIS CHAPTER

Planning ahead for your first weeks of breastfeeding

Designing your breastfeeding spaces

Buying bras, shirts, and gowns

Making your first attempt at breastfeeding

Chapter 2

Delving Deeper into Breastfeeding

I f you're reading this chapter, you've probably weighed the positives and negatives of breastfeeding and have decided to at least try it. This chapter helps you look at your post-delivery schedule and how breastfeeding will fit into your life, offers advice on how to set up a functional nursery, and makes a few wardrobe and paraphernalia suggestions that can make breastfeeding easier and more comfortable. This chapter also helps you through the first breastfeeding after delivery.

Evaluating Your Postpartum Schedule — Realistically!

What do you imagine happening after you deliver your baby? If your life were a TV show, you might find yourself in a dreamy haze, sitting in a rocking chair with your baby sleeping peacefully in your arms. Perhaps you'd wear a long dress and have your hair pulled back in a soft, matronly style. Your baby would be dressed in a rose pink (or sky blue) handmade outfit. The hard work would be over, and you'd finally be able to relax.

Well, forget it. The end of pregnancy is the start of your new, sleep-deprived existence. And if you plan on returning to work, you have to consider how to breastfeed while you work.

Time management tips

Yes, new motherhood is an exciting, sweet time, but then there's all the rest. Many women go wrong by setting themselves on a post-delivery course that no woman could possibly maintain without a staff of four to help.

TIP

The time to consider postpartum time management techniques is long before you ever feel the first labor pain. Consider these examples:

» You may be feeding the baby every two to three hours when you first get home, so don't plan to host a major event — your parents' 40th anniversary party or a Cub Scout Jamboree — in your house for at least several weeks.

» If you have older children in school or daycare and belong to a carpool, try to beg off for a few weeks. If your child's nursery school has after-school care, consider utilizing it a day or two each week so you can catch up on sleep — or at least get the kitchen cleaned.

» Ask your partner to take time off work if his workplace offers paternity leave. If that's not possible, ask your mom, sister, or best friend to help out for a few days.

» If your church or another social group has a program that provides meals for the sick, take advantage of it; a casserole or two may last through the better part of the first week home.

» Hire a cleaning service once a week for the first few weeks. Looking at dust and clutter can push you over the edge when you're sleep deprived.

» Don't view your maternity leave as a wonderful time to get major household projects done, such as remodeling the bathroom. You may think you'll have lots of time for this sort of thing, but you won't!

» Sleep whenever possible. Really.

The need to rest can't be overemphasized, so don't try to jump right back into your old routine the minute you get home. Too much running around decreases your milk supply, slows your healing, and makes you cranky!

Considering your return to work

The last thing you may be thinking about as you prepare to deliver your baby is what life will be like when you have to go back to work. But continuing to breast-feed after you return to work is a challenge, so you'd be wise to consider your situation before you go on maternity leave.

Ask yourself these questions:

» Where is the best place to pump? An office with a door that locks is ideal, but if you don't have that luxury, you'll need to get creative.

» Are your supervisors and coworkers supportive of breastfeeding? If you don't know the answer to that question, now is the time to start having conversations about your plans.

» Can you arrange your schedule to go home at lunchtime and nurse?

» Has anyone in your office ever breastfed? If so, ask that person for advice.

Arranging Your Space and Amassing Supplies

When you start arranging your nursing space, you'll probably set up two areas. First, of course, is the baby's room. You'll probably do most of your night feedings here, and visitors usually want to see this space first so they can oooh and ahhh over the cute decorating job. During the day, you may spend most of your time in your family room or living room.

Nesting in the nursery

Curtains that match the crib sheets are very nice and will satisfy your *form over function* needs, but other items are more essential for a comfortable breastfeeding experience:

» Topping the list is a comfortable place to sit, whether you prefer an uphol-stered chair, a wooden rocker, or a glider.

>> A footstool or ottoman elevates your feet and knees, bringing the baby closer to your breasts. This position can reduce neck, shoulder, and back strain. Some ottomans are too high for comfort, so you may want to look for a special nursing stool. Alternately, you can get creative and make your own from a kitchen step stool.

>> A table by your chair is a must, because you need burping cloths, baby wipes, a clock, and receiving blankets within arm's reach. And having a drink next to you at each feeding is a great reminder to keep your fluid intake up while you're breastfeeding.

Setting up space in the family room

Hide and seek is fun when you're 10 but not when you're a new mom and you have to disappear into the nursery to breastfeed every time company arrives. Arranging your nursing space in the family room is the start of public breastfeeding. Setting up a comfortable spot allows you to feed the baby discreetly and still be part of the action in the house.

REMEMBER

Having a nursing spot set up in the middle of the action is good only if you're comfortable with it. When you first come home from the hospital, you may feel comfortable nursing only in front of your partner — and maybe not even him! Be direct about your needs for privacy, even if that means kicking everyone out of the family room for a while. Ask your partner for help telling your family and friends to give you space; he may enjoy having an active role to play as "keeper of the gate."

If you have other children, you need to decide if you're comfortable nursing in front of them. Of course, depending on their ages, you may not have a choice.

TIP

If you have toddlers, arrange your nursing area so they can sit next to you. That way, they won't climb on top of the kitchen cupboards every time you nurse. Have favorite books or puzzles handy, prepare a snack for them before you begin nursing, and encourage them to watch the baby make funny faces.

If you plan to nurse in front of your children or other people, you may want to arrange the furniture in your family room so your nursing chair isn't center stage. Perhaps set your table and chair behind the couch or in a corner. Unless you want all eyes on you, definitely don't put your chair right next to the TV! Keep in mind, also, that as the baby grows, he'll be distracted by what's going on around him. He may nurse better if you're away from the action.

Your furniture and equipment needs for the family room are similar to those in the nursery:

>> A comfortable chair is still a must, although you may choose to use the corner of the couch. Your impulse might be to go for a great overstuffed chair, but be warned: Many overstuffed chairs are too deep to sit in comfortably, unless you're tall. If you're short, your feet will stick straight out in front of you — not comfortable for the long haul!

>> A table within easy reach will hold not only the breastfeeding essentials but also the remote control, a magazine, and a snack or two!

>> Lots of extra pillows are helpful, especially when you're just learning how to nurse.

Breastfeeding in your bedroom

If you choose to share your room with your baby, at least for the first few months, keep the following in mind:

TIP

>> An overstuffed reading pillow provides back and arm support for feedings. You'll also need pillows under your arms to help lift the baby up to the breast.

>> A bedside bassinet helps you scoop up the baby easily. Many bedside cribs are designed to line up at the same level as your bed so you can reach the baby without any barriers.

Breastfeeding paraphernalia

In addition to a comfy chair and a quiet place, you need a few more things to stock your breastfeeding nursery.

A breast pump

Every nursing mom, whether staying at home or going back to work, should have a breast pump. How exotic the pump is up to you. You can buy a manual, battery operated, or electric breast pump:

>> **Manual pump:** Manual pumps may work for occasional pumpers. They're easy to find and easy to assemble, but they're not always easy to use. The big plusses of manual pumps are that they're inexpensive, compact, portable, and quiet. They don't have moving parts that could break, and they don't require

electricity or batteries to operate. They're also easy to find; most pharmacies have them in stock. The downside? Many women are able to get only a scant amount of milk using a manual pump, and some pumps can bruise or scrape your nipples.

>> **Battery-operated pump:** These tend to have more disadvantages than advantages. Their energy is supplied by AA batteries, so you may need to buy stock in a battery company. It takes eight to ten seconds to build up suction, so a battery-operated pump takes longer to use than a regular manual pump. They're also slower than electric pumps because they have less power. The advantage of a battery-operated pump is it's easier to maneuver than a manual pump and just as portable. If you don't think that you'll need to pump on a regular basis, a battery-operated pump may work for you.

>> **Electric pump:** If you pump frequently, an electric pump is the only way to fly! It requires only one hand to use; imitates your baby's sucking action, even down to number of sucks per minute (48 to 60); and comes in models that allow you to pump both breasts at one time. Most women find electric pumps more effective than other pumps in getting milk out of their breasts. The disadvantages? They're larger, making them less portable and more conspicuous; they're more expensive than others ($200 to $300 isn't uncommon); and they're not quiet. These pumps are work horses, and they often sound like it!

If possible, don't start pumping until your milk supply is well established — at least four weeks after delivery.

Discuss pumps with a lactation consultant before purchasing one; she'll probably recommend that you get your feet wet with breastfeeding before investing in a pump. Pumps can be expensive, and you can't return them after they've been used, so you want to make as informed a decision as possible. The consultant can also provide information about renting a pump; be sure to ask.

Resting on nursing pillows

To be comfortable while nursing, you'll probably want to tuck pillows behind you for back support and under your arms to help support the baby. A pillow on your lap brings your baby closer to the breast. You can use plain bed pillows for this purpose, or you can splurge with special nursing pillows.

Make sure the pillow you use is firm; if it's too soft, the baby will sink into it and not get any higher on your lap. A plastic cover over the pillow is essential. (No matter how much disposable diapers improve, they still can leak!) Most nursing pillow covers are washable, and some pillows are as well.

Stocking Your Wardrobe

No one ever said nursing shirts and nursing bras were glamorous, but they've made great strides over the last 20 years. Whether you're a stay-at-home mom or chair of the board, you need to get dressed in the morning in clothes that are comfortable and conducive to nursing.

Trying on nursing bras

REMEMBER

Wearing the proper nursing bra provides breast support and makes you more comfortable. You should buy two or three *all cotton* nursing bras in the final weeks of your pregnancy. At this time, your cup size will be its closest to your post-delivery size.

Most maternity shops, department stores, and undergarment specialty stores carry nursing bras. Wherever you go, make sure that the person helping you knows how to measure and fit you. Proper fit is the key to comfort with any type of bra.

TIP

When you try on a nursing bra, bend over and gently "shake" your breasts into the cups. A well-fitted bra should cover the entire breast; no part of the breast should spill out. The bottom band should be snug, but the bra shouldn't put pressure on your breasts. If the bra is too tight, it could cause a milk duct to become plugged or *mastitis* (infection) to develop. The bra shouldn't ride up in the back, and the straps should keep your breasts elevated without cutting into your shoulders.

REMEMBER

When considering cup size, keep in mind that you may need room for a breast pad or breast shell. For band size, buy a bra that you can fasten on the inside row so you have more hooks to expand to after your milk comes in.

Make sure your bra flaps are easy to open and close. You don't want a bra that requires neighborhood assistance to open! Opening the flap should be a one-hand operation; you want to be able to hold your baby in one arm and slip up your top and undo the flap with the other. Some bras have clips, and some have snaps to hold the flap up; you may want to try them both to see which is easier for you to manage.

Nursing bras can be expensive but are worth the investment. Don't be surprised if you need to buy bras in different sizes as time goes by. You may even find yourself back in your regular bra months down the road. At this point, you can use the *lift and load* routine — just *lift* your bra up off the breast and *load* the baby on.

You don't have to wear a bra. Some women like that *born free* (or *hang free*, at least) feeling. But wait until you're an advanced breastfeeder before ditching your bra. Your breasts need support in the beginning — at least for the first month. Some women even wear their bras to bed in the beginning because it's more comfortable.

Looking chic in nursing shirts

Nursing shirts (and gowns) can be helpful, especially at first. When you wear a nursing shirt, you don't have to bare all to feed the baby. There's a slit in the front of the shirt; you just slide the slit over your breast to give the baby access. The time may come when you feel so comfortable with nursing that you wouldn't care if the President of the United States were in the same room with you. But until then, these "peek-a-boob" aids are helpful.

Of course, you don't need special shirts to nurse. If you're comfortable, just place a receiving blanket over your baby, and he'll cover the rest.

Using pads, shields, shells, and creams

Breast pads, nipple shields, and breast shells all fit into your bra, but they have very different functions. The simplest and the one almost everyone needs? Breast pads.

Stopping leaks with breast pads

In the first few weeks of nursing, you may experience a considerable amount of leakage! Breast pads are absorbent cotton pads that collect milk that leaks out of the nipple until your let-down reflex (see Book 5, Chapter 1) is better controlled. Breast pads (also called *nursing pads*) bear a strong resemblance to sanitary napkins, which can actually be cut down to size and used for this same purpose.

You can purchase boxes of disposable breast pads, or you can choose washable cotton pads, which are more cost-effective if you don't mind adding to your laundry pile.

Some pads are contoured, and some are more like flat circles. If you buy contoured, keep in mind that the contour of the pad may not fit your particular contour! On the other hand, flat pads slide around more easily and are more noticeable through your shirt. Some brands come with sticky strips to hold them in place in your bra.

Covering your nipples with a shield

Nipple shields are sometimes recommended to help draw out flat or inverted nipples (refer to Book 5, Chapter 1) or protect sore nipples. The shields are made of soft plastic or silicone and fit over the entire areola. You need to moisten the back of the shield to help it adhere to your skin. You wear the shields while breastfeeding. Nipple shields should be used only as a last resort.

REMEMBER

Most lactation consultants agree that sore and cracked nipples are caused by poor positioning and/or improper latch-on (see Book 5, Chapter 1). Nipple shields are only a temporary measure to help your nipples heal or help your baby latch on when all else fails. Using shields for long periods may decrease your milk supply, so use them only under the supervision of a lactation consultant or physician.

Wearing breast shells

Breast shells are quite different from nipple shields. Shells are never worn while nursing; they're used between feedings or before the baby arrives to help draw out flat or inverted nipples or to collect leaking milk.

Shells come in several pieces, as shown in Figure 2-1. The piece that fits next to the breast puts gentle compression to help draw out flat or inverted nipples (discussed in Book 5, Chapter 1). The outer piece fits over the top and usually has air holes to allow circulating air to keep the nipple drier. Leaking milk collects in the shell; some brands have a little spout you can use to pour the milk into a bag or bottle if you're storing breast milk.

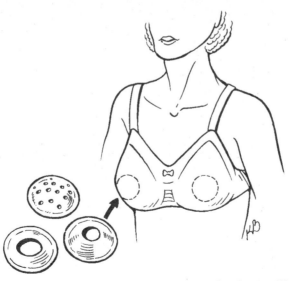

FIGURE 2-1:
Breast shells can help you collect and store milk.

Illustration by Kathryn Born, MA

Unless you're able to dump the milk immediately after it leaks, don't save it. Milk that sits in the shell may grow bacteria.

Make sure the spout points upward when you put the shell on, or milk will pour all over you when you remove it! Also make sure the air vents are at the top; if they're on the bottom, milk comes right back out through the little holes.

During nursing, you can wear a breast shell on the breast you're not using, to prevent you from getting soaked during let-down and also to help collect milk.

Coating your nipples with creams

Sometimes all you need to heal sore nipples is a little air drying; other times, you may need lotions or creams. Most creams are food grade and lanolin-based. *Food grade* means the cream doesn't need to be removed before you feed the baby.

One disadvantage to creams is that they're often yellow and somewhat greasy, meaning they can stain your clothes. Wear a breast pad, unless you're not concerned with staining your nursing bras, and try to keep the baby's clothes away from the cream. You need to use only a tiny dab of cream; it spreads a little easier if you warm it by rolling it between your fingertips before applying.

Some types of creams absolutely should not be used on your breasts when nursing. Among them are alcohol-based products, which make nipples more prone to crack; petroleum-based products, which don't allow the skin to breathe; and vitamin E-based products, which may be toxic to the baby. Look for ultra-purified lanolin ointment, which is pharmaceutical grade and safe for breastfeeding.

AVOIDING NIPPLE CONFUSION

Nipple confusion may arise when a breast-fed baby is fed with a bottle or given a pacifier. Breastfeeding requires a strong coordinated suck. The tongue is placed below the nipple, and the jaw muscles are used to massage the milk ducts to keep milk flowing. When the baby stops sucking, the milk flow stops. If you watch your baby when he nurses, you can see the muscles in his face moving.

If you give your baby a bottle, the milk flows quickly and constantly. The baby grasps only the nipple to suck and uses his tongue to compress the nipple to stop the milk flow.

Because milk from a bottle flows much faster, the baby may learn to prefer the bottle and refuse to nurse, or he may not nurse as strongly. This is why you should avoid using bottles or pacifiers for at least the first four to six weeks, if possible.

TIP

One of the best things you can use to help heal your nipples is free: your own breast milk! Dab a little of your milk on sore nipples and let it dry thoroughly.

Nursing for the First time: Breastfeeding at the Hospital

In some hospitals (or if you deliver at home), your baby is placed on your naked abdomen immediately after delivery. With your doctor, nurse, partner, and mom all staring expectantly at you, you try to position the baby to nurse. Watch out — he's slippery! What on earth is your doctor doing down there? Is that the placenta? This tender moment may be a little awkward, with everything else that's going on distracting your efforts.

Starting off on the right foot

TIP

Try to ignore everything else going on around you and concentrate on the baby. Eye-to-eye and skin-to-skin contact are the best ways for you and the baby to get acquainted. If possible, don't be rushed. Sometimes nurses want to give you a one-minute token bonding session and then grab the baby away to be weighed, measured, eye-dropped, cleaned, and brought back after the doctor has put you back together. Sometimes space is tight in labor and delivery, and two or three more couples are waiting for your room.

Obviously, if your baby isn't breathing well or needs to be evaluated immediately, you won't be able to hold him right away. But if at all possible, hold him for a little bit. He may or may not be ready to nurse right after delivery; watch for clues, such as *rooting* (turning his head looking for the nipple) or sucking his hands, which show he's ready to start nursing. Doing so may save you from some frustrating first attempts to nurse before he's ready.

If your baby is taken to the warmer to be cleaned up first because that's the way things are done at Rules-Oriented Hospital, don't get upset. When the nurses finish, they'll bring the baby back to you.

TIP

If you're too distracted by the doctor pulling and tugging as he sews up your episiotomy or any tears, wait to start breastfeeding until he's finished. Try to concentrate on one major event at a time. Some women are uncomfortable and afraid to hold the baby while the doctor is stitching; if that's the case, ask your partner to hold the baby close to you so you don't have to worry about dropping him.

Sooner or later your doctor will finish putting you back together, and you can concentrate on the baby. After a minute or two of gazing into each other's eyes, you're ready for the big moment: your first breastfeeding.

Positioning the baby for comfort

Right after delivery, a healthy baby who is left alone will crawl up to his mother's breast, find his own position, latch on, and begin suckling. If you're giving birth in a hospital, your baby probably won't be given that opportunity.

Most likely, a nurse will hand you your baby after the initial weighing and measuring rituals are out of the way. Unless you've had a cesarean delivery (refer to Book 2, Chapter 5), you'll probably be sitting up or semi-reclining, and you'll naturally cradle the baby in the crook of your arm to get ready to breastfeed.

REMEMBER

You can position the baby for breastfeeding in many different ways, and changing positions helps the baby empty different duct areas in the breast. The positions described here are most common, but as you become more experienced, you can certainly try others.

The cradle hold position

The cradle hold (or *Madonna position*) is the traditional baby holding position. With the cradle hold, the baby's head rests on the crook of your arm, and you support his legs and back with your forearm (see Figure 2-2). If you're using the left breast, his head is in your left arm. Turn the baby toward you, chest to chest. (Skin to skin is wonderful if you can manage it.) You may want to put a pillow under the baby to support his weight and bring him up to breast level. Fold a pillow in half and place it under your arm, with the fold up along your side. This keeps your arms at breast level and supports them comfortably during the feeding. Use your free hand to position and support your breast.

The cross cradle hold

With the cross cradle (or *reverse cradle*) hold, the baby's head is supported with the left hand if you use the right breast. The baby's body is supported by the rest of your arm (see Figure 2-3). If you're feeding off the right breast, your right hand supports the breast. Turn the baby toward you, chest to chest. This position works well for a baby who has trouble latching on, because you have control of his head and can see his mouth better. This is also a good position if your baby arrives early; a preterm baby's head is big in relation to the rest of his body, and his neck muscles are weaker.

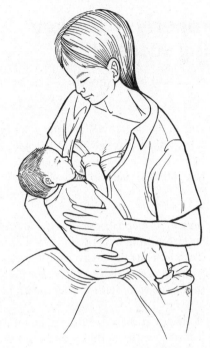

FIGURE 2-2:
The cradle hold,
or Madonna
position.

Illustration by Kathryn Born, MA

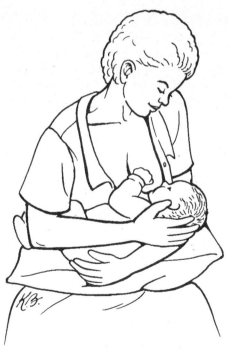

FIGURE 2-3:
The cross cradle
position gives you
better control of
the baby's head.

Illustration by Kathryn Born, MA

Latching on properly — the key to breastfeeding success!

Getting the baby to latch on to your breast properly is crucial. Latching on properly helps prevent sore nipples and ensures that your baby gets enough milk.

Make sure you're comfortable in the bed. If you're lying at a funny angle or don't have a good grip on the baby, adjust yourself. Hold the baby on his side so he doesn't need to turn his head to reach the nipple. You and the baby should be chest to chest. Bring the baby close to your breast, with his nose lined up with your nipple.

You may need to use your fingers to support your breast and make it easier for the baby to grasp the nipple. Place your thumb on the top of your breast and, forming a C, place your other four fingers below the breast to lift up. Make sure your fingers and thumb are resting on the breast tissue, not on the areola. If your breasts are very large, place a rolled-up towel in the fold underneath to give support.

TIP

Don't touch both the baby's cheeks at the same time in an effort to turn his head in the right direction. He'll turn toward anything touching his cheek, and if you touch both, you'll confuse him. Tickle his lips with the nipple; don't try to force it into his mouth.

Some babies bobble their heads back and forth wildly, looking for the nipple; others find the nipple easily but don't seem all that interested in sucking. Try to calm the bobbler down by teasing his lower lip with the breast so he'll turn toward it. If you have a bobbler, try using the cross cradle hold, which gives you better control to guide his head where it needs to go. If he finds the nipple but doesn't seem all that interested, give him a little time. Some babies want to lick the nipple for a few minutes before they nurse.

When your baby opens his mouth wide, move his mouth toward the nipple. Move the baby, not the breast. If you have a perfect baby who's read all the books, he'll turn slowly toward the nipple, open his mouth wide, pull the areola and the nipple into his mouth, and begin sucking. More likely, he'll find the nipple, open his mouth halfway like a guppy, and get frustrated and turn away because he can't get it into his mouth. Or he'll root wildly, passing the nipple a dozen times but never grabbing onto it. Keep trying — it'll happen eventually!

When the baby is latched on well, an inch or so of the areola is in his mouth. His lips are rolled out, his tongue is under the breast, and his chin is touching your breast. His nose should be resting on top of your breast, not buried in it. Figure 2-4 shows what a proper latch-on looks like.

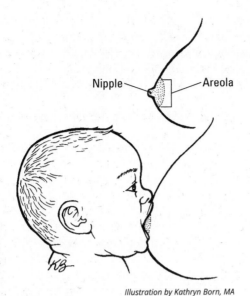

FIGURE 2-4:
Latching on
properly is the
key to successful
breastfeeding.

Illustration by Kathryn Born, MA

Several things need to take place in a perfect latch-on:

» The baby needs to open his mouth wide.

» He needs to close his mouth on the areola, not just the nipple.

» He needs to begin sucking so that the nipple and areola are pulled into his mouth to form a teat. The nipple makes contact with a spot where the baby's hard and soft palate meet; touching this spot stimulates more sucking.

» The baby needs to coordinate his ability to suck and swallow.

Removing the baby from the breast

TIP

If you need to remove the baby from your breast, break the suction by inserting your finger between your breast and the baby's mouth. Press gently on the areola and remove the nipple from the baby's mouth. If you pull the baby off without breaking the suction first, you could injure your nipple.

Feeling frustrated? It's normal

If your baby hasn't read any of the books and doesn't seem to understand the concept of nursing at all, don't worry. If your baby is the wild man type, throwing his head back and forth like the MGM lion but never getting near the nipple, don't worry. If she just brushes past the nipple without even opening her mouth, don't worry. Immediate success is nice, but it's not essential.

Try not to get upset at yourself or the baby. You're both brand-new at this, and breastfeeding is a coordinated, learned activity. Remember how long it took you to learn to ride a bike? Think of nursing the same way.

Relaxing during the first feeding

The point of the first nursing is for you and your baby to get to know each other. You're not going anywhere, and neither is the baby. You don't absolutely need to complete the first feeding in the first hour after delivery, although the baby may be very alert in the first hour or two and then sleep deeply for several hours.

REMEMBER

If you feel as though you're accomplishing nothing in your first feeding, rest assured that's not the case. You're establishing contact; the baby begins to know your smell. You're starting the bonding process. If your baby nurses well, he gets some high-calorie colostrum to carry him through the next few hours and begins to learn the mechanics of breastfeeding. Even if the baby just licks the nipple, you're starting to stimulate milk production, and you're stimulating your uterus to contract.

All that, on top of labor and delivery! You've had a busy day, so have something to eat and drink and take a nap. Your next nursing attempt will go better if you're taking care of yourself.

Chapter 3

Common Concerns and Challenges

Rarely does a woman breastfeed without experiencing some problem along the way. Most problems, like sore nipples, are easily solved. But others can be complicated to manage. This chapter discusses some of the challenges that nursing moms encounter most often and tells you how to deal with them. It also looks at the problem of not producing enough milk — or producing too much! — and the difficulties of handling a baby who doesn't nurse well, no matter what you do.

Dealing with Engorgement

When first-time moms-to-be ask, "How will I know that I'm really in labor?" women who've been there before almost always give the same answer: "Believe me, you'll *know*." The same can be said about breast engorgement.

If you haven't delivered yet, your breasts probably seem humongous, and you may think they can't possibly get any bigger. The day or two after delivery, your breasts will feel fuller. As your milk comes in, this fullness can quickly turn into engorgement.

The "before" of engorgement

Almost every new mom experiences some degree of engorgement. Engorgement begins from two to five days after you deliver and lasts 24 to 48 hours if you treat it by nursing your baby frequently. Engorgement signals that *colostrum*, your baby's first food, is turning into a more mature milk.

Before your milk comes in, you produce about 1 to 2 ounces of colostrum a day. As your regular breast milk comes in, this increases to about 20 ounces a day. In addition, your breasts have an increased blood flow and enlarged milk ducts.

You may feel like you're producing milk up to the top of your chest and into your armpits. Your breasts may be hot, hard, and shiny. This is all normal, and feeding your baby frequently resolves it.

The "during" of engorgement

Engorgement occurs whether you breastfeed or not; in fact, engorgement is usually worse in moms who don't nurse. To help minimize engorgement,

>> Begin breastfeeding as soon as you can, preferably in the delivery room.

>> Breastfeed 8 to 12 times in a 24-hour period to prevent milk from accumulating in the breasts. Nurse at least 10 to 15 minutes on one breast (and as much as 30 minutes) before switching sides. The baby may need to nurse for longer time periods in the first few days because your milk volume is low.

>> Initially, breastfeed from both breasts at each feeding; alternate the side you start with.

>> Make sure your baby empties your breasts. If she doesn't, use a breast pump to complete the job. Contrary to previous beliefs, experts now say that pumping after nursing if you're engorged does not stimulate more milk production and may help keep your milk production from decreasing due to increased swelling in the ducts.

>> Before you leave the hospital, have a lactation consultant or another nursing expert confirm that your baby is latching on correctly.

>> Avoid supplemental feedings in the beginning. Your resulting engorgement may not be worth the night's sleep that you get. If you miss a feeding, pump both breasts so they aren't twice as full for the next feeding.

Treatments for aching breasts

Although the steps in the preceding section can minimize symptoms of engorgement, they probably won't eliminate them. Following are suggestions to make you more comfortable when you're engorged:

>> Apply a hot towel to your breasts for five minutes or so, or take a warm shower. This softens the breast tissue and makes latch-on easier. A hot towel also helps get your milk flowing and catches dripping milk; the resulting increase in comfort will help with your let-down reflex.

>> Give yourself a gentle breast massage or hand-express some milk in order to improve your milk flow. Try these techniques before you start nursing; sometimes a few drops of milk on your nipple remind the baby what she's supposed to be doing. Continue the massage while you nurse your baby, massaging the breast the baby is nursing from. Massage the breast during the pause she takes between sucks.

REMEMBER

Milk production is directly related to milk emptying. If you don't take it out, Mother Nature won't put it back.

>> Wear a good supportive bra, but make sure it's not too restrictive. A too-tight bra could decrease your milk flow and cause a blocked milk duct or mastitis (see Book 5, Chapter 1).

>> Use deep-breathing techniques to relax and increase let-down. Maybe you thought you were done with breathing techniques after delivery, but they may work better for you here than they did in labor. Sometimes, when the baby first latches on, you'll feel a pain akin to his twisting your nose off your face. This can last until your milk starts flowing.

TIP

>> Cabbage leaves aren't just for Mr. McGregor's garden anymore! Place cold cabbage leaves on your breasts to reduce swelling in the breast tissue. You can put them directly on your breasts for 10 to 15 minutes before you nurse. Leaving them on longer may reduce your milk supply. Don't use cabbage leaves if you're allergic to cabbage or sulfa drugs or if you develop a rash.

>> Take ibuprofen to relieve discomfort and decrease inflammation in the breast tissue. But don't take it on an empty stomach.

>> To reduce breast swelling, use cold compresses after you nurse. Keep them on for no more than 20 minutes. You can use an ice pack, but something as simple as a bag of frozen peas often works better because it molds to the shape of your breast.

WARNING

Left untreated, engorgement can lead to *mastitis,* an inflammation or infection of the milk ducts or gland tissue that develops from incomplete emptying of the breast (see the later section "Developing Mastitis").

Knowing If You're Nursing Enough

If your baby eats every hour for an hour, you'll probably suspect that she's nursing too much. But what if the opposite is true, and you have to wake her up every five hours to eat? You may be tempted to pat yourself on the back for your baby's wonderful sense of timing, even though you know in your heart she should be eating more. How much is too much — or too little — when it comes to breastfeeding in the first few weeks at home?

REMEMBER

Unless your baby hasn't regained her birth weight after two weeks, you don't need to be preoccupied with how much she's getting at each feeding. If she's gaining well, she's eating enough. If you're still not sure, read on for suggestions on how to judge how much your baby's eating.

Weighing the baby

If you're really, *really* concerned about your milk supply, you can weigh the baby before and after a feeding to see how much she took in. This requires a precise scale (not your bathroom scale, which varies up to 5 pounds, depending on whether you lean forward or backward when you stand on it). You need a scale that weighs in ounces as well as pounds, because your baby's certainly not drinking a pound of milk at a time. You can buy a baby scale that weighs in ounces if you just have to know, but after a day or two, you'll probably get bored with weighing.

TIP

Most pediatricians have a very accurate scale, and if you ask nicely, yours may let you come in to weigh the baby, then nurse the baby, and then weigh the baby again. Keep in mind that you can't change the baby's clothes or diaper between weighings; everything has to be exactly the same so that the only variable is the breast milk.

REMEMBER

Any time you feel that the baby doesn't seem satisfied or that she shows symptoms of dehydration (see the next section), take her to the pediatrician's office for a weight check. This doesn't mean you're obsessive; it means you're an observant parent.

FEEDING ON DEMAND

Are you always starving when you eat? Do you put food in your mouth only when you absolutely need to eat? If you're like most of people, the answer is no. Sometimes, you eat because you need something else, like comfort, or you want to fill some need you can't even explain.

In your first few weeks at home, let your baby set the schedule. If you feel like you're meeting yourself coming and going at Mom's Milk Bar, remind yourself that this, too, shall pass.

Imposing a nursing schedule on a newborn may result in some of her needs not being met. For one thing, breast milk is digested quickly — much more quickly than formula. So while it may seem as if your baby can't possibly be hungry an hour or two after her last feeding, the truth is that she can be. Don't you sometimes dig through the freezer for ice cream an hour after you finish dinner?

Also, an infant has few comfort resources when something seems not quite right in her world. *You* are her primary comfort resource! She may not be hungry when she starts rooting, looking for a nipple. She may just need a little comfort.

Another reason to avoid imposing a strict nursing schedule on your baby is that her nutritional needs aren't always the same. When your baby goes through a growth spurt, she may need to nurse much more often than she normally does. Growth spurts usually occur when your baby is 2 to 3 weeks old, again when she is 6 weeks old, and around the age of 6 months. You may notice your baby wanting to nurse frequently for two or three days. The best way to handle growth spurts is to let the baby nurse as often as she needs; she'll soon settle back into her established nursing pattern.

Tip: Don't wait until your baby cries to feed her. Watch for early signs of hunger, such as turning her head as if looking for a nipple, putting her fist in her mouth, or making sucking motions.

Rest assured that as the baby gets older, she won't always want to nurse when she's unhappy. Maybe she'll respond positively to a change of scenery, a little attention, a position change, or a diaper change. Chances are you'll get her on a nursing schedule in a few months, but in the first few weeks, listen to her needs.

Common Concerns and Challenges

Checking for dehydration

A dehydrated baby shows some obvious signs. A baby who is severely dehydrated

>> **Is lethargic:** A dehydrated baby lies still and shows little interest in eating or anything else.

>> **Has skin that "tents" when you pinch it:** Instead of springing back, dehydrated skin remains somewhat folded after you pinch it.

>> **Has a sunken fontanelle and sunken eyes:** The *fontanelle* is the soft spot on the top of the baby's head.

>> **Has a slightly dry mouth:** The mouth and lips look parched.

>> **Has fewer wet diapers than normal:** Most newborns urinate frequently, up to ten times a day. Today's disposable diapers are so absorbent that you may not notice a decrease in wetness at first. If you're concerned that the baby may be dehydrated, use a cloth diaper so you can be sure she's urinating enough.

Counting dirty diapers

Newborns often pass stool every time they eat. (The good news is that breast-fed babies have slightly more fragrant diapers than bottle-fed babies!) The typical newborn breastfed baby has

>> Between 3 and 12 stools a day

>> Stools that are soft, seedy, or curdy

>> Yellowish to brownish-greenish stools

As breast-fed babies get older, they tend to have less frequent but still soft stools. Stool patterns often change at around 6 weeks of age, when the baby may have one stool each day or may have a stool every three to four days. As babies get older, they become more efficient at using more of your milk, so they create less waste. Constipation is rarely a problem for the breast-fed baby.

Soothing Nipple Issues

Nipple problems can make or break breastfeeding. Many women experience soreness in the beginning; after all, your nipples have probably never gotten this much use! Look at possible causes as soon as any soreness develops so you can try to prevent cracking, bleeding, and scabbing.

Identifying sources of pain

TIP

If your nipple begins to get sore, especially at the start of a feeding, the most important thing you can do is make sure your baby is properly latched on and that you're holding him correctly during nursing. If not, the result may be the baby pulling on your nipples and causing damage. Refer to Book 5, Chapter 2 for a detailed discussion of proper latch-on and to review breastfeeding positions.

The fungal infection *thrush,* discussed in the later section "Sharing Yeast Infections," can also cause nipple pain. Discomfort from thrush occurs throughout the feeding, not just at the beginning, and is often described as a burning sensation. If you suddenly develop this type of discomfort when you had been nursing without pain, chances are you have a yeast infection.

Coping with soreness

Beyond making sure your baby is latching on correctly, you can try the following tips:

TIP

>> Massage your breast before having the baby latch on to help soften the areola and encourage your let-down reflex. Pumping or hand-expressing a little milk prior to feeding softens the areola, which can help the baby latch on.

>> Don't just pull your baby off the breast when you're done nursing. Use your finger to break the suction so he doesn't cause nipple trauma.

   If the baby wants to keep sucking after he's had enough to eat, you can use your finger— rather than your breast — as a pacifier until the soreness decreases. (You'll know the feeding is finished when you hear long pauses between short bursts of light sucks. If he still wants to suck, offer him your finger.)

>> If you notice that your nipples are starting to get sore, try nursing more frequently but for a shorter duration (10 to 15 minutes instead of a half hour, for example).

>> Dry your nipples after each feeding. Always pat your nipples to dry them; don't rub. Air drying works best. If you can expose them to the sun without getting arrested, that's even better!

>> Avoid using soaps that can dry out the nipples and ultimately cause cracking or even eczema.

>> After a feeding, rub some of your breast milk on each nipple and let it dry. Then apply a coat of a purified lanolin cream (assuming you don't have an allergy to wool products).

>> Feed your baby on the side that is less sore, at least until your milk lets down.

>> If you use breast pads to absorb milk leaks (see Book 5, Chapter 2), make sure they don't have plastic liners, and change them frequently so bacterial growth doesn't occur.

If soreness progresses to nipple cracking or bleeding, add these measures to your arsenal:

>> Continue to nurse, even if your nipples are bleeding; your baby won't be harmed. If your nipples start to scab, soften the scabs by hand-expressing some milk, rubbing it on your nipple, and letting it dry before putting your bra or clothing on. Use a purified lanolin cream after nursing.

>> Place ice on your nipples right before nursing, but keep it there only for very short periods so your nipples don't become numb. (Numbness can interfere with let-down.)

>> If ice doesn't help you, try a warm compress (a hot wet washcloth) for a few minutes right before you nurse.

>> If you're in considerable pain, try hand-expressing or pumping for a day, and feed your baby the expressed milk.

>> Use a breast shell (see Book 5, Chapter 2) to keep pressure off a sore nipple when you're wearing clothing, but use it only for short time periods. Make sure that your bra isn't rubbing against your nipples.

>> After you nurse, rinse your nipples with a saline solution. Mix ⅓ teaspoon table salt in 1 cup warm water. You can also buy packaged saline solutions at pharmacies. Spray the solution on the nipple area with a squirt bottle, and then pat it off.

>> Contact a health professional or lactation consultant if you're not seeing any improvement or if you develop a fever, which could mean a more serious infection. Ask about topical antibiotics, which can be thinly applied. A triple antibiotic like Polysporin (an over-the-counter medication) is better than Neosporin (an antibiotic ointment containing neomycin), which could cause a rash around your baby's mouth. Some recommended topical antibiotics are available by prescription only. Always discuss antibiotic use with your doctor or lactation consultant first.

Developing Mastitis

You don't have to be a nursing mom to develop *mastitis*, a breast inflammation, but nursing mothers are more prone to mastitis, because bacteria that cause the inflammation usually enter the breast through cracks or fissures in your nipples.

Mastitis occurs most often in the first month of breastfeeding, but it can occur at any time. Sometimes the first sign of mastitis is feeling like you've got the flu. You may run a fever (over 100.4° F), have chills, or feel achy or ill. Another obvious sign of mastitis is having red, hot, or swollen areas on your breast. Usually only one breast is affected — more often the left than the right.

TIP

A plugged duct — when milk becomes clogged in a duct — may feel like a tender lump in your breast, but it differs from mastitis because it's not usually accompanied by a fever or flu-like symptoms. If not treated, a plugged duct can lead to mastitis.

Realizing risk factors

WARNING

If you're rundown and stressed, or if your immune system isn't functioning properly, you're more likely to develop mastitis. Other risk factors for mastitis are

>> **Incomplete emptying of the breast:** Milk ducts can become blocked if the baby doesn't remove enough milk from the breast, because the milk sitting in the ducts thickens. Blocked ducts increase the risk of mastitis.

>> **Missed feedings:** If you supplement, make sure you pump enough to compensate for the missed feeding.

>> **Sustained pressure on your breast:** This pressure can be from wearing a too-tight bra, carrying a heavy purse or diaper bag, using a baby carrier, sleeping on your stomach, or sleeping with the baby lying on top of you.

>> **Poor latch-on:** If the baby isn't properly positioned, he won't empty the milk ducts thoroughly.

>> **History of breast surgery or trauma:** Women with this type of history may be prone to developing blocked ducts and mastitis. Women with *fibrocystic breasts* (breasts that contain cysts) may also have this problem.

>> **Sudden weaning:** If you stop breastfeeding suddenly, you're more likely to develop blocked ducts. If you have to wean suddenly, pump your milk until you can gradually decrease the supply of milk you're making.

>> **Yeast infections:** If your baby has *thrush* (a yeast infection in the mouth, discussed in the later section "Sharing Yeast Infections") or if you have a yeast infection, it can lead to mastitis.

Treating the infection

If you experience the common symptoms of mastitis, see your doctor. Most likely, she'll prescribe antibiotics. You should feel better and see an improvement in the breast within 48 hours after starting the prescription; if you don't, call your doctor because you may need a different antibiotic. Make sure you finish all the medication, or the infection may return — and it may be worse than it was initially.

TIP

You can take pain relievers such as ibuprofen or acetaminophen as needed. Alternating hot and cold packs may also help relieve the discomfort. Gently massaging the affected area can increase blood flow and loosen plugs in the ducts.

Following are other helpful steps to take:

>> **Drink lots of fluid.** Staying hydrated helps you feel better and recover faster. This is especially important if you run a high fever.

>> **Get lots of rest.** Remember that you're sick. You need to lie down as much as possible. Doing so helps your immune system fight off the infection.

>> **Go braless or wear a loose-fitting bra.** Put as little pressure as possible on the breasts.

>> **Nurse in different positions.** Vary the holds you use while nursing so that all the ducts get thoroughly emptied.

Continuing to nurse

If you have mastitis, you should continue to breastfeed. Otherwise, the infection could turn into an *abscess,* an isolated pocket of pus that would need to be drained surgically.

If possible, start each feeding with the affected breast to make certain the ducts are being drained completely. You may find this too painful; if you do, start with the unaffected side and switch after your milk lets down. Nursing is usually more comfortable after let-down occurs.

REMEMBER

Some babies may refuse to nurse on the affected side because the milk tastes more salty than normal due to the inflammation. If that's the case, you'll have to thoroughly pump the affected side to make sure the infection doesn't worsen.

Nursing with mastitis is not dangerous for the baby. Either the bacteria that caused the infection came from the baby's mouth to begin with, or you passed the bacteria on before you realized you had the infection. Continuing to nurse ensures that the baby benefits from the antibodies you're developing to fight the bacteria.

Having mastitis more than once

Some women are prone to mastitis, developing it several times. Not only is this frustrating and debilitating, but it may also make you question whether breast-feeding is right for you.

If this happens to you, you need to look carefully for the cause. In addition to those listed earlier, causes of mastitis include the following:

» **Not finishing the complete course of antibiotics.** Many people stop taking antibiotics as soon as they start feeling better, figuring they don't need them anymore. This allows more resistant and stronger strains of bacteria to infect you again. Make sure you finish all your medication!

» **Are you run down?** Make sure you're eating well and resting enough and that you aren't anemic. Keep taking your prenatal vitamins to help supply nutrients you may be missing. Don't try to be superwoman, maintaining five carpools and two PTA positions as well as spackling the bathroom and refinishing the deck while nursing with one hand. Sit down and enjoy the experience of nursing!

Sharing Yeast Infections

Perhaps you've experienced a vaginal yeast infection — the incredibly itchy, cheesy white growth you can get from taking antibiotics or wearing nylon under-wear. When you're nursing, yeast can grow on your nipples or in your baby's mouth, causing problems for both of you.

Realizing the origins of Candida

All of us carry some forms of microorganisms on our skin. *Candida* is a yeast (a fungus) carried by half the population. Normally, microorganisms such as *Candida* cause no problems at all. However, if the normal balance between good and bad microorganisms in your body is upset, the harmless yeast fungus can overgrow, causing symptoms such as painful red skin, itching, and a white appearance.

Yeast usually flourishes for one of two reasons: Either the good bacteria that keep problem-causing organisms like yeast under control are destroyed (as is the case when you take antibiotics), or an area that is usually fairly dry becomes more moist than normal. Yeast thrives in dark, warm, moist areas — a yeast infection can be in your vagina, under your breasts, in the baby's diaper area or mouth, or even under your fingernails!

Wearing wet breast pads for extended times can also give *Candida* a nice, warm growth area, especially because the fungus grows well in the sugar found in breast milk.

REMEMBER

Both you and your baby need to be treated any time one of you has a yeast infection so you don't keep passing it back and forth to each other. Yeast is tenacious! Be sure to ask both your obstetrician and the baby's pediatrician for medication to treat both of you. Your partner can also develop a yeast infection on the head of his penis; he may need to be treated as well.

Thrush little baby, don't say a word

Thrush generally affects babies in one of two ways: as a mouth infection called *oral thrush* or as a diaper rash. Both are uncomfortable, and oral thrush can interfere with nursing.

Oral thrush usually shows up as white patches inside the baby's mouth, including on the tongue. If you wipe the white area off, you can see reddened, irritated skin underneath. The baby may refuse to nurse, or he may nurse only a short time before crying. He may be especially gassy (a side effect of yeast). Before the patches show up, you may notice that the baby's saliva and the insides of his cheeks have what's been described as a *pearly* appearance.

The baby may or may not have yeast in the diaper area at the same time. Diaper rash is especially common if the baby is heavy; yeast grows in the moist crevices. Instead of white spots, you may see a bright red, bumpy rash; the affected skin may be cracked and oozing clear fluid and blood.

If you suspect that your baby has thrush, consult your pediatrician for treatment.

Battling your own yeast infections

You may have a yeast infection and not even know it. With all the discomforts of late pregnancy, a yeast infection may go unnoticed.

REMEMBER

You probably associate yeast with vaginal infections, but yeast can grow anywhere the conditions are right. Pregnancy can foster yeast growth for several reasons: You may develop extra folds of skin under your enlarged abdomen and breasts; you may experience increased perspiration; and your hormone levels spike. Even your chocolate cravings can contribute to the problem, because yeast thrives in a sugar-laden environment!

If you receive antibiotics after a cesarean delivery, you can easily develop a yeast infection, because killing off the good bacteria along with the bad allows yeast to overgrow. You can infect your nipple with yeast by touching another yeasty area, such as your vagina, and then your nipple, or the baby can infect you with thrush from his mouth.

Yeast on your nipples may not be visible at all; your first symptom may be sharp, stabbing pain in the nipple. Sometimes infected nipples crack, itch, burn, or turn bright red. You may even experience shooting pains in the breast.

TIP

If your nipples are infected, your first treatment should be to always wash your hands before touching them. Also, rinse your nipples after each feeding, using either plain water or a vinegar solution made with a tablespoon of vinegar per cup of water. This changes the pH of your skin to make it less hospitable for the yeast to grow.

To cure the fungus, first try a local treatment. After each feeding, apply an anti-fungal cream to your nipples and areola. Gently wipe off any excess if you can still see it before the next feeding.

If topical solutions don't work, consult your doctor, who can prescribe a medication to take care of the problem. Also, be sure to talk to your lactation consultant. She may have additional information on how to help you treat thrush.

Knowing When Crying Becomes Colic

Do you recognize this baby? She's sleeping peacefully in her infant seat as you stir the spaghetti sauce for dinner. Suddenly, she wakes up, draws her knees up to her chest, and begins to howl. You try feeding her, rocking her, carrying her in the sling, putting her in the swing, singing to her, and jiggling her up and down, but she just cries. And cries. By the time your partner walks in, two hours later, you and the baby are both sobbing. You shove the baby at him, pour the burned spaghetti sauce down the disposal, and collapse in a heap on the nearest chair.

The first time this happens, you may chalk it up to a bad day. By the fourth or fifth day in a row, your worst suspicions are confirmed: Your baby has colic.

Recognizing the signs

Distinguishing a crying infant from a colicky infant isn't difficult. Both babies are trying to tell you something, but with the crying baby, you can usually figure out what it is. A colicky baby is just as confused as you are, uncertain about why she's feeling this way.

The word *colic* comes from the Greek word *kolikos*, which translates roughly into "colon." Colic has long been thought to be a gastrointestinal problem. Unfortunately, no one is really sure what colic is or why it happens. One thing that everyone involved knows is that it can bring parents as well as babies to tears.

Colic attacks start early, at around 2 weeks old. Colic occurs in about 20 percent of babies, occurring equally in boys and girls, whether breast-fed or bottle-fed. It generally reaches a peak at around 6 weeks but may continue until 4 months of age. The worst part of this early infancy condition is that there's no known cause and no specific treatment. This is what makes a colicky baby so frustrating.

Colic seems to occur most often in first-borns. Perhaps that's due to first-time parents being nervous about their parenting skills. We can attest that parenting skills become more fine-tuned with each baby, resulting in calmer, more relaxed parents. But beware: Even if your first three babies are angels, the fourth one may have colic.

As quickly as it comes, colic can disappear, or the good days may slowly replace the bad ones. However it ends, by the time it goes away, everyone in your household will be exhausted, frazzled, and praying that your baby will soon go off to college.

REMEMBER

Colic-type symptoms occasionally indicate a more serious problem. If your baby develops colic, notify your pediatrician to rule out any potential serious conditions that the colic symptoms could camouflage.

Avoiding foods that upset baby

Sometimes what you eat can aggravate colic. If you suspect this may be the case, experiment with eliminating certain foods from your diet to see whether the colic improves.

If your baby's colic is worsened by what you eat, cow's milk is the most likely culprit. Gas can form inside her bowel from the protein in the cow's milk, causing cramping, diarrhea, abdominal pain, or vomiting. Sensitivity to cow's milk doesn't happen overnight. It usually takes about two to three weeks before a colicky reaction shows up.

To test for cow's milk sensitivity, completely eliminate dairy products from your diet for at least two weeks. If dairy products are the culprit, you'll see a much happier baby within four to five days. If you don't see an improvement in a week or so, dairy is probably not the culprit.

REMEMBER

Lactose intolerance and milk protein allergy aren't the same thing. Lactose intolerance is rare in infants, usually developing after age 2. People of Asian, African, or Hispanic descent have a higher chance of being lactose intolerant. If you're a member of one of these ethnic groups, you may be surprised to find that you feel better yourself when you lower your dairy intake.

Some foods — such as cabbage, broccoli, and beans — have a reputation for causing intestinal problems or for giving your milk a flavor that the baby may refuse. Spicy foods and foods that give you gas may cause your baby to have an upset stomach. Then again, they may not!

TIP

Before dismissing things like corned beef and cabbage permanently from your diet, try them one at a time. Doing so can help you figure out whether your baby reacts negatively when you eat them.

Another common culprit is caffeine, which can make you and your baby more restless and irritable. Try to limit yourself to two caffeinated drinks per day.

WARNING

Watch out for foods that you or your partner is allergic to, because allergies sometimes run in families (although more commonly, it's the tendency toward allergies rather than a specific allergy that's inherited). In addition to cow's milk, common allergenic foods include peanuts, eggs, wheat products, soy, citrus foods, corn, and fish. An allergy could cause colic symptoms, or it could take the form of asthma, diarrhea, or eczema. Babies exposed to allergens at an early age are more likely to develop allergic reactions to them later in life.

Nursing through colic

Nursing from both breasts at each feeding may result in the baby getting too much foremilk and not enough hindmilk. The *hindmilk* — the creamier milk that appears after the baby has been eating for several minutes — has a high fat content that is needed to satisfy her hunger. If the baby doesn't get the hindmilk, she needs to nurse more often. This means she takes in more foremilk, which contains more sugar. The sugar load, without the fat to balance it, can cause gas and explosive bowel movements.

TIP

If your baby's distress seems to be accompanied by loose green bowel movements, she may be getting too much foremilk. Try letting her nurse as long as she wants on one breast so she gets enough hindmilk to keep her satiated longer. When she nurses again, start on the opposite side and repeat the process.

Common Concerns and Challenges

REMEMBER

Colic-type symptoms are not a reason to give up breastfeeding. Chances are that your baby's symptoms would worsen if you switched to formula. Colic symptoms should resolve within four to six months.

Getting an Uncooperative Baby to Nurse

Your baby needs to nurse frequently in order for you to develop a good milk supply. In the first couple days of life, most babies are sleepy and nurse only six to eight times a day. By day three, they're waking up and eating more frequently. Try to nurse every two to three hours after the first few days (count the time from the start of one feeding to the start of the next), or 10 to 12 times in a 24-hour period. This is your full-time job right now, and the job description is simple: Get to know your baby and build up your milk supply.

But what if your baby hasn't read the job description and is too sleepy, too uninterested, or too frantic at feeding time? Don't get discouraged. Trust that perseverance will win out.

Looking for hunger signs

Newborns haven't quite mastered the art of letting you know when it's time to eat. Your baby's hunger signs may be subtle, such as

>> Sucking his lips, his tongue, his fingers, or his fists

>> Starting to fidget (which indicates he's not in a deep sleep anymore)

>> Turning toward your breast (especially if his mouth is open)

REMEMBER

Crying is a late sign of hunger. Try to read these earlier hints so your baby doesn't get too hungry. If he starts crying, you may have a harder time calming him down and getting him to nurse.

Feeding the uninterested baby

If they're not medicated, most babies are interested in breastfeeding shortly after delivery. However, if you need pain medication during labor or require a cesarean delivery, your baby may not be as alert or interested in feeding immediately after delivery. It may take a while before your milk comes in and he's interested in actively breastfeeding. During this period (which can be as long as 10 days), your baby may seem uninterested and distant. Although this is very frustrating, remember that many babies react this way.

REMEMBER

Some moms feel rejected by this lack of interest. Keep in mind that your baby isn't consciously deciding he isn't interested in breastfeeding, and he isn't rejecting you or your milk.

Some babies won't nurse right after delivery if they've been suctioned vigorously and have an aversion to anything placed in their mouths. If your baby had some fluid in his nose and mouth that needed to be suctioned out right after delivery, he may not appreciate a nipple in his mouth, but this lack of interest will be short-lived. Keep in mind that pacifiers will draw the same response. If someone jabs a pacifier into the baby's mouth too hard or too early when he's not ready to suck, he may feel startled and upset, setting up a negative reaction to mouth stimulation.

Remember also that, like you, the baby's been put through a complicated physical experience. Maybe his neck was at a funny angle during delivery and the position you're holding him in is uncomfortable. Try changing positions before you throw in the towel on breastfeeding.

You can also set the mood for nursing. Here are some things you can do to encourage him to relax and breastfeed:

>> **Talk to him.** Make eye contact.

>> **Unwrap him so he's not quite as warm and cozy.**

>> **Keep the lights dimmed.** He's very much like the sleepy baby who is retreating from activity.

>> **Lie on your side to nurse.** This encourages you both to relax.

>> **Take some time to stroke your baby.** Gently rub his body. Skin-to-skin contact is a great way to entice and interest your baby.

>> **Let him suck on your finger initially, stimulating his upper palate.** When he seems ready to nurse, try to put him on the breast.

>> **Tease him with some drops of expressed milk on his lips.** Remind him what you're both doing here.

>> **Encourage your let-down reflex.** Some babies get frustrated quickly — if the milk isn't pouring into their mouths, they're going to go somewhere else, like to sleep! Place a warm washcloth on your breasts to get your let-down engine running. Use breast massage while you nurse. Some babies start nursing eagerly but lose interest when the flow decreases; gently massaging the ducts helps keep a steady flow coming.

>> **Try short, frequent nursing sessions.** Nurse whenever you can. If he seems even the slightest bit awake and alert, try to get him on the breast. Remember, this frequent nursing is necessary only until he gets with the program.

If he stays uninterested for more than 24 hours, you'll have to pump to get your milk to come in, and you may have to feed him the expressed milk through a cup, bottle, or lactation aid. If you persist in trying every few hours or so, he should get with the program.

If none of these suggestions helps, get the assistance of a lactation consultant or La Leche League leader.

Calming the frantic nurser

Some babies seem quite anxious to nurse but can't seem to grasp the mechanics. They brush past the nipple, mouth open, over and over until they become frustrated and start crying. This turns into a vicious cycle: The baby cries because he can't grasp the breast, and he can't grasp the breast because he's crying. What can you do to stop this merry-go-round without joining him in the frustration?

First, don't feed the fire. Take a deep breath and try to keep calm. Babies are very sensitive to their surroundings. (This is a good thing to remember throughout motherhood.) If you get upset about his behavior, he'll become tenser.

TIP

If he works himself into a real frenzy, help him calm down and start again. Try the following suggestions:

>> **Walk around the room with him.** Babies love movement. He's used to it — he walked with you for nine months.

>> **Cuddle him in the cradle position or bundle him snugly with a lightweight blanket so his arms and legs are close to his body.** Some babies miss the tightly held feeling they had in the womb, so try to recreate it.

Many times a baby becomes frantic because he missed his early hungry stage while he was sleeping. When he wakes up, he's overly hungry. To prevent this, feed your baby when you see early hunger signs; don't wait for him to cry. Nursing him more frequently also helps by preventing your baby from getting to the frantic stage if it's caused by hunger.

If you're certain that your baby isn't overly hungry but he's still frantic, explore other possibilities. Try changing his position; he may have a sensitive neck or a sore throat after delivery, or he may just prefer another position. Support his neck so his head doesn't wobble. It sounds simple, but sometimes simple things work.

REMEMBER

As you attempt to soothe your baby, make sure you're not stroking both cheeks. Babies have a rooting reflex that causes them to turn their heads toward the source of the stroking. If you're touching both cheeks, you'll confuse and frustrate him.

Focusing on Baby's Weight

Weight loss in a newborn is normal within certain limits. If you breastfeed frequently, and if your baby latches on properly and nurses long enough to get the *hindmilk* (the creamier milk that comes later in a nursing session), she'll regain weight very quickly.

Some babies, however, are a little slower to regain weight than others. If your baby is gaining weight slowly, ask a professional to assess her nursing skills. Together you can make sure your baby is

>> Nursing often and long enough (at least every 2 hours, lasting at least 15 to 20 minutes on each breast)

>> Sucking vigorously enough to cause a let-down reflex in your breasts; you should hear and see swallowing

>> Latching on properly to stimulate milk production

>> Emptying the breasts with each feeding and appearing satisfied after nursing

>> Looking healthy, bright-eyed, active, and alert

A weight gain of 4 to 7 ounces per week or an ounce a day is considered normal for the breast-fed newborn. However, this is an average: Babies don't gain weight back in a textbook-perfect format.

REMEMBER

Babies who are larger at birth tend to regain weight at a slower pace. They should, however, regain and surpass their birth weight by 14 days. Baby boys gain weight a little faster than baby girls.

6

Special Conditions

Contents at a Glance

Chapter 1

Pregnancies with Special Considerations

No two pregnancies are exactly alike. If you're like most women, you figure out pretty early in the game that your experience is different in some way from every friend and relative you talk to. You're not as nauseous as your sister was during the first three months — or your morning sickness is 20 times worse than your best friend's. You feel comfortable exercising throughout your pregnancy, although your cousin Jennifer was put on bed rest. Plenty of variation occurs within the boundaries of what's considered to be a "normal" pregnancy. But some special kinds of pregnancies come with their own particular characteristics and challenges. This chapter focuses on them.

Figuring Out How Age Matters

Whether you're a prospective father or mother, age can make a difference. Special problems and issues arise for men and women in their late 30s and older. Teen moms also face unique challenges. This section covers these challenges.

Over-30-something moms

Long gone are the days when almost all pregnant women were in their early 20s (and many were in their teens). Now, a greater number of women postpone having families until they've not only finished their education but also had time to become established in their careers. These days, too, divorce is more common, and many women find themselves having children with a second husband — often when they're well into their 30s or 40s (and sometimes 50s).

How old is too old? The answer used to be when you reach menopause — or even some years earlier — when your body no longer produces healthy eggs that can be fertilized to become embryos. But today, because of advances in assisted reproductive technologies like in vitro fertilization (IVF), which may use eggs donated by another woman, even women who are past the age of menopause can become pregnant. Also, over the last few years, there have been incredible advances in *egg freezing*, so even if you aren't ready to have children, eggs can be frozen and stored until the time is right.

REMEMBER

Today, a more useful question is "At what age do you need to watch out for special problems?" And here, the answer is more specific. Any woman who is at least 35 years old during her pregnancy falls into the medical category of *advanced maternal age,* or AMA. (An impersonal term, to be sure, but perhaps less insulting than the alternatives that are also used: *older gravida, mature gravida,* and the particularly unfortunate *elderly gravida.*) The reason for singling out older mothers with any special term at all is that the incidence of certain chromosomal abnormalities increases with advancing maternal age. At age 35, the risks begin to increase significantly, as shown in Figure 1-1.

Doctors formerly concluded that at age 35, the risk of the fetus carrying some chromosomal abnormality was great enough to equal the risk of pregnancy loss after undergoing amniocentesis (about 0.5 percent at that time, although now the risks are thought to be much lower, 1/300 to 1/500 or even lower). Genetic testing — either amniocentesis or chorionic villus sampling — was routinely offered for pregnant women older than 35 in the United States. Some practitioners still adhere to the traditional age-35 dictum, but the American Congress of Obstetricians and Gynecologists now recommends women of all ages be offered the option of screening for Down syndrome — either by nuchal translucency screening, chorionic villus sampling, or amniocentesis (see Book 2, Chapters 1 and 2).

Maternal Age and Chromosomal Abnormalities (Live Births)		
MATERNAL AGE	RISK FOR DOWN SYNDROME	TOTAL RISK FOR CHROMOSOME ABNORMALITIES*
20	1/1667	1/526*
21	1/1667	1/526*
22	1/1429	1/500*
23	1/1429	1/500*
24	1/1250	1/476*
25	1/1250	1/476*
26	1/1176	1/476*
27	1/1111	1/455*
28	1/1053	1/435*
29	1/1000	1/417*
30	1/952	1/384*
31	1/909	1/384*
32	1/769	1/322*
33	1/602	1/286
34	1/485	1/238
35	1/378	1/192
36	1/289	1/156
37	1/224	1/127
38	1/173	1/102
39	1/136	1/83
40	1/106	1/66
41	1/82	1/53
42	1/63	1/42
43	1/49	1/33
44	1/38	1/26
45	1/30	1/21
46	1/23	1/16
47	1/18	1/13
48	1/14	1/10
49	1/11	1/8

FIGURE 1-1: As maternal age rises, so do the risks of chromosomal abnormalities.

*Source: Data of Hook (1981) and Hook et al. (1983). Because sample size for some intervals is relatively small, confidence limits are sometimes relatively large. Nonetheless, these figures are suitable for genetic counseling. *Excluded for ages 20–32 (data not available).*

Recently, noninvasive prenatal screening (NIPS, or noninvasive prenatal testing, NIPT) has become available for women 35 and older. This actually identifies fetal DNA in Mom's blood and has a high detection rate for Down syndrome and disorders involving an extra chromosome 13 or 18. This can also tell the sex of the baby. It's important to remember that NIPS is still a screening test and not a definitive test. Currently, the test isn't available to women carrying multiple gestations, although research over the next few years may determine its utility in these situations.

The good news is that except for this increase in certain chromosomal abnormalities, babies born to women older than 35, or even older than 40, are as likely as any other babies to be healthy. The moms themselves do stand a higher-than-average risk of developing preeclampsia or gestational diabetes (see Book 6,

Chapters 2 and 3), and they stand an increased risk of delivering early or needing a cesarean delivery. Additionally, and for reasons not quite understood, women over age 35, and especially over age 40, are at a higher risk for stillbirth. Some doctors recommend closer surveillance in the last month of pregnancy and even earlier delivery at about 39 weeks. Still, these risks aren't terribly high. Naturally, an older woman's experience with pregnancy depends to a large extent on her underlying health. If a woman is 48 years old or even 50 but she's in excellent health, she's likely to do extremely well.

Not-so-young dads

As mentioned earlier, pregnancies in older women call for some special scrutiny because of the increased risk of genetic complications. To some extent, pregnancies involving older dads should likewise be singled out for observation. There's no absolute age cutoff for "advanced paternal age," but many people use 45 or 50 (although some argue it should be 35, just as it is for women).

A WORD ABOUT ALTERNATIVE CONCEPTIONS

Thanks to assisted-reproductive technologies, more and more women older than 40 are becoming pregnant, some even with twins or triplets. Although many of these women conceive with their own eggs, many others conceive with someone else's. These women have unique issues to deal with, including what to tell their future children, friends, and family. Some, when they're pregnant, experience internal conflicts about the baby's genetic identity; they worry about the fact that their baby is biologically related to someone else and what that may mean. But often, these concerns disappear when the woman begins to feel her baby moving around inside her — and if not then, as soon as the baby is born.

Parents — even parents of children conceived the old-fashioned way — often discover after they meet their new baby in person that each child's identity is unique and that the exact genetic ancestry doesn't matter nearly as much as they thought it would. So it makes sense that women who've had children conceived with donor eggs typically find that, after only a few days of caring for the new baby, they feel every bit as maternal as any biological mother would. The same is true of fathers of children who've been conceived with donor sperm. As the number of people having children with donated eggs or sperm grows, the whole experience is likely to become more comfortable for everyone involved.

Whereas for women the main genetic risk is having a fetus with a chromosomal abnormality (most commonly an extra chromosome), for men the risk is spontaneous gene mutations in the sperm, which can lead to a child with an autosomal dominant disorder, such as *achondroplasia* (a type of dwarfism) or neurofibromatosis. It only requires an abnormal gene from one parent to cause this kind of problem. (In so-called recessive genetic disorders — cystic fibrosis and sickle-cell anemia, for example — both parents must provide an abnormal gene for the problem to occur.) Autosomal dominant disorders are very rare, however, and many are impossible to test for, which is why no routine testing exists for advanced paternal age. Also, some studies suggest a slightly higher risk of autism with older dads, but again, the exact age at which this risk increases isn't quite clear, and it's still an unusual factor in this disorder.

Very young moms

Pregnancy in teenage women raises a different set of concerns. Although this age group doesn't sustain any increase in chromosomal abnormalities, these women may experience a higher incidence of some birth defects. Because teenage moms tend to have less-than-optimal nutritional habits, they also experience a higher incidence of low-birth-weight babies. Teenage moms are also at a higher risk of developing preeclampsia, are more likely to deliver by cesarean delivery, and are less likely to breastfeed. Due to their unique situation, young moms need special guidance and counseling. If you're a teenage mom, make sure you receive adequate prenatal care, follow a healthy diet, and consider the benefits of breastfeeding (see Book 5, Chapter 1).

Having Twins or More

Having twins may seem simple — to someone who's never faced the reality of it. It's either "double the pleasure" or a living nightmare (twice the work and only half the sleep). Twins are complicated, as any mother of twins can tell you — for hours and hours, if you're willing to listen. A sizable part of having twins, triplets, or more is the experience of pregnancy.

If you're having triplets or more, what applies to twins generally applies to triplets (and more), only to a much greater extent.

Although the vast majority of twin pregnancies proceed smoothly and result in the birth of two beautiful, healthy babies, some risks are involved for both the fetuses and the mom. As a result, most practitioners want women who are pregnant with twins to have checkups more frequently than other moms, and they may schedule plenty of extra ultrasound exams.

THE ODDS (AND ODDITIES) OF HAVING TWINS, TRIPLETS, OR MORE

The number of twins conceived is much larger than the number of twins who are actually born. Many pregnancies that begin as twin pregnancies end as single births because one of the fetuses never develops. In many cases, one of the fetuses disappears before the pregnancy is even diagnosed (the so-called *vanishing twin*). The incidence of twin births is usually estimated to be close to 3 percent of all births. However, the incidence is rising, mainly due to the increasing use of fertility techniques.

The incidence of spontaneous triplets is much rarer — about 1 in 7,000. Spontaneous quadruplets or more are exceedingly rare. However, with the increasing use of infertility treatments, the incidence of triplets has increased tenfold over the past few decades. Fortunately, though, the rate of increase is slowing because of refinements in infertility treatments.

Ethnic background and family history can increase your chances of having twins; certain women are constitutionally more likely to ovulate more than one egg in a cycle. If twins occur in your family, let your practitioner know.

This section takes a closer look at several questions and issues you may have if you're pregnant with twins.

Looking at types of multiples

Twins can be either identical or fraternal. These old-fashioned terms don't completely describe how twins occur.

>> *Identical* twins look very much alike and are always the same sex. They come from a single embryo, meaning they're a product of the union of one egg and one sperm. (In other words, they're *monozygotic* — they come from the same zygote.) They have exactly the same genes as each other, which explains their resemblance. In the United States, roughly one-third of all twins are identical. An egg can split into three, leading to identical triplets, but it's very unusual.

>> A woman conceives *fraternal* twins when she ovulates more than one egg, two different sperm fertilize two eggs, and the resulting zygotes implant in her uterus at the same time. These twins — who arise from two zygotes and are thus *dizygotic twins* — don't share an identical set of genes. Instead, their genetic makeup is as similar as that of any pair of children born of the same

parents. They're just born at the same time. They can be the same sex, or they can be of opposite sexes. Roughly two-thirds of all twins conceived spontaneously in the United States are fraternal. If three eggs are fertilized, the result is fraternal triplets. A triplet pregnancy can also consist of two fetuses that are monozygotic and one from a second fertilized egg — leading to two babies who are identical and one who's fraternal.

TECHNICAL STUFF

The chances that a woman will have identical twins increases after she reaches the age of 35. The chances a woman will have fraternal twins (because she ovulates more than one egg in any given month), on the other hand, rise until about the age of 35 and then drop off. Some families have more than their statistical share of fraternal twins. Some women are predisposed to ovulating more than one egg at a time, and that can lead to fraternal twins. If a woman has a history of twinning on her mother's side, she may stand a higher chance of twinning. Fraternal twinning also becomes more likely when a woman takes fertility drugs, because these medications boost her chances of ovulating more than one egg. Of course, a woman who takes fertility drugs can still produce an egg that gets fertilized and then splits in two to form identical twins.

Determining whether multiples are identical or fraternal

Many women who are pregnant with twins ask their doctor or sonographer during an ultrasound exam whether her twins are fraternal or identical. In some cases, the technician or your doctor can tell: If the babies are two different sexes, they're fraternal. If they're the same sex, they may be fraternal or identical. If they're the same sex or if the fetuses' sexes aren't yet visible, other findings on ultrasound can suggest whether the twins are identical:

>> An egg that splits very early after fertilization, within the first two or three days, results in two embryos that have separate placentas and separate amniotic sacs. This situation is called *diamniotic/dichorionic* (see Figure 1-2a). On ultrasound, they look no different from fraternal twins who come from two separately fertilized eggs. So with twins who have separate placentas and are of the same sex, it's impossible to tell on ultrasound if they're identical or fraternal.

>> If an egg splits between the third and eighth day after fertilization, the resulting twins are in two separate amniotic sacs but share a single placenta (see Figure 1-2b). Your doctor may use the term *diamniotic/monochorionic* to describe this situation. If, on ultrasound, your doctor or sonographer can see that a set of twins shares a single placenta, chances are they're identical. (Keep in mind, though, that sometimes determining whether there's one placenta or

two that are very close together is difficult on ultrasound.) The thickness of the membrane separating the sacs gives another clue — with two separate placentas, a thick membrane separates the two sacs, whereas with one placenta, the membrane is very thin.

>> An egg that splits sometime between 8 and 13 days after fertilization results in twins that not only share a placenta but also are in a single amniotic sac (see Figure 1-2c). Twins like these are called *monoamniotic/monochorionic*. If your doctor does an ultrasound examination and sees twins sharing the same amniotic sac, she can be sure that they're identical. This is pretty rare (1 percent of all twins, or 1 in 60,000 pregnancies).

>> An egg that splits after the 13th day of gestation results in conjoined or "Siamese" twins, which are exceedingly rare.

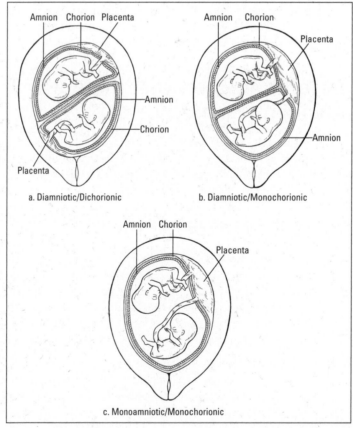

FIGURE 1-2:
Your practitioner can often tell which type of twins you're having by viewing the placenta(s) and amniotic sac(s) during an ultrasound exam.

Illustration by Kathryn Born, MA

An expert sonographer can use subtle signs to help differentiate the various types of twins, although sometimes it still may be hard to be certain. The sonographer establishes whether the twins have two separate placentas and, of less importance, whether they're actually fraternal or identical. Establishing the type of placentation (monochorionic or dichorionic) is easier in the first trimester than in the second or third trimester.

REMEMBER

Because different types of twins are associated with different problems and risks, trying to figure out which type of twinning is present is important. If the ultrasound signs are ambiguous and the medical situation suggests that determining the type of twinning is especially important, special tests can be performed to answer this question. These tests are called *zygosity* studies and require an invasive procedure, such as amniocentesis, chorionic villus sampling (CVS), or fetal blood sampling (see Book 2, Chapter 2).

Screening for Down syndrome in pregnancies with twins or more

For many years, the most common way of screening pregnancies for Down syndrome was by measuring different markers in the mother's blood at 16 weeks of pregnancy (see Book 2, Chapter 2). The accuracy of this test with twins is fair, but with triplets or more, it doesn't help at all. The newer method of Down syndrome screening in the first trimester (*nuchal translucency;* see Book 2, Chapter 1) appears to work pretty well for moms with multiple gestations because the doctor can obtain a nuchal-translucency measurement for each fetus, thus determining each fetus's individual risk of having Down syndrome.

Using the nuchal translucency and Mom's blood markers, doctors can detect about 70 to 75 percent of all cases of Down syndrome in twins. This is a little lower than the detection rate in single fetuses but still pretty good. With triplets or more, using the nuchal-translucency measurement alone tends to be the most helpful approach, because it's difficult to determine how to use the mother's blood markers in this situation.

Conducting genetic testing in pregnancies with twins or more

Chorionic villus sampling and amniocentesis are a little trickier with twins or more. The two main challenges are to make sure each fetus is sampled separately and that none of the tissue taken from one fetus contaminates the tissue taken from the other. In the case of identical twins, this issue isn't as critical, because the fetuses have the same genetic makeup. If you find a genetic abnormality (or lack of any genetic abnormalities) in one, the same is almost always true for the other. With fraternal twins, triplets, or more, testing each one separately is critical.

Amniocentesis

Amniocentesis (see Book 2, Chapter 2) is the most common way to do genetic testing in multifetal pregnancies. This method requires inserting a separate needle into the uterus for each fetus being tested. Of course, the amniocentesis is done under ultrasound guidance. After the doctor removes some fluid from the first fetus's amniotic sac, she may leave the needle in place to inject a harmless organic blue dye (called *indigo carmine*) into that fetus's amniotic sac. (Don't worry — you won't give birth to a Smurf. This blue dye is absorbed over time.) Then, if the fluid from the second needle comes out clear (not blue), the doctor knows that she has sampled the second sac. If you're carrying more than two fetuses, the doctor adds a few drops of blue dye to each consecutive sac after she taps it.

Chorionic villus sampling

Chorionic villus sampling, or CVS (see Book 2, Chapter 1), can be somewhat complicated in multifetal pregnancies, but experienced doctors can usually handle the job. In some cases, the placentas are positioned in such a way that CVS is technically impossible. In these cases, the mother has the option of having an amniocentesis a little later in the pregnancy, at about 15 to 18 weeks (rather than 10 to 12 weeks for CVS).

PATIENTS WANT TO KNOW . . .

Q: "Is doing an amniocentesis or CVS for twin or triplet pregnancies riskier than for singleton pregnancies?"

A: Although scientists have conducted little research on this question, it appears the chances of complications aren't substantially greater in multifetal pregnancies if the person performing the procedure is experienced in doing it with mothers carrying twins or more.

Keeping track of which baby is which

Your doctor designates your babies before birth as Twin A and Twin B (or Triplets A, B, and C). These designations enable your doctor to communicate to you and others (nurses and other medical personnel) which baby is which and to follow the progress of each baby separately and consistently throughout the pregnancy. By convention, the fetus closest to the cervix (the opening to the womb) is designated as Twin A (or Triplet A). This baby is usually born first. In a triplet pregnancy, the highest triplet (closest to your chest) is designated as Triplet C. (Some patients come up with their own clever names.)

Living day-to-day during a multiple pregnancy

If you're pregnant with multiples, don't ignore everything else written in this book. In many ways, your pregnancy proceeds like any other. The difference, as you may already know, is that your experience is more intense in various ways: You grow a larger belly more quickly, your nausea may be worse, your amniocentesis (if you have one) is a bit more complicated (as described earlier in this chapter), and the birth may take longer. With triplets or more, these physical changes and symptoms are even more exaggerated. In addition, certain complications are more frequent in multiples than in singletons. The following list describes many of the ways your experience may be somewhat different:

>> **Activity:** In the old days, doctors recommended women with twins be placed on bed rest beginning at 24 to 28 weeks. However, data shows women placed on bed rest appear to be no less likely than others to experience preterm delivery or have babies of low birth weight. Whether you need to reduce your activity depends on your prior obstetrical history as well as on how smoothly your pregnancy goes from week to week. If you develop preterm labor or have problems with fetal growth, your doctor may recommend you take it easy. With triplets or more, the benefit is unclear, but many obstetricians routinely recommend bed rest starting in the second trimester.

>> **Diet:** Many experts recommend women carrying twins consume an extra 300 calories a day above what is required for a singleton (in other words, an extra 600 calories per day above their pre-pregnancy intake). For triplets and more, no consensus exists, but obviously your food intake should be somewhat greater.

>> **Iron and folic acid:** Women carrying twins, triplets, or more stand a greater chance of developing anemia, which is due to dilutional anemia (see Book 1, Chapter 3) as well as greater demands for iron and folic acid. Doctors recommend supplemental iron and folic acid for women carrying two or more fetuses.

>> **Nausea:** Most women carrying two or more fetuses definitely have more nausea and vomiting in early pregnancy than women with only one. This nausea may be related to higher levels of hCG (a pregnancy hormone) circulating through the bloodstream. The good news is that nausea and vomiting for mothers of multiples, as for mothers of single babies, usually goes away by the end of the first trimester.

>> **Prenatal doctor visits:** Your practitioner is likely to follow pretty much the same routine she uses for mothers of single babies. That is, you have your blood pressure, weight, and urine checked at each visit.

But because you have more than one fetus, your practitioner may ask you to come in more frequently. Some practitioners perform routine pelvic exams to make sure your cervix isn't dilating prematurely; others may suggest your cervix be checked with an ultrasound exam. On the other hand, if you don't have any preterm labor symptoms, your doctor may decide you don't need these extra exams. (See the later section "Monitoring for preterm labor in twins" for details.)

>> **Ultrasound examinations:** Most practitioners suggest that mothers of twins or more have ultrasound examinations every four to six weeks throughout their pregnancy in order to check fetal growth. If you have any problems, these exams may need to be more frequent.

With more than one fetus, your doctor can't use fundal height measurements to evaluate the growth. And because women with twins, triplets, or more are at a higher risk of having problems with fetal growth (see the "Intrauterine growth restriction" section later in this chapter), these periodic ultrasound exams are very important. Some doctors also monitor the cervix every two weeks by transvaginal ultrasound during the second trimester to look for an increased risk of preterm birth. (For more on this, see the later section "Monitoring for preterm labor in twins.")

>> **Weight gain:** The average weight gain for a twin pregnancy is 35 to 45 pounds (15 to 20 kg). But the exact amount you gain depends on your pre-pregnancy weight. The Institute of Medicine recommends that mothers with twin pregnancies gain about 1 pound per week during the second and third trimesters.

Recent studies show that you can achieve the optimal growth rates by taking into account your body mass index (see Book 1, Chapter 3) prior to pregnancy and show that weight gain in the first two trimesters may be especially important. Doctors recommend weight gains of 45 to 50 pounds (20 to 23 kg) by 34 weeks for triplets and more than 50 pounds (23 kg) for quadruplets.

>> **Delivery:** If you're carrying dichorionic twins and everything is going smoothly, many practitioners recommend delivery by 38 weeks, 0 days to 38 weeks, 6 days because this has the best outcome for your babies. If you're carrying uncomplicated monochorionic twins, doctors recommend delivery earlier, somewhere between 34 weeks, 0 days and 37 weeks, 6 days.

Going through labor and delivery

Although some studies have suggested that in very specific situations and with very strict criteria, vaginal delivery of a triplet pregnancy may be possible, almost all triplets are delivered by cesarean. This section on birth positions and delivery is addressed to women carrying twins.

Often, pregnancy goes smoothly for mothers of twins, but labor and delivery can still be complex. For this reason, women carrying more than one fetus should deliver in a hospital, where extra personnel are present to handle any complications that may arise.

Assuming the babies are full-term, your babies can be in different positions. Basically, their positions fall into one of three possibilities:

>> Both fetuses can be head-down (vertex), as they are in about 45 percent of twin pregnancies (see Figure 1-3a). Vaginal delivery is successful 60 to 70 percent of the time when the babies are in this position.

>> The first fetus can be head-down and the second not (see Figure 1-3b), as is the case about 35 percent of the time, making a cesarean delivery more likely unless your practitioner can turn the second baby to a head-down position. Whether trying to manipulate the baby in this way makes sense is a matter of some debate among practitioners. Your doctor's choice of trying to turn the baby around or delivering the baby breech depends on her training, experience, and professional bias.

>> The first fetus can be breech or transverse (lying horizontally across the uterus), and the second can be breech, head-down, or transverse. This positioning occurs about 20 percent of the time (see Figure 1-3c).

With any of these combinations of positions, if the babies are preterm, the options may be different. In any case, discuss the possibilities with your doctor before the time of delivery.

Covering special issues for moms with multiples

If you're pregnant with twins or triplets (or more), your doctor puts you under closer surveillance because the risk of certain complications is greater in multifetal pregnancies. The following topics are some of the things she's watching out for.

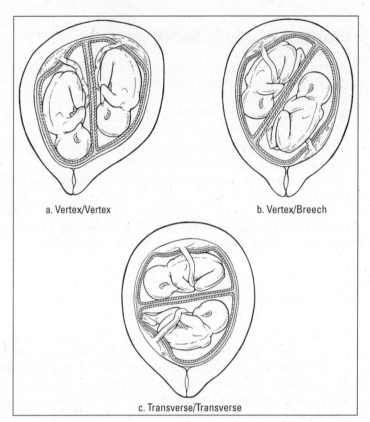

FIGURE 1-3:
Three possible
positions of twins
before delivery.

a. Vertex/Vertex

b. Vertex/Breech

c. Transverse/Transverse

Illustration by Kathryn Born, MA

REMEMBER

Don't let this list scare you. Just be aware of potential problems so that if they develop, you and your practitioner can recognize them early and manage them appropriately.

Preterm delivery

The biggest risk you face in carrying more than one baby is that you may have preterm labor and delivery. The average length of pregnancy for a singleton is 40 weeks, but for a twin pregnancy, it's only about 36 weeks; for triplets, 33 to 34 weeks; and for quadruplets, about 31 weeks. A pregnancy is full-term if it lasts 37 weeks or more. Preterm delivery is technically between 24 and 37 weeks, but most babies born at 35 or 36 weeks are generally as healthy as babies delivered after 37 weeks.

About 80 percent of mothers carrying triplets and 40 percent of those with twins experience preterm labor, but not all deliver early. (See details about preterm labor and delivery in Book 6, Chapter 2.)

Chromosomal abnormalities

When you have more than one fetus and they aren't identical, the chances that either one of them has a genetic abnormality are somewhat higher. After all, each baby has its own individual risk of some abnormality, and the risks add up. Mothers of single babies are considered to be of advanced maternal age (AMA) at 35, as described earlier in this chapter, but in twin pregnancies derived from two separate eggs, AMA may be as early as 33, and for triplets, 31 or 32. This all becomes relevant for women considering the genetic testing mentioned earlier.

Diabetes

Because the incidence of gestational diabetes is higher with twins or more, many practitioners recommend all women carrying more than one fetus be screened for this condition. (See Book 6, Chapter 3.)

Hypertension and preeclampsia

Hypertension (high blood pressure) is more common in multifetal pregnancies. The risk is proportional to the number of fetuses present. Some women develop hypertension alone, without other symptoms or other physical signs. Others develop a condition unique to pregnancy called *preeclampsia*, which involves high blood pressure in association with spilling protein in the urine *(proteinuria)*, or if proteinuria is absent, the presence of some other abnormalities (see the description of preeclampsia in Book 6, Chapter 2). Forty percent of mothers carrying twins and 60 percent or more carrying triplets develop some form of hypertension during pregnancy. For this reason, your practitioner keeps a close eye on your blood pressure.

Intrauterine growth restriction

Problems with fetal growth occur in anywhere from 15 to 50 percent of all twins. The problem is even more common in triplets and in fetuses that share the same placenta. In the case of a single placenta, the blood may not be distributed equally, which may cause one twin to get more nutrients than the other. In multiples that have different placentas, growth restriction can result when one placenta is implanted in a more favorable position within the uterus and therefore provides better nourishment than the other. Your doctor is likely to schedule periodic ultrasound exams during your pregnancy to check that both (or all three) fetuses are growing properly.

Twin-twin transfusion syndrome

Twin-twin transfusion syndrome is specific to twins who share a single placenta. In some cases, the single placenta contains blood vessels that interconnect between the two fetuses. This connection enables the two fetuses to exchange blood — and allows the blood to become distributed unequally. The fetus who gets more blood grows bigger and produces extra amniotic fluid, whereas the one who gets less blood may suffer impaired growth and have significantly decreased amniotic fluid in his or her sac. This situation can be very serious, but fortunately, it affects only 10 to 15 percent of monochorionic twins.

Multifetal pregnancy reduction

Some doctors perform the multifetal pregnancy reduction procedure to decrease the number of fetuses a woman is carrying in order to improve the chances that she delivers healthy babies. Doctors more commonly use it in women who have at least three viable fetuses resulting from fertility treatments because of the high risk of preterm delivery if they try to carry all the fetuses. Also, some women carrying twins want to reduce their pregnancy to a singleton, and this is becoming increasingly common. Usually a maternal–fetal medicine specialist performs a multifetal pregnancy reduction between 10 and 13 weeks in a special center. The risk involved is acceptably low when an experienced physician specifically trained in this procedure performs it. The important thing is to find out about all possible options so you have as much information as possible to make the best decision for you.

Selective termination

A selective termination procedure can be used in a multifetal pregnancy to terminate one of the fetuses when that fetus has a significant abnormality. A maternal–fetal medicine specialist can perform this procedure if the fetuses have separate placentas so that the medication used can't cross over and affect the normal fetus. In the case of identical twins who share a single amniotic sac, some other options are available (ask your doctor). In the latter case, only a few centers in the United States perform this procedure.

Monitoring for preterm labor in twins

Doctors aren't sure what exactly causes labor to start in any pregnancy, but it has something to do with how distended the uterus is. With twins, the uterus becomes larger much earlier than it does with a single fetus, so the risk of going into labor early — as well as delivering early — is increased. As mentioned earlier, the average gestational age when a single fetus delivers is 40 weeks. The average gestational age for the delivery of twins is 36 weeks.

Doctors have come up with ways to try to prevent premature births in twin gestations. Some approaches include putting in a *cervical cerclage* (a stitch sewn into the cervix to try to keep it closed) and using progesterone to keep the uterus from contracting. Unfortunately, neither of these two treatments has been shown to change the rate of premature delivery in twins.

Although no surefire treatments exist to prevent premature birth in twins, doctors have focused on trying to come up with strategies to predict which patients with twins are at the highest risk for delivering early. If your risk is high, your doctor may decide to admit you to the hospital for more intensive observation and to make sure you don't have preterm labor that is unrecognized. Your doctor may also give you steroid shots between weeks 24 and 34 to help your babies' lungs mature sooner in the event that you do deliver early.

Two factors that are indicators of early delivery can be examined via transvaginal ultrasound:

>> **The length of the cervix:** The cervix usually gets progressively shorter prior to delivery. Cervical length measurements are most helpful in twins between 16 and 24 weeks of pregnancy, but sometimes they're continued after that time if the situation warrants.

>> **Whether the cervix is dilating:** Early dilation is sometimes called *funneling* because the cervix looks like a funnel on ultrasound.

The frequency of the measurements depends on your own situation, but they're typically taken about every two weeks. If your cervix is long and not dilated, your chances of a premature delivery are low. If it's short or showing signs of early dilation, your doctor will probably step up the frequency of your visits or even admit you to the hospital.

Another test to predict the likelihood of delivering early involves determining the level of *fetal fibronectin* (see Book 6, Chapter 2). This substance is found in vaginal secretions obtained by using a special swab. Fetal fibronectin levels are higher in women with twins who are at an increased risk for early delivery. Even if your cervix is closed and you aren't in premature labor, if your fetal fibronectin test is positive, your doctor may decide to give you steroids.

Getting Pregnant Again

Doctors and parents haven't come to a consensus on the optimal time to get pregnant again. Probably the most important consideration is your overall health. If you can get back to your pre-pregnancy or ideal body weight quickly after you deliver, and if you can replenish any lost nutrients and vitamins (particularly folate, iron, and calcium) from your last pregnancy, you can probably consider getting pregnant again fairly soon — in about 12 to 18 months. A recent large study showed getting pregnant again in less than 18 months was associated with an increased risk of adverse pregnancy outcomes. If you've had a complicated pregnancy, a difficult delivery, or excessive loss of blood, wait until you're in better shape before trying again.

TIP

Also ask yourself what you consider to be the ideal age difference in your children. Some people feel having children close in age is better. That way, the older child doesn't have so many years to settle into the role of only child and therefore may not feel so jealous when the new baby comes. Others feel spacing the children further apart so that the older child is mature enough to handle the introduction of a new sibling is better. Most important is how you and your partner feel and how ready you are to take on another child. The decision may involve emotional and financial issues as well as physical ones. Ask yourself whether you can handle the pressure and the expense and can do the work that having another child takes.

Realizing how each pregnancy differs

Naturally, any mother compares her second pregnancy with her first, but every pregnancy is different. If your last pregnancy went smoothly, you may think any little thing out of the ordinary that happens in the next pregnancy is a signal that things aren't going well. By the same token, if your first pregnancy was difficult, you needn't assume the same complications are going to happen again. And no matter what anybody tells you, remember that different symptoms don't mean the second baby will be a different sex from your first child.

These are some of the ways in which you may experience pregnancy differently the second (or third or fourth) time around:

>> Many women feel that they're showing sooner or are at least more bloated and distended. This condition may be because their abdominal muscles have been stretched by their previous pregnancy and are now more lax.

>> Many women find that nausea isn't as severe as it was the first time around, and others find that it's worse.

>> You can usually identify fetal movement earlier.

>> Labor is usually shorter, and delivery is easier.

>> Many women find they feel Braxton-Hicks contractions earlier and more frequently than with their first child. (See Book 2, Chapter 3 for more on Braxton-Hicks contractions.)

>> Most women are less anxious the second time around.

One thing remains the same: As hard as it may be to believe, you will love your second child as much as your first.

REMEMBER

In their third pregnancy, many women commonly experience a special kind of worry: They feel that because their first two pregnancies were healthy and problem-free, the third one's bound to have complications. Many feel that they were lucky twice in a row and that going for a third time is pushing their luck. If you feel this way, believe us, you aren't alone. Keep in mind the chances of trouble aren't inherently greater in a third pregnancy, even if the first two went smoothly.

Giving birth after a prior cesarean delivery

If you've had a cesarean delivery and you get pregnant again, you may wonder whether you can deliver vaginally this time or need another cesarean. To some extent, the answer depends on which of the following kinds of cesarean you had:

>> **Low transverse:** Most cesarean deliveries are done through a low-transverse incision (across the floor in the lower part of the uterus) — see Figure 1-4a. Women who have this kind of incision usually can deliver vaginally in a subsequent pregnancy as long as they have no other complicating factors. The risk of uterine rupture is lowest with this kind of incision.

>> **Classical:** If you have what's known as a *classical cesarean*, in which a vertical incision is made in the upper portion of the uterus (see Figure 1-4b), don't try to have a vaginal delivery in a subsequent pregnancy, because this type of incision is more likely to rupture. Vertical incisions are sometimes performed in cases of very preterm birth or placenta previa (see Book 6, Chapter 2) or when the mother's uterus is an abnormal shape or has large fibroids.

>> **Low vertical:** A low-vertical incision (see Figure 1-4c) is performed less frequently than a low-transverse incision, but it does enable the mother to attempt labor and delivery in a subsequent pregnancy.

REMEMBER

The incision made on your skin doesn't reflect the type of incision on your uterus. In other words, you may have a transverse incision on your skin (a bikini cut) but still have a vertical incision on your uterus.

Doctors used to think that after a woman had a cesarean delivery, all her babies would have to be delivered the same way and that trying a vaginal delivery risked the uterus rupturing through the old cesarean scar. But studies have demonstrated that the risk of such a rupture is quite low — less than 1 percent. Discuss the issues of uterine rupture with your doctor. Other recent studies show that 70 percent of the time, women can successfully deliver a baby vaginally after they've had a cesarean.

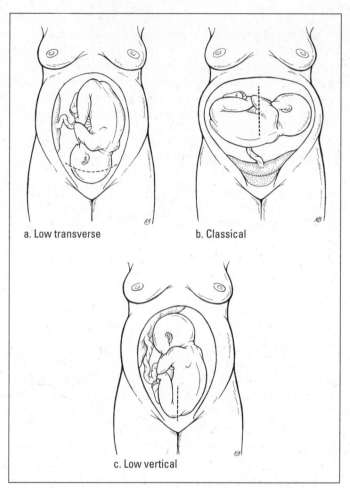

a. Low transverse   b. Classical

c. Low vertical

FIGURE 1-4:
Various kinds of
uterine incisions.

Illustration by Kathryn Born, MA

Of course, the likelihood of success depends to some extent on why a cesarean was performed in the first place. If your doctor performed it because the baby was breech, the chances that the next baby can be delivered vaginally are nearly 90 percent. If the cesarean was performed because the baby was too large to fit through the mother's pelvis, the chances of a future vaginal delivery fall to 50 to 60 percent. Some smaller hospitals are unable to offer VBAC (*vaginal birth after cesarean*) to their patients because they don't have the capacity to meet the special requirements needed to do so (like 24/7 availability of an anesthesiologist).

Why would you want to deliver your next baby vaginally? The main benefit is that if you're successful, your recovery is much shorter. Another potential benefit from a vaginal birth is that it's often associated with less postpartum pain. However, although most patients find the pain associated with vaginal birth to be less than that associated with cesarean delivery, some vaginal births have painful complications of their own. See Book 2, Chapter 7 for more information.

Other benefits of a vaginal birth include the following:

>> A lower risk of the kind of complications associated with abdominal surgery, including

- Anesthesia problems

- Inadvertent injury to adjacent organs

- Infection

- Possible blood clots from being immobile for a longer period of time

>> For some women, a psychological benefit from experiencing a vaginal birth

>> A shorter hospital stay

>> The possibility, indicated by some studies, that the baby clears her secretions more efficiently if born vaginally

However, you do have some risk: If you try labor and then end up with another cesarean, studies show that the complication rate is higher than if you went straight to a repeat cesarean without labor. Additionally, your recovery may be longer than if you had elected to have a repeat cesarean.

If You're a Nontraditional Family

Single women and gay or lesbian couples bearing children are becoming more and more common. If you fall into one of these categories, discussing your situation with your practitioner is important. Don't worry that your doctor may judge or ridicule you. Practitioners are trained to be sensitive to all patients' needs, and you're no different. If your practitioner does seem to have a problem with your situation, move on to someone who's more understanding — the sooner, the better.

In many single-mother and lesbian pregnancies, the father of the baby isn't physically present. Still, try to have information about the father's family history and ethnicity so you and your practitioner can go over any genetic implications (see Book 2, Chapter 1).

If the father isn't going to be around for the whole process, build your own support network. If you're a single mom, you may choose one or more people (family members or close friends) to share your pregnancy, labor, and delivery. If you're part of a lesbian couple, the nonpregnant partner can assume the primary support role. If the father is a male friend, include him as support. No matter the case, having your support people accompany you to any prenatal visits or prenatal classes and having them around for the labor and delivery process is completely appropriate.

Preparing Your Child (or Children) for a New Arrival

Many parents look forward to having a second child specifically because they want to provide a sibling for the first one. But your first child may not easily understand this reasoning. She may feel completely content about being the only child, and it may be months or years before the first one appreciates the second one. For those of you who are having your second child — or third or fourth (or more!) — the following sections offer a few ideas about how to help prepare the older one(s) for the new arrival. Many hospitals now offer sibling classes to help your child acclimate. Contact the hospital in which you plan to deliver for information.

Explaining pregnancy

The ease or difficulty you may have introducing a new baby sister or brother depends quite a bit on how old the elder sibling is. Explaining a new baby to a 15-year-old is easy; getting the concept across to a 15-month-old can be tricky. And the challenge begins at the time you tell the first child that you're pregnant. A 2-year-old has little concept of time and may not understand that Mom is pregnant for months before the baby comes. She may be frustrated the baby can't come immediately. So delay telling a very young child about your pregnancy until the second or third trimester, unless you don't mind being hounded every day about when the new baby is coming.

If your child is old enough — at least 2 or 3 years old — you may want to bring her along to prenatal doctor visits, ultrasound examinations, or shopping trips for baby items. (While you're doing that shopping, consider getting a small present for your child so she doesn't feel neglected.) A child who is old enough may also like to join in discussions about what to name the new baby.

TIP

If you anticipate moving your child to a new room or having her graduate from a crib to a bed, make the change before the baby is born. This change allows your older child to have a chance to acclimate so she doesn't associate the new situation directly with the new baby's arrival.

As you near the end of your pregnancy, don't be surprised if your child starts to act up or becomes unusually clingy and dependent. Many children get a sense that things are about to change when they see their mother getting physically bigger or when they overhear conversations about the impending arrival. During this time, be supportive and loving. Include your child in the preparations as much as possible. And remember that although having a new sibling affects almost all children in certain predictable ways, each child is unique, and how yours reacts depends in large part on her personality.

Making babysitting arrangements for your delivery

Obviously, you need to plan on having someone take care of your child when you and your partner go to deliver the new baby. If your delivery is scheduled (that is, you're having a planned cesarean or an elective induction), making arrangements is relatively easy. But most women don't know exactly when the big moment will arrive. And you still need to be ready beforehand.

If you go into labor spontaneously in the middle of the night, you want your child to be prepared in advance for what will happen and who will show up to take care of her while you're gone. Reassure your child you will be okay and that she can come to see you and the new baby in the hospital very soon. If possible, phone your child at home while you're in the hospital to tell her that you're doing well, especially if your labor is unusually long. Many hospitals now have special sibling visiting hours, and you may want to check out the details ahead of time.

TIP

Pack a couple of gifts to take with you to the hospital — one for your child to give to the new baby and one for the baby to give to the child.

Coming home

During the first few days that the new siblings live together, you may be amazed at how well-adjusted, happy, and excited your older child is. Part of this attitude is genuine enthusiasm. But keep in mind that part of it may also be your older child's attempt to share the limelight with the new baby. Some children have a short period of difficulty coping; others do fine at first but develop longer-lasting sibling rivalry.

Don't be surprised if your child begins to regress in terms of some developmental milestones. A previously potty-trained child may resort to bed-wetting, for example. Or a child may resume thumb-sucking or have difficulty sleeping. You may notice your older child gets especially jealous while you're breastfeeding. During this period, understand your child may need extra reassurance that you still love her and the new baby hasn't replaced her in your heart at all.

TIP

Explain that your heart is big enough to love more than one child. If possible, allow your elder child to help care for the baby. How much "help" your child is capable of providing depends on her age, but even small children can fetch a diaper if you need one or help give the baby a bath. Don't be surprised if at times your child expresses aggression toward you or the baby. Usually, these acts of aggression are harmless, but during this early stage of adjustment, don't leave your child alone with the baby unsupervised. She may not realize certain ways of handling the baby may be harmful.

REMEMBER

Several months may pass before your older child feels secure, but eventually most children do deal with the change successfully. Quite often friends, neighbors, and family shower the new baby with gifts. Again, having a stash of inexpensive new toys for your older child to prevent excessive jealousy may be a good idea. It's also a good idea to occasionally spend some one-on-one time with the older child to maintain your special bond with one another. With extra love and understanding, you can help your child through what can be a difficult period.

Chapter **2**

When Things Get Complicated

The vast majority of pregnancies are smooth, uncomplicated affairs — perfectly well managed by Mother Nature alone. Sometimes, though, your pregnancy can get a little complicated. Even when problems arise, ultimately both baby and mother are healthy in most cases. If you have no major medical problems going into your pregnancy and it remains uncomplicated, you may just as well skip this chapter. If, on the other hand, you're the type of person who wants to know about every possibility — and this kind of knowledge doesn't drive you nuts — you may find this chapter interesting.

This chapter's information is meant to either reassure you that your pregnancy is safe or, if you do have some particular problem, provide useful information to help you understand the situation better.

Dealing with Preterm Labor

Normally, during the second half of pregnancy, the uterus contracts intermittently. As the end of your pregnancy approaches, these contractions grow more frequent. Finally, they become regular and cause the cervix to dilate. When contractions and dilation occur before 37 weeks of gestation, labor is considered *preterm*. Some women notice periods of regular contractions prior to 37 weeks. If the cervix doesn't dilate or efface, however, the condition isn't considered preterm labor.

Of course, the earlier preterm labor occurs, the more troublesome it can be. The problems that a premature baby has if he is born after about 34 weeks are usually much less worrisome than those he faces if born at only 24 weeks. Prior to about 32 weeks, the main problem is that the baby's lungs may still be immature, but other complications may exist as well. Nevertheless, the majority of babies born at 26 to 32 weeks do just fine, especially if they have access to modern neonatal intensive care.

Premature babies stand a higher risk of contracting an infection, they may experience problems with the gastrointestinal tract (stomach and intestines), or they may experience an *intraventricular hemorrhage,* which is bleeding into an area in the brain.

The following can be signs and symptoms of preterm labor:

>> Constant leakage of thin fluid from the vagina

>> An increase in mucous-like vaginal discharge

>> Intense and persistent pressure in the pelvis or vaginal area

>> Menstrual-like cramps

>> Persistent lower-back pain

>> Regular contractions that don't stop with rest or decreased activity

Focusing on high-risk categories

Nobody knows for sure what causes premature labor, but clearly, some patients are at higher risk for developing it. If you fall into one of the high-risk categories, your practitioner probably will want to follow you more closely than usual. Here are some factors that put you at risk for preterm delivery:

>> An abnormally shaped uterus

>> Bleeding during pregnancy, especially during the second half (not including occasional spotting during the first trimester)

>> A prior preterm delivery

>> Some infections, like bacterial vaginosis, periodontal disease, or a kidney infection

>> Smoking

>> Abuse of certain illicit drugs

>> Being African-American

>> Poor nutrition and/or a low pre-pregnancy weight

>> Being pregnant with twins or more

A lot of women ask whether certain working conditions can increase the risks of preterm birth. There does seem to be some association between premature birth and physically demanding work, prolonged standing, shift or night work, and significant fatigue. However, having a demanding job doesn't make preterm labor a certainty by any means.

TIP

The following suggestions can decrease your chances of preterm labor:

>> **Stop (or decrease) smoking.** See Book 1, Chapter 2 for more on how smoking affects your baby.

>> **Avoid illicit drugs and alcohol.** To find out more about the risks posed by the use of these substances, turn to Book 1, Chapter 2.

>> **Reduce occupational fatigue.** Limit work to less than 42 hours per week, and minimize standing to less than 6 hours per day.

>> **Make sure you're getting adequate nutrition and hydration.** Check out Book 1, Chapter 3 for the details of a healthy diet.

>> **Try 17-hydroxyprogesterone caproate.** If you have a history of spontaneous preterm delivery in a prior pregnancy, talk to your doctor about starting a medication called 17-hydroxyprogesterone caproate. See the later section "Preventing preterm labor" for information on this medication.

Some interventions that haven't been shown to be helpful in lowering your chances of preterm labor are

>> Bed rest and hospitalization

>> Avoiding intercourse

>> Taking medications that are typically used to stop premature labor after it has set in (called *tocolytics* as a group — see "Stopping preterm labor" later in this chapter) as a preventive step to keep it from starting

>> Taking antibiotics unnecessarily

Although studies show these things haven't been shown to be beneficial, they're still sometimes prescribed in individual situations in the hope that they may help.

Checking for signs of preterm labor

Practitioners have various ways of detecting preterm labor, although the techniques aren't always effective. The most common methods are for your practitioner to check your cervix by performing an internal exam and to monitor you for contractions.

TECHNICAL STUFF

Some practitioners look for symptoms of preterm labor using transvaginal ultrasound. A small ultrasound probe is placed into the vagina next to the cervix in order to measure the length of the cervix. Measuring cervical length can help predict whether you're at an increased risk of delivering prematurely. If you're found to have a shortened cervix and are considered high risk for preterm birth, vaginal progesterone may be helpful in decreasing your chances of delivering prematurely. The routine use of cervical ultrasound for the prediction of preterm birth in women without any symptoms or risk factors is controversial. More studies are needed to show doctors how best to use transvaginal ultrasound.

Interestingly, some researchers have found that a specific type of *pessary*, which is a device placed in the vagina and around the cervix, may also help decrease preterm delivery in singletons.

TECHNICAL STUFF

A test called *fetal fibronectin* is probably the best available predictor of who is *not* likely to have preterm delivery. The test involves swabbing the back of the vagina with a cotton swab. A negative result on this test is a good indicator that delivery is unlikely within the next few weeks. A positive result, however, doesn't necessarily mean that you're going to deliver prematurely.

Stopping preterm labor

Depending on how far along you are when you develop preterm labor, your doctor may attempt to stop your contractions (assuming he believes in this practice), and you may be admitted to the hospital. Your doctor may use several medications (called *tocolytics*) to block preterm labor.

TECHNICAL STUFF

Doctors have never come to widespread agreement that these medications are useful in the long run, although they have been shown to help for a few days to a week. Most tocolytics have side effects on the mother. Terbutaline is a medication that was commonly used until 2011, when the U.S. Food and Drug Administration (FDA) issued a warning regarding its use to treat preterm labor. The side effects of terbutaline include flushing and a feeling that your heart is racing. It can also make it easier for you to develop a serious condition known as pulmonary edema, in which water accumulates in your lungs. The data suggest that the use of terbutaline should be limited to short-term in-patient use to stop preterm labor. Two other types of medications have side effects as well: Magnesium sulfate may cause nausea, flushing, or drowsiness, and indomethacin is well-tolerated, but it can't be used for too long because of some effects on the fetus with long-term use. Nifedipine has recently become the first line of treatment for many doctors because it appears to have few side effects and there are no restrictions on the length of use.

If your doctor thinks your preterm labor may lead to premature delivery prior to 34 weeks, he'll probably recommend you receive an injection of steroids, which have been shown to decrease the risk of respiratory problems and other complications in the premature newborn. The risks to the mother of taking these drugs are negligible, and large studies have shown that the steroids are beneficial to the baby for about a week. Patients who continue to be at risk for preterm delivery a week after the steroids were first administered may be given a second course of steroids under certain circumstances. In particular, if you're less than 28 weeks along and still at risk for preterm birth, a repeat course may be beneficial to the baby. Recent data suggests that using a lower dose of steroids for the second course is still beneficial and may have fewer long-term side effects.

Recently, magnesium sulfate has been used not for its anti-contractive effect but for its effectiveness in protecting the preterm fetal brain. Studies have shown that magnesium sulfate given to mothers shortly before delivering infants prior to 32 weeks reduces the chances of infant death as well as cerebral palsy.

Preventing preterm labor

Several recent studies indicate that women who are at an increased risk for a preterm delivery (see the earlier section "Focusing on high-risk categories") may have a reduced chance of delivering preterm if they take a specific type of progesterone during their pregnancies. The studies looked at both progesterone injections and progesterone vaginal suppositories.

The injections involve weekly doses of a medication called 17-hydroxyprogesterone caproate (17-P) starting at 16 to 20 weeks and continuing until about 36 weeks. The suppositories involve placement of a tablet or gel into the vagina nightly starting at 16 to 24 weeks and continuing until 36 weeks.

At this time, progesterone injections seem effective for women with a history of a prior preterm birth and possibly for women with abnormally shaped uteruses or cervical insufficiency. Recent studies suggest that high-risk women diagnosed with a shortened cervix may also benefit from progesterone therapy. Vaginal progesterone — either 90 mg gel or 200 mg suppository — can help reduce preterm birth in women with singleton gestations, without a history of a prior preterm birth, and with a short cervix found on ultrasound prior to 24 weeks. There currently isn't good enough data to recommend progesterone to women carrying twins or more.

Delivering the baby early

Sometimes delivering a baby early makes sense. When a woman experiences preterm labor at 35 or 36 weeks, for example, letting her go ahead and deliver is usually wise because the outlook for the baby is so good that there's no reason to subject the mother to the side effects of medications to forestall labor. Regardless of the gestational age, premature delivery may also be the best option in cases where the baby has a condition that doctors can't treat inside the uterus or when the mother has a condition that is worsening, such as preeclampsia (see the next section), and continuing the pregnancy would be risky.

FOR PARTNERS: NAVIGATING THE NICU

The *neonatal intensive care unit* (NICU) is like nothing you've ever seen before. Although hospitals put more emphasis than they used to on keeping NICUs quiet, they are, by necessity, fairly noisy and busy, with alarms going off, lights on day and night so hospital personnel can see what they're doing, and at the center of it all, your little baby. She may be hooked up to just a single monitor or perhaps so laden down with medical equipment and IV lines that you can scarcely find her.

The best way to deal with the NICU is to focus on your little part of the world. Get to know your baby's nurses and stay near your baby's incubator. Asking what's wrong with other babies is really bad etiquette, and the nurses won't (or shouldn't) tell you, anyway.

Preterm babies are often moved from the hospital where they're born to a level 3 nursery with advanced technology to handle complicated preterm issues. This can make your life difficult, especially if the new hospital is some distance from your house, but your baby's care is ultimately worth it.

Some hospitals with large, regional NICUs have facilities that allow parents to stay overnight for a small charge or for free. Ronald McDonald houses are examples of facilities available near some hospitals.

If your partner is still in the hospital and can't see the baby right away, make sure you take lots of pictures — not just of the baby but also of the neonatal unit and, if possible, of the people taking care of her. That way your partner can get a real sense of where the baby is and picture her in an actual place. Some regional NICUs provide a video feed to community hospitals so that moms who are separated from their babies can maintain a connection until they have a chance to see the baby in person.

Handling Preeclampsia

Preeclampsia — also known as *toxemia* or *pregnancy-induced hypertension (PIH)* — results when a woman experiences elevated blood pressure along with some other laboratory abnormalities or symptoms after about 20 weeks of gestation. This condition isn't all that uncommon, occurring in about 7 percent of pregnancies. Women having their first child are especially susceptible. Preeclampsia usually occurs late in pregnancy, but it can develop in the late second or early third trimester. The condition goes away after delivery.

Making a diagnosis

Doctors have different criteria for diagnosing the condition, but in general, blood pressure that stays above 140/90 is considered elevated if you have no history of blood pressure problems prior to pregnancy.

Recently, the criteria to diagnose preeclampsia have changed. Following are the current criteria:

>> **Recurring high blood pressure:** Systolic blood pressure ≥ 140 mm Hg or diastolic blood pressure ≥ 90 mm Hg on two occasions at least 4 hours apart after 20 weeks in a patient without any history of chronic hypertension

>> **Protein in the urine (proteinuria):** Protein in the urine of ≥ 0.3 g in a 24-hour urine specimen or protein/creatinine ratio of ≥ 0.3 mg/dL or a dipstick urine protein of 1+

>> **Other factors:** In a patient with new-onset hypertension without proteinuria, the new onset of any of the following is also diagnostic of preeclampsia:

  • Platelet count < 100,000/microliter

  • Serum creatinine > 1.1 mg/dL or doubling of serum creatinine in the absence of other renal disease

  • Certain liver enzymes at least twice normal

  • Pulmonary edema (fluid in the lungs)

  • Cerebral or visual symptoms

The presence of one or more of the following criteria is a feature of severe preeclampsia:

>> Symptoms of central nervous system dysfunction

>> New-onset cerebral or visual disturbances, severe headache, or altered mental status

>> Liver abnormalities

>> Severe persistent pain just under your rib cage on the right or in the middle just under your breastbone (sternum)

REMEMBER

Many of these symptoms can occur harmlessly during any pregnancy. Unless they happen in combination with elevated blood pressure or protein spillage in the urine, they're quite normal. If one day you have a headache, or if for a second you see spots, don't jump to the conclusion that you have preeclampsia. If the symptoms persist, though, tell your doctor.

Examining risk factors

No one knows exactly what causes preeclampsia, but it probably involves a combination of maternal, fetal, and placental factors. Some women are at a higher risk of developing it than others. Here are risk factors for preeclampsia:

>> Existing chronic hypertension

>> First pregnancy

>> History of preeclampsia in a prior pregnancy

>> Long-standing diabetes

>> Mother older than 40

>> Significant obesity

>> Medical problems such as serious kidney or liver disease, lupus, or other vascular diseases

>> Triplets or more (twins also but to a much lesser extent)

Considering treatments

Despite extensive ongoing medical research on preeclampsia, no one knows exactly how to prevent it. Some data suggests that taking a low dose of aspirin daily starting at 12 to 14 weeks may help reduce the incidence of preeclampsia or delay its onset for women at moderate to high risk of developing the condition. Other treatments have been tried with varying degrees of success, including the following:

>> **Calcium supplementation and antioxidant therapy:** Like low-dose aspirin, calcium hasn't been shown to prevent preeclampsia in low-risk women; however, there may be some benefit to women at high risk.

>> **A combination of vitamins C and E:** Although initial studies suggested a benefit, more recent data shows not only no benefit but also a higher risk of certain complications.

>> **Fish oil:** This has been investigated, but it hasn't been shown to be helpful in lowering the incidence of preeclampsia.

Ultimately, the only real treatment for preeclampsia is delivering the baby. When to deliver depends on how severe the condition is and how far along you are in your pregnancy. If you're close to your due date, induced delivery may be the wisest approach. If you're only 28 weeks along, your doctor may try close observation of you and the baby, either at home or in the hospital. Doctors weigh the risks to the mother's health against the risks to the baby of preterm delivery.

Understanding Placental Conditions

Two problems with the baby's placenta can occur in the latter part of pregnancy: placenta previa and placental abruption. This section describes both.

Placenta previa

Placenta previa occurs when the placenta partially or completely covers the cervix, as shown in Figure 2-1. Doctors typically diagnose patients with placenta previa during a routine ultrasound exam, but sometimes women find out about the problem only when they begin bleeding late in the second trimester or early in the third.

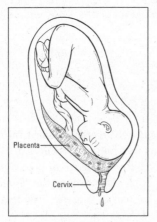

FIGURE 2-1:
Placenta previa.

REMEMBER

In early pregnancy, having the placenta positioned near the cervix or even partially covering it is common and usually poses no danger to the mother or the baby. In fact, this condition occurs in as many as one out of five pregnancies. In the vast majority of women (95 percent), the placenta rises as the uterus enlarges with the growing baby, which is why you have no reason to worry about the placenta covering the cervix early in pregnancy.

Even if the situation persists through the late second trimester and into the third, it can be harmless. Many women who have placenta previa never bleed at all. However, the possibility of heavy bleeding is the main concern with placenta previa. Sometimes bleeding leads to preterm labor. In this case, your practitioner attempts to stop the contractions, which often stops the bleeding. If bleeding is severe and can't be stopped, the baby may have to be delivered.

If you're in your third trimester and you have placenta previa, your practitioner may want you to have regular ultrasound examinations to see whether the placenta will eventually move out of the way. These are usually transvaginal ultrasounds and are safe to use with a placenta previa in experienced hands. Your doctor may tell you to avoid intercourse and not undergo internal (digital) examinations in order to lower the risk of any bleeding. If the condition persists until 36 weeks, he'll most likely recommend a cesarean delivery because the baby can't come through the birth canal without disrupting the placenta, which can lead to heavy bleeding.

Placental abruption

In some women, the placenta separates from the uterine wall before pregnancy is over. This condition is called *placental abruption* (it's sometimes also called *abruptio placentae* or *placental separation*). Figure 2-2 shows you what it looks like.

Placental abruption is a common cause of third-trimester bleeding. Because blood is an irritant to the uterine muscle, it can also cause premature labor and abdominal pain. An abruption is difficult to see on an ultrasound exam unless it's quite large, so in many cases, doctors can make the diagnosis only after they rule out every other possible cause of bleeding. Rarely, a placental abruption occurs suddenly, and if the separation is large enough, it may necessitate rapid delivery. See Book 2, Chapter 3 for other causes of third-trimester bleeding.

If you experience a small placental abruption, your practitioner may recommend you try bed rest. He'll also start to observe your pregnancy more closely to make sure the problem has no harmful side effects on the fetus.

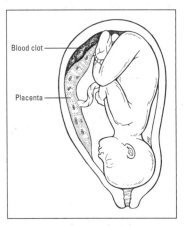

Blood clot

Placenta

FIGURE 2-2: Placental abruption.

Illustration by Kathryn Born, MA

Recognizing Problems with the Amniotic Fluid and Sac

As you know, the fetus grows within a "bag of water" known as the *amniotic sac*, which contains the amniotic fluid. This fluid increases in volume throughout the first part of pregnancy and reaches its maximum level at 34 weeks. After that, the volume gradually declines. Medical science hasn't yet discovered exactly what mechanism regulates the amniotic fluid volume, although it is known that the fetus plays some role in how much fluid the sac contains. During the second half of pregnancy, the amniotic fluid comprises mainly fetal urine. The fetus urinates into the sac and then swallows the fluid. The fluid circulating around the fetal lungs aids in lung development.

Sometimes, a practitioner may suspect that the amount of amniotic fluid is above or below average, and he may do an ultrasound examination to see what's happening. Minor increases or decreases in the amount of amniotic fluid usually aren't a problem. But large variations in amniotic fluid volume may be a symptom of some other problem. This section describes what happens when problems with the amniotic fluid or sac occur.

Too much amniotic fluid

The medical term for too much fluid is *polyhydramnios* or *hydramnios.* This situation occurs quite frequently, in about 1 to 10 percent of pregnancies. Often the increase in volume is small. Doctors don't always know what causes it, but they do know that a small increase usually isn't a problem. Larger increases may be associated with a medical condition in the mother — diabetes or certain viral illnesses, for example. In some rare cases, the excess fluid may be due to certain fetal problems. The fetus may be having difficulty swallowing the fluid, for example, so more of it accumulates inside the sac.

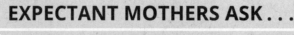

EXPECTANT MOTHERS ASK . . .

Q: "Is the amount of amniotic fluid determined to any extent by the amount of water I drink?"

A: No. The mother's fluid intake has little to do with it. Some recent studies suggest a mother can cause small increases in the amount of amniotic fluid by drinking plenty of liquids, but the effect isn't that great. Nevertheless, stay well hydrated.

Usually the fluid isn't increased to the point where it causes significant problems, but on rare occasions there can be massive accumulations of fluid to the point that it becomes difficult for the mom to breathe and causes the uterus to contract prematurely (premature labor). If this happens and Mom is near her due date, then her doctor will most likely recommend delivery to relieve the discomfort. If, however, she is remote from her due date, then doctors can remove some of the fluid during an amniocentesis to make Mom more comfortable. Also, indomethacin has occasionally been used in this setting because one of the side effects of indomethacin is that it causes amniotic fluid volume to decrease.

Too little amniotic fluid

A woman who has too little amniotic fluid has *oligohydramnios.* As mentioned earlier, amniotic fluid volume normally decreases after 34 to 36 weeks. If yours starts to fall below a specific range, however, your practitioner may want to observe the fetus more closely by performing certain tests. One common cause of low amniotic fluid is a rupture of the membranes, which allows fluid to leak out.

A fluid level that drops significantly prior to 34 weeks may indicate a problem with the mother or the baby. For example, some women with hypertension or lupus may have less blood flow to the uterus and, consequently, less blood flow to the placenta and the baby. When the baby receives less blood, the baby's kidneys make less urine, and that results in lower levels of amniotic fluid.

If the reduction in fluid is mild or moderate, the baby is watched carefully and undergoes tests of fetal well-being. Sometimes, oligohydramnios is a sign that the baby's growth is restricted (see the later section "Describing Problems with Fetal Growth") or, rarely, that there are abnormalities in the baby's urinary tract. Sometimes it's a sign the placenta isn't functioning optimally.

If you have decreased amniotic fluid, your doctor may suggest you get more rest and try to stay off your feet. By doing so, you may promote more blood flow to the uterus and placenta and thus increase the baby's urine output. (Just be glad you don't have to change all the diapers yet!)

Rupture of the amniotic sac

Premature rupture of the membranes or amniotic sac, sometimes called PROM, occurs when a woman's water breaks sometime before labor starts. When it happens close to your due date, it's referred to as *term PROM.* If you're less than 37 weeks at the time, it's called *preterm PROM.*

>> **If you experience term PROM:** Your practitioner may simply wait until you go into labor on your own. Or he may induce labor in order to avoid the risk of an infection developing inside the uterus.

>> **If you experience preterm PROM:** You may or may not go into labor, depending on how far along you are. If you're very far from your due date and don't appear to have an infection in your uterus, your doctor may use some medications (antibiotics, tocolytics, and steroids) to prolong the pregnancy as long as possible and to help your baby's chances of lung development. Your doctor will probably perform frequent ultrasound exams and monitor the fetal heart rate to ensure the baby is managing okay.

WARNING

If you think your membranes may have ruptured and you're preterm, let your practitioner know immediately or go to the hospital. He can perform tests to definitively let you know whether the membranes have ruptured.

Describing Problems with Fetal Growth

One of the main reasons to get prenatal care is to ensure that your baby is growing well. A practitioner typically gauges growth by measuring the fundal height (see Book 1, Chapter 2). As a general rule (in a singleton pregnancy), the measurement in centimeters from the top of the pubic bone to the top of the uterus roughly equals the number of weeks gestation. If your practitioner finds this measurement is greater or less than expected, he may recommend you have an ultrasound exam to more precisely assess the baby's growth.

During the exam, the technician measures various fetal body parts to come up with an approximate fetal weight. That estimate is then compared with the average weight for fetuses at the same gestational age and assigned to a certain percentile. The 50th percentile is average. But because fetuses (like babies, toddlers, children, teenagers, and grown-ups) come in different sizes, there's a range of normal weights. Anything between the 10th and the 90th percentiles is considered normal (see Book 2, Chapter 3 for more information about fetal weight).

REMEMBER

These upper and lower limits are somewhat arbitrary. They do imply that 10 percent of the population is larger than normal and that 10 percent is smaller, but this statement isn't exactly true. Most fetuses below the 10th percentile or above the 90th percentile are completely normal. On the other hand, some of them may not be growing normally and may need extra surveillance.

Smaller-than-average babies

A fetus whose estimated weight falls below the 10th percentile may have *intrauterine growth restriction* (IUGR). IUGR can lead to the birth of a baby who is small for gestational age (SGA). IUGR has many possible causes, including the following:

>> **Normal variations:** The baby is measuring small but is otherwise normal. Just as healthy adults come in all sizes, so do fetuses.

>> **Chromosomal abnormalities:** This cause is most common with early-onset IUGR, which occurs in the second trimester.

>> **Environmental toxins:** Cigarette smoking causes a decrease in birth weight between ¼ and ½ pound, on average. Chronic alcohol consumption (at least one to two drinks a day) and cocaine use also can cause low birth weight.

>> **Genetic factors:** Some genetic factors cause the fetus to grow less than average.

>> **Heart and circulatory abnormalities in the fetus:** Examples include a congenital heart defect or umbilical cord abnormalities.

>> **Inadequate nutrition for the mother:** Proper nutrition is especially important in the third trimester.

>> **Infection such as cytomegalovirus (CMV), rubella, or toxoplasmosis:** Book 6, Chapter 3 provides more information.

>> **Multiple gestation:** Fifteen to 25 percent of twins, and an even higher percentage of triplets, have IUGR. Twins grow at the same rate as singletons until 28 to 32 weeks, when the twin growth curve drops off.

>> **Placental factors and uterine-placental problems:** Because the placenta provides nutrition and oxygen to the fetus, if it's functioning poorly or if the blood isn't flowing smoothly from the uterus to the placenta, the fetus may not grow properly. Women with antiphospholipid antibody syndrome (a blood-clotting problem), recurrent bleeding, vascular diseases, or chronic hypertension are at risk for IUGR because those conditions cause poor placental function. Preeclampsia (described earlier in this chapter) may also impair placental function and lead to IUGR.

The way your practitioner responds to IUGR depends on your individual situation. Fetuses with mild IUGR, normal chromosomes, and no evidence of infection are likely to be fine. Sometimes early delivery is warranted, however, because the fetus may grow better in the nursery than inside the uterus. The way your practitioner responds to signs of IUGR depends on both the cause of the problem and the gestational age at which it's diagnosed. He may recommend more frequent office visits, periodic ultrasound examinations, fetal heart rate exams (known as NSTs — see Book 2, Chapter 3), or other tests such as a biophysical profile (an ultrasound assessment of fetal well-being) and measurement of blood flow through the umbilical cord called *Dopplers.* If the problem is severe but the pregnancy is far enough along, your doctor may recommend delivery.

In many cases, SGA babies turn out to be perfectly normal. Unfortunately, though, severe cases have been associated with learning difficulties later in life and even fetal death, which is why having your practitioner conduct some form of fetal surveillance is important.

Larger-than-average babies

A baby whose estimated weight is above the 90th percentile may have *macrosomia* ("big body") and end up being large for gestational age, or LGA. The risk factors of having an exceptionally large baby include the following:

>> The mother has previously delivered a large baby.

>> The mother has gained an excessive amount of weight during the pregnancy.

>> The mother is obese.

>> One or both of the parents were born very large.

>> The pregnancy lasts longer than 40 weeks.

>> The mother has poorly controlled diabetes.

The mother's main risk, naturally, is that the delivery is more difficult. If she delivers vaginally, she may suffer increased trauma to the birth canal, and she has an increased chance of needing a cesarean delivery. The main risk to the baby, likewise, is injury during delivery. Birth injury is more likely when a large baby is delivered vaginally, but it can also occur during a cesarean delivery. Most commonly, birth injury involves excessive stretching of the nerves in the baby's upper arm and neck resulting from shoulder dystocia (see Book 2, Chapter 5) during delivery.

REMEMBER

If your practitioner thinks your baby may be exceptionally large, based on either an ultrasound estimate of fetal weight or an abdominal exam, and it appears your pelvic bones may make for a tight fit, he'll discuss your delivery options with you.

Looking at Blood Incompatibilities

If a baby's parents have different blood types, the baby's blood type can differ from the mother's. Usually this situation creates absolutely no problem for the mother or the baby. In some rare cases, these blood-type mismatches warrant special consideration. Even then, however, there's hardly ever a significant problem.

The Rh factor

Most people are Rh-positive, which means they carry the Rh factor on their red blood cells. Those who don't carry the Rh factor are considered Rh-negative. If an Rh-positive man and an Rh-negative woman conceive, the fetus may be Rh-positive, thereby creating a mismatch between the baby and mother.

This kind of mismatch usually isn't a problem and is almost never a problem in a first pregnancy. If, however, any of the baby's blood leaks into the mother's circulation, her immune system may form antibodies to the Rh factor. And if any such antibodies reach a significant level in a future pregnancy, they can cross through the placenta into the baby's circulation and begin to destroy the baby's red blood cells.

The problem sounds scary, but it isn't insurmountable. The doctor usually gives the mother an injection of anti-D immune globulin at certain times to prevent the formation of antibodies. Rhogam and Rhophylac are two common preparations of anti-D globulin. If your baby's father is Rh-positive and you're Rh-negative, your doctor may recommend that you receive anti-D immune globulin at the following times:

>> Routinely at about 28 weeks gestation (as a precaution, just in case any passage of blood across the placenta has already occurred) and again 12 to 13 weeks later, if you haven't already delivered

>> After amniocentesis, CVS (chorionic villus sampling), or any invasive procedure (see Book 2, Chapters 2 and 3)

>> After a miscarriage, abortion, or ectopic pregnancy (see Book 2, Chapter 1 for more on ectopic pregnancy)

>> After significant trauma to your abdomen during pregnancy, if your doctor thinks that some of the baby's blood may have leaked into your circulation

>> After significant bleeding during pregnancy

>> Within 72 hours of delivery (either vaginal or cesarean); a nurse gives you the injection after delivery to prevent problems in future pregnancies

In unusual circumstances — either when the anti-D immune globulin wasn't given but should have been (very rare) or when it didn't work effectively (exceedingly rare) — a mother produces antibodies to the Rh factor. Then, if she becomes pregnant again, an Rh-positive fetus may be at risk of developing anemia (not enough red blood cells), depending on the levels of antibodies in the mother's blood and how they interact with the baby's blood. The anemia may be mild, requiring only that the baby be placed under special lights in the nursery to clear any extra *bilirubin* (a pigment that's released from red blood cells that are destroyed). If you've been sensitized and have developed these antibodies, your doctor can perform tests on amniotic fluid to check the baby's Rh status. If the fetus is Rh(D)-negative, he isn't at risk of anemia, even though the mother has the antibodies.

In moderate cases, frequent ultrasound exams may be necessary to assess the situation's severity. Recently, a new technique using ultrasound to measure the blood flow through one of the blood vessels in the fetus's brain (the middle cerebral artery, or MCA) has emerged as the best method for predicting fetal anemia in at-risk pregnancies. If the mother is close to her due date, her practitioner may recommend an early delivery. In the most severe cases, the baby may need to have a blood transfusion while he's still inside the uterus. The procedure is called a *fetal blood transfusion,* and a maternal–fetal medicine specialist performs it. A transfusion is the worst-case scenario, but even if things become this severe, a baby who has transfusions in a timely fashion can be born healthy. However, this procedure is associated with some risks.

Determining the baby's Rh(D) status by detecting fetal DNA in the mother's blood is now possible. Practitioners in Europe routinely use this method, and it will probably become part of the routine prenatal care of Rh(D)-negative women in the future in the United States. This test allows sensitized women to avoid invasive procedures for determining the fetal blood type, and it allows some women who aren't sensitized to avoid the anti-D immune globulin injection.

Other blood mismatches

Other kinds of blood mismatches are possible. Kell, Duffy, and Kidd are a few examples of blood factors that can differ between mother and baby. Fortunately, all these factors are very rare. No Rhogam-like medications are available to treat these mismatches, but if a problem does occur, your practitioner can provide care for the baby in the other ways described for Rh incompatibility (special lights, early delivery, or blood transfusion). And these babies, too, are usually born healthy.

Finally, some blood group antibodies — Le, Lu, and P, for example — can be mismatched but have no harmful effects on the fetus. Usually, no special action is needed.

Dealing with Breech Presentation

A baby is in a so-called *breech* position when her buttocks or legs are down, closest to the cervix. Breech presentation happens in 3 to 4 percent of all singleton deliveries. A woman's risk of having a breech baby decreases the further along she goes in her pregnancy.

The fetus is more likely to assume a breech position for one of the following reasons:

>> The fetus is preterm or especially small.

>> An increased amount of amniotic fluid exists (all the more room to turn around in).

>> A congenital malformation of the uterus is present, such as a bicornuate (T-shaped) uterus.

>> Fibroids that impinge on the uterine cavity are present.

>> You have placenta previa (described earlier in this chapter).

>> You're having twins or more.

>> Your uterus is relaxed from having had several babies already.

If your baby is in a breech position, your will doctor talk with you about the potential risks and benefits of a vaginal breech delivery versus version (turning the baby) or cesarean section. Special concerns about a breech delivery include the following:

>> Trapping the baby's head (which comes out last in a breech delivery) in a cervix that has been incompletely dilated by the passage of the baby's body, which is smaller than the head (this situation is especially troublesome if the baby is very small or premature)

>> Trauma resulting from an *extended fetal head* (meaning the head is tilted back)

>> Difficulty delivering the arms, which can lead to arm injuries

Because of these potential problems, many practitioners recommend that all breech babies be delivered by cesarean section. However, some fetuses in breech position are actually good candidates for vaginal delivery. Conditions that should be present for you and your doctor to consider a vaginal breech delivery include the following:

>> Estimated fetal weight is between 4 and 8 pounds.

>> The baby is in a *frank* breech position, which means the buttocks, not the feet, are positioned to come out first.

>> The buttocks are engaged in the pelvis.

>> Your doctor doesn't detect (by physical exam or by X-ray) any problem with the baby's head fitting through the birth canal.

>> Ultrasound shows the fetal head is either flexed (chin to chest) or in the *military* position (looking straight ahead, not tilted back).

>> Immediate anesthesia is available so that cesarean delivery can be done in an emergency.

>> The doctor is experienced in vaginal breech deliveries.

A few recent large studies have shown that breech babies delivered vaginally are at a higher risk for certain complications. In fact, the information is so compelling that most obstetricians have stopped performing vaginal breech deliveries. However, studies show that while the short-term complications were higher in the babies born vaginally, there was no difference in long-term problems (combined death and neurodevelopmental delays) at 2 years of age.

If you and your practitioner decide that a vaginal breech delivery isn't right for you, another option is *external cephalic version*, a procedure in which the doctor tries to turn the baby into normal delivery position by externally manipulating the mother's abdomen, which is a common and usually safe procedure. Sometimes it's fairly uncomfortable, but it works in about 50 to 70 percent of cases. The use of spinal or epidural anesthesia for the version may decrease the discomfort for the mother and improve the chances of successfully turning the baby.

There are certain conditions in which external cephalic version isn't advisable, such as bleeding, low amniotic fluid level, or multiple gestations.

Pondering Post-Term Pregnancy

The average pregnancy lasts about 40 weeks (or 280 days) after the last menstrual period, but only about 5 percent of women deliver on their due date. Some deliver a couple of weeks earlier, and some, a couple of weeks later, and all are considered to be "at term." Here are the most recent definitions of term pregnancy:

>> **Early term:** 37 $^6/_7$ weeks through 38 $^6/_7$ weeks

>> **Full term:** 39 $^0/_7$ weeks through 40 $^6/_7$ weeks

>> **Late term:** 41 $^0/_7$ weeks through 41 $^6/_7$ weeks

>> **Post term:** 42 $^0/_7$ weeks and beyond

Why should you or your practitioner care whether you go past your due date? Because the chances of certain complications rise as time goes on. From 40 to 42 weeks, the increased risks are small, but after 42 weeks, they climb into a range that's more worrisome. The worst complication is perinatal death (also called perinatal mortality). The chances of perinatal death start to increase after 41 to 42 weeks and double by 43 weeks.

REMEMBER

This situation isn't as scary as it may sound, though, because the actual number of deaths is so low. The vast majority of late babies are born healthy. Even at 44 weeks (the point at which perinatal mortality rates quadruple), 95 percent of babies are fine if appropriate testing is done. Your doctor can help you make the best decision for you as to the safe timing of delivery.

The increase in mortality rates in post-date pregnancies involves several factors, including the following:

>> **The placenta can function efficiently for only a finite length of time — about 40 weeks.** Fortunately, most placentas have some amount of "reserve," and they still work well beyond 40 weeks. But in a few rare cases, they don't last as well. If a placenta can't get enough nutrients to the baby, the baby may actually lose some weight by remaining inside the uterus.

>> **In a post-term pregnancy, the volume of amniotic fluid may decrease.** As mentioned earlier in this chapter, amniotic fluid volume peaks at about 34 to 36 weeks gestation and starts to slowly drop after that. Most of the time, adequate fluid is left after 40 weeks. Sometimes, however, the fluid level drops into a range doctors consider too low. In this situation, the umbilical cord has a chance of becoming compressed, and doctors may recommend that labor be induced.

>> **Babies sometimes pass their first bowel movement while they're still in the uterus.** The longer a pregnancy lasts, the more likely this is. In rare instances, the baby breathes in this thick *meconium* before or during birth, which can cause problems with breathing in the first few days or weeks after birth (for more information, see Book 2, Chapter 6).

>> **In a post-term pregnancy in which the placenta continues to function normally, the baby keeps growing.** These late babies are more likely to be very large, or *macrosomic* (see the earlier section "Describing Problems with Fetal Growth").

Practitioners use various strategies to manage post-date pregnancies, none of which is inherently better than another. Some doctors want to be sure all babies are delivered as soon after 40 weeks as feasible and induce labor to ensure that they are. (See Book 2, Chapter 4 for information on labor induction.) Others are willing to wait longer for spontaneous labor. The argument for the first approach is that you don't have to worry about any of the aforementioned complications. With the second approach, on the other hand, you may have less chance of needing a cesarean delivery.

Chapter 3

Pregnancy from Sickness to Health

Pregnancy may give you a "maternal glow" and make you feel as if something magical is happening to your body. But face it: Pregnancy doesn't make you superhuman. You're still susceptible to all the illnesses and other health problems that can affect anyone who's not expecting a baby. When illnesses arise during pregnancy, they can have special consequences. This chapter explains how a variety of medical conditions affect pregnant women.

Getting an Infection While Pregnant

Try as you may, avoiding every person who's carrying an infection during your pregnancy may be impossible. Keep in mind that most infections don't hurt the baby at all; they just make life more uncomfortable for you for a while. This section covers the most common infections as well as some of the more unusual ones.

Bladder and kidney infections

Bladder infections come in two basic types: with and without symptoms. *Silent* (symptom-free) bladder infections are common, occurring in about 6 percent of pregnant women. The other kind, called *cystitis,* comes with symptoms that include

>> Constantly feeling that you need to urinate

>> Discomfort above your pubic bone (where the bladder is)

>> More frequent urination

>> Pain with urination

If you develop either type of bladder infection, your doctor treats it with antibiotics.

If left untreated, a bladder infection can progress into a kidney infection, also known as *pyelonephritis.* A kidney infection produces the same symptoms as cystitis, plus a high fever and *flank pain* — pain over one or both kidneys (see Figure 3-1). Flank pain also can occur in someone who has kidney stones. The difference: A kidney infection causes a constant pain, whereas kidney stones produce more-severe but intermittent pain. Also, kidney stones are more often accompanied by small quantities of blood in the urine.

If your practitioner diagnoses you with pyelonephritis, she may want to admit you to the hospital for a few days so you can get intravenous antibiotics. Because kidney infections tend to recur during pregnancy, your practitioner may also want to keep you on a daily antibiotic for the remainder of your pregnancy.

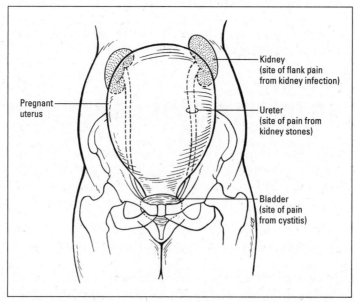

FIGURE 3-1:
Bladder infections, kidney infections, and kidney stones have their own unique symptoms.

Illustration by Kathryn Born, MA

Chickenpox

The varicella-zoster virus causes chickenpox. The first time someone comes down with an infection caused by this virus, usually in childhood, she gets chickenpox. Chickenpox is pretty rare in adults, and pregnant women stand no greater risk of contracting this virus than women who aren't pregnant.

If you've already had chickenpox, you aren't likely to get it again because your body has produced antibodies that make you immune. Even if you've never had chickenpox, you have a good chance of having these protective antibodies in your blood because you've probably had some exposure to the virus in the past, even though it didn't produce any illness. However, if you know that you've never been exposed to chickenpox and you haven't recently been vaccinated, or if you're unsure about your prior exposure, have your blood checked to see whether you're immune. Most of the time, antibodies to the varicella virus are checked at the first prenatal visit with all the rest of the routine prenatal labs.

REMEMBER

Because the chickenpox vaccine is relatively new, there's very little information about how safe it is for pregnant women, which is why the vaccine's manufacturer recommends that pregnant women be given it after delivery. The recommendation is that women wait three months after receiving the vaccine before they get pregnant. If you get the vaccine and then suddenly find out you were pregnant at the time, let your doctor know. The little experience that pregnant women have had with the vaccine suggests that it probably doesn't increase the chances of birth defects, nor has it led to any cases of congenital varicella syndrome in the baby (see the bulleted list that follows).

WARNING

If you aren't immune to chickenpox and you're exposed to someone with the infection while you're pregnant, let your practitioner know immediately so you can receive an injection known as VZIG *(varicella-zoster immune globulin)*, which may reduce the risk of infection to you and the baby. Get this injection within three days of exposure, if possible. If you contract chickenpox within several days of giving birth (before or after), your baby should receive VZIG.

Chickenpox can cause three potential problems during pregnancy:

>> It can make the mother ill with flu-like symptoms, plus produce the infamous skin rash (lots of little red blemishes). In rare circumstances, pneumonia develops two to six days after the rash appears. If you have chickenpox and you develop symptoms like shortness of breath or a dry cough, let your doctor know right away.

>> If you contract chickenpox during the first four months of pregnancy, the fetus has a small chance of developing the infection, too, leading to *congenital varicella syndrome.* With this syndrome, the fetus can have scarring (the same kinds of scars that little kids get on their bodies from chickenpox), some abnormal development of the limbs, problems with growth, and developmental delays.

REMEMBER

Fortunately, congenital varicella syndrome is very rare. It happens in less than 1 percent of cases in which the infection occurs in the first trimester, 2 percent if in the early second trimester.

>> If you contract chickenpox within the interval from five days before to five days after giving birth, the baby is at risk for developing a serious varicella infection in the newborn period. You can greatly reduce this chance by giving the baby VZIG.

The same varicella-zoster virus that causes chickenpox can also produce a recurrent form of the infection called *shingles* or *herpes zoster.* Most babies born to pregnant women who develop shingles are completely normal. Because shingles is much less common than chickenpox in pregnancy, doctors don't really know how common birth defects are after a pregnant woman develops this condition, although the incidence is thought to be less than the 1 to 2 percent seen with chickenpox.

WARNING

If you know that you're susceptible to chickenpox, avoid direct contact with anyone who has shingles or herpes zoster; the lesions contain the varicella-zoster virus and can cause a chickenpox infection in susceptible women.

EXPECTANT MOTHERS ASK . . .

Q: "Is getting the flu vaccine safe while I'm pregnant?"

A: Yes, the vaccine is completely safe. In fact, not only is it safe, but it's recommended that pregnant women get vaccinated for flu season. This is because pregnant women who get the flu can become much sicker than nonpregnant women. There's no evidence that additives in the vaccine cause any problems for the baby (like birth defects or autism). Remember, the vaccine doesn't protect against all flu viruses, only the ones that researchers believe will be common in your area.

Colds and the flu

REMEMBER

Most people get a cold about once a year, so the fact that most women get one during pregnancy isn't surprising. Nothing about pregnancy makes you more vulnerable to a cold virus, but the fatigue and congestion that go along with pregnancy can make a cold seem worse. In any case, the common cold is perfectly harmless to the developing fetus. As everyone knows, there's no cure for a cold, so the only option is to treat the symptoms. Contrary to popular belief, most cold medications — antihistamines, cough suppressants, and the like — are safe for pregnant women when taken in the recommended doses.

Following are a few suggestions for dealing with cold and flu symptoms:

>> **Drink fluids, fluids, and more fluids.** All viral illnesses promote dehydration, and being pregnant only makes the problem more extreme. If you're normally hydrated, your urine will be a pale yellow color or colorless, and you'll typically urinate every four to six hours. If you go for hours without urinating or notice dark yellow or orange urine, then you're probably dehydrated.

To keep from getting dehydrated when you have a cold or the flu, drink plenty of water, juice, or soda. Try to stay away from milk; many pregnant women complain that it makes the nausea often associated with the flu feel worse. If you think you may be dehydrated, you can try some of the over-the-counter oral rehydrating electrolyte solutions sold at your drugstore (like Rehydralyte or CeraLyte), but if you don't notice that your urine is turning lighter quickly or that you're going to the toilet at more typical intervals, then you should contact your healthcare provider for advice.

>> **Take a fever reducer.** Taking acetaminophen (Tylenol) in the recommended doses is okay to help bring a fever down. This action alone helps some people feel better. If your fever persists for more than a few days, however, call your doctor.

>> **Take a decongestant.** Pseudoephedrine (Sudafed) is the decongestant of choice during pregnancy. No evidence suggests that Sudafed taken in normal doses after the first trimester has any harmful effects.

>> **Try nasal spray, but not for long.** Nasal spray decongestants are okay if you use them only short-term (the same is true for people who aren't pregnant). Used intermittently, decongestant sprays may allow you to breathe more comfortably. Used day after day, they may only make the problem last longer. Saline nasal sprays are fine long-term, but they often aren't as effective in reducing congestion.

>> **Eat some comfort food.** Last but certainly not least, eat some chicken soup. Scientific studies have shown that chicken soup has properties that help cold sufferers feel better, even though no one knows exactly what those properties are.

You can use the same treatments for the common cold and for influenza infections. If you get the flu while you're pregnant, you're likely to have the same experience as when you're not pregnant.

Many patients ask about the use of echinacea during pregnancy. People in Asia have used this herb for centuries to fight inflammation and the common cold. Typically, people use a preparation or supplement containing echinacea when they feel the first signs of a cold coming on. No evidence suggests that echinacea causes a problem during pregnancy. In a study that included only a small number of patients, no adverse effects were found; however, drawing any conclusions from such a limited study is difficult.

WARNING

If your fever persists for more than a few days or if you develop a cough with greenish or yellow phlegm or have difficulty breathing, call your doctor to make sure that you're not developing pneumonia.

Seasonal allergies and hay fever

People commonly take antihistamines to treat seasonal allergies. The older, first-generation medications, such as chlorpheniramine (Chlor-Trimeton or Sinutab), have been around for a long time, and most obstetricians are comfortable with their use in pregnancy. The newer antihistamines, such as Claritin or Zyrtec, have an additional benefit of not causing as much drowsiness. Researchers haven't studied these newer medications as much in pregnancy. A third, very effective option is a nasal spray containing cromolyn or low-dose steroids.

Cytomegalovirus (CMV) infections

Cytomegalovirus (CMV) is a viral illness that's common among preschool-age children. The symptoms are very similar to the ones you get with the flu — fatigue, malaise, and aches. In most cases, though, an infection produces no symptoms at all. By the time they're old enough to have children, more than half of women have already had a CMV infection at some time in their lives, as evidenced by antibodies present in their blood.

Most practitioners don't routinely test for antibodies because of the very small chance that a woman would acquire the infection during pregnancy. Also, the infection doesn't usually cause any symptoms, so a woman would have to be repeatedly tested to see whether she develops the infection during her pregnancy. However, checking for susceptibility to the infection (that is, checking for antibodies) in women who are at higher risk — for example, women in close contact with preschool-age children — may be useful.

The importance of CMV infection during pregnancy is that the virus can pass to the fetus and cause a congenital infection. Actually, congenital CMV is the most common cause of an infection inside the uterus, and it occurs in 0.5 to 2.5 percent of all newborns. However, most of the time, babies born with this infection are healthy at birth.

REMEMBER

If you do develop CMV during pregnancy (and only 2 percent of susceptible pregnant women do), the infection is transmitted to the fetus only about one-third of the time. Options for diagnosing the fetal infection include undergoing amniocentesis to check for evidence of infection in the amniotic fluid and having ultrasound exams. Even in those babies who contract CMV, 90 percent have no symptoms of the infection at birth (although a small percentage experience symptoms later in life, such as hearing loss or developmental problems).

If your baby contracts CMV in utero, the chances of the baby having serious problems vary according to the following:

>> The baby's gestational age when the infection occurs

>> Whether the mother comes down with CMV for the first time during pregnancy (a primary infection) or whether she's had it in the past (a recurrent infection)

If the mother comes down with the infection after the second trimester or if it's a recurrent infection, the chances of serious problems in the newborn are much lower.

Severe symptomatic congenital CMV is rare and occurs in only about 1 in 10,000 to 20,000 newborns. It can lead to hearing impairment, visual problems, and even some mental deficiencies. Because CMV is a virus, antibiotics don't help.

German measles (rubella)

The rubella virus causes German measles, which are the only kind that have any significant impact on pregnancy. If you contract rubella within the first trimester, the baby has about a 20 percent chance of developing congenital rubella syndrome. The chances of this, however, vary even within the first trimester from the first month to the third month. Fortunately, acute rubella infection during pregnancy is extremely uncommon because most people in the United States are vaccinated at childhood.

Hepatitis

Various types of hepatitis affect the mother and baby in different ways:

>> **Hepatitis A** is transmitted by person-to-person contact or by exposure to contaminated food and water. Serious complications from hepatitis A in pregnancy are rare. The virus isn't passed to the developing baby. If you're exposed during pregnancy, take immune globulin within two weeks after exposure. Hepatitis A isn't transmitted in breast milk, so it's okay to breastfeed after you've had hepatitis A.

>> **Hepatitis B** virus is transmitted through sexual contact, intravenous drug use, or through a blood transfusion. A small percentage of women with hepatitis B infection have a chronic condition, which can lead to liver damage. Women who have high amounts of the virus in their blood or who became pregnant while on therapy should discuss antiviral therapy with their doctors. Although not that common, hepatitis B infection can be transmitted to the fetus. If you're positive for hepatitis B infection, inform the baby's pediatrician after delivery so that the baby can receive the appropriate immunizations and be a candidate for breastfeeding.

>> **Hepatitis C** is transmitted in the same way as hepatitis B. Less than 5 percent of hepatitis C–positive women transmit the infection to their baby. The CDC, American Congress of Obstetricians and Gynecologists, and American Academy of Pediatrics all support breastfeeding in a mom who has hepatitis C. They recommend not breastfeeding only when Mom's nipples become sore and cracked to the point that they bleed.

Hepatitis D, E, and G are much less common. Ask your practitioner if you want information on these conditions.

Herpes infections

Herpes is a common virus that infects the mouth, the throat, the skin, and the genital tract. If you have a history of herpes, rest assured that the infection poses no risk to the developing fetus. The main concern is that you may have an active genital herpes lesion when you go into labor or when your water breaks. If you do, there's a small risk of transmitting the infection to the baby as she passes through the birth canal. If it's your first herpes infection, the chance of the fetus contracting the virus is greater because you have no antibodies to the virus. Studies show that women with a history of recurrent herpes may lower the chance of having an active herpes infection at delivery by taking a medication called *acyclovir* or *valacyclovir* in the last month of pregnancy.

REMEMBER

If you have active genital herpes lesions at the time of labor or ruptured membranes, let your practitioner know. She's likely to perform a cesarean delivery to avoid infecting the baby. If you see no lesions but you feel as if you may be developing them, also tell your doctor. In this case, having a cesarean may also be advisable.

Human immunodeficiency virus (HIV)

Over the past few years, studies have shown that some of the medications used to treat HIV infection can dramatically reduce the chance of the virus being transmitted from a mother to her baby. For this reason, doctors recommend that women undergo HIV testing early in pregnancy; if a woman is HIV-positive, they suggest that she receive these medications during pregnancy as well as during labor. Some states even require that every pregnant woman be tested, and if the testing hasn't been performed, that her newborn be tested prior to discharge from the hospital. HIV testing is often repeated at about 35 weeks to see whether the infection was contracted during the pregnancy so that treatment during labor can be initiated.

To decrease the chances your baby will become infected with HIV, avoid any invasive procedures that can cause bleeding, such as amniocentesis or CVS, unless they're required. Most doctors recommend that the mother receive IV doses of antiviral medications immediately before these procedures to minimize the chances of infecting the fetus.

WARNING

Depending on your individual situation, most experts recommend that you not breastfeed if you're infected with HIV because you may transmit the virus to your baby. Whatever form of birth control you choose, the additional use of condoms is necessary.

If you're HIV-positive, maintain close contact with HIV specialists so you may benefit from the ever-improving treatments.

Listeria

Many women ask us about whether they can eat "soft" cheese. What they're usually concerned about is an infection called *listeriosis,* which is caused by eating food contaminated with the bacterium *Listeria monocytogenes. Listeria* is a cause for concern because it can lead to fetal infection, miscarriage, or preterm birth. When infection occurs during pregnancy, antibiotics given promptly can often prevent infection of the fetus or newborn.

Listeria can be found in a variety of different foods — packaged salads, hot dogs, luncheon meats, cheeses, and raw fruits and vegetables. Cheese is a concern because some outbreaks of *Listeria* have been reported with certain unpasteurized cheeses. In the United States, all cheese that is sold is supposed to be either pasteurized or, if it's raw, aged for 60 days (the aging process prevents the growth of the bacteria). The good news is that it really is quite uncommon. Your chances of contracting *Listeria* during pregnancy are about 0.12 percent.

TIP

Because of the rarity of infection and the ubiquity of the bacteria — and because you can't avoid eating everything! — try to limit your exposure to the highest-risk foods:

>> Don't eat hot dogs from the fridge without heating them completely.

>> Make sure the cheese you eat is either pasteurized or aged.

>> Wash all raw fruits and vegetables well.

Lyme disease

Lyme disease is an infection transmitted through a deer tick bite. Pregnancy doesn't predispose you to getting Lyme disease or make it any worse if you get it. The great news is that no evidence suggests that Lyme disease causes any harm to the fetus. The main problem is that it may make you sick.

WARNING

If you think a deer tick has bitten you, let your practitioner know. She may want to draw blood to see whether you've contracted Lyme disease and possibly start you on antibiotics to prevent long-term effects.

Parvovirus infection (fifth disease)

Parvovirus is a common childhood infection that comes with a fever and a characteristic "slapped cheek" rash. In adults, the infection can bring on flu-like symptoms — fever, aches, sore throat, runny nose, and joint pain — but may not cause a rash at all. Or it may come without any symptoms whatsoever. Three-fourths of all pregnant women are immune to parvovirus, so even if they're exposed to someone who has it, no problems come of it.

TIP

If you aren't immune to parvovirus or don't know whether you are and you come in contact with an infected person, let your practitioner know so you can be tested. Pregnant women who spend a great deal of time around school-age children (teachers or daycare workers, for example) may undergo routine testing before pregnancy or in the early first trimester.

Even if you contract this illness, chances are very good that your baby will be born healthy. No evidence indicates that parvovirus causes any birth defects. However, in rare cases, it can increase the risk of early miscarriage or the development of anemia in the fetus. For this reason, your practitioner may recommend that you have periodic ultrasound exams to look for signs of fetal anemia and to measure blood flow in a particular blood vessel in the brain, which can also indicate fetal anemia. (These are called *MCA* or *middle cerebral artery* Dopplers and are usually done on a weekly basis for 12 weeks after exposure.) If anemia does occur, doctors can perform a fetal blood transfusion (see Book 2, Chapter 2) while the baby is still inside you or suggest that the baby be delivered, if you're nearing the end of pregnancy.

The ultimate good news: Recent studies show that babies infected with parvovirus during pregnancy, even if they develop anemia, are likely to be born as healthy as any other baby if they're adequately treated.

Stomach viruses (gastroenteritis)

A bout of stomach flu can occur any time, regardless of whether you're pregnant. Symptoms include stomach cramps, fever, diarrhea, and nausea, with or without vomiting, and they last anywhere from 24 to 72 hours. The viruses that cause gastroenteritis usually don't harm your baby.

REMEMBER

Don't worry that your baby won't get adequate nutrition if you can't eat for a few days. Fetuses do just fine even when their mothers miss a few meals.

TIP

If you get a stomach virus, make sure that you drink plenty of liquids. Dehydration can lead to premature contractions and can contribute to fatigue and dizziness. Try chicken soup as well as other liquids — water, ginger ale, tea, or broth. Take care of yourself in the same way you would if you weren't pregnant. If your symptoms persist for more than 72 hours, call your doctor.

Toxoplasmosis

Toxoplasmosis is an infection caused by a parasite that lives in raw meat and in cat feces. If the parasite enters a person's bloodstream, it may lead to flu-like symptoms or, in some cases, no symptoms at all. This type of infection is very rare in the United States, and infections in pregnant women are rarer still, occurring in only 2 out of every 1,000 women, whereas in France, infection is more common.

If a pregnant woman is infected, the chances that she will transmit the infection to her baby, and the effects it may have, depend largely on when she contracts it. If she contracts it during the first trimester, the chances of the baby becoming infected are less than 2 percent. Later on in pregnancy, the chances of the baby being infected are greater, but the effects of infection are less severe. In a fetus, early toxoplasmosis infection can cause abnormalities of the central nervous system and in vision.

TECHNICAL
STUFF

If you've had the infection in the past and therefore have antibodies in your blood, you're highly unlikely to get the infection again. If a screening indicates that you may have been recently infected, your practitioner is likely to have your blood tested by a special laboratory to confirm that the positive test result was real. (Many initial tests produce false positives.) If the result still comes back positive and you appear to have contracted the infection after you became pregnant, your practitioner can give you special antibiotics to reduce your fetus's chances of infection. Then, in the second trimester, your practitioner may perform an amniocentesis to find out whether the fetus has been infected. If so, taking additional antibiotics for the rest of the pregnancy is necessary. Your practitioner may advise you to consult a maternal-fetal medicine specialist to discuss all your options.

If you get toxoplasmosis, keep in mind that recent studies from France indicate that the vast majority of fetuses who are infected with the parasite and are treated with appropriate antibiotics have an excellent prognosis.

TIP

No vaccine exists to prevent toxoplasmosis. The best way to avoid the disease is to minimize your exposure to raw or undercooked meat. Skip the carpaccio. Order your steaks cooked at least medium. Also avoid cat feces. If you have an outdoor cat, ask someone else to change the litter. (Indoor cats that have never been outdoors and never come in contact with mice or rats are extremely unlikely to have the parasite.) If no one else can change the litter, wear rubber gloves when you do it. Also wear gloves if you work in a garden that neighborhood cats may play in.

Vaginal infections

Bacteria and other organisms, when given half a chance, readily make themselves at home in a vagina, where the conditions — warm and moist — are perfect for them to grow and reproduce. A woman can get an infection at any time, even when she's pregnant.

Bacterial vaginosis

Bacterial vaginosis (BV) is a common vaginal infection. Symptoms include a whitish-yellow, odorous discharge that gets worse after sexual intercourse.

Research has linked BV to a slightly higher risk for premature delivery, which is why some practitioners screen for BV in patients known to be at risk for preterm delivery. Treatment includes oral antibiotics or vaginal antibiotic creams.

Chlamydia

Chlamydia is one of the more common sexually transmitted diseases. It often comes with no symptoms. Some practitioners routinely perform a culture from the cervix to check for chlamydia at the same time they do a Pap smear. If you have a positive culture, your doctor will prescribe a medication to treat the infection. Chlamydia can be passed to your newborn during vaginal delivery, increasing the chances your baby will develop conjunctivitis (an eye infection) or, less likely, pneumonia. Most hospitals routinely place an ointment in a newborn's eyes shortly after delivery to prevent conjunctivitis, regardless of whether the mother is infected with chlamydia.

Yeast infections

Yeast infections are very common in pregnancy. The large amounts of estrogen that circulate in the bloodstream during pregnancy promote the growth of yeast in the vagina. Symptoms of an infection are vaginal itching and a thick, whitish-yellow discharge. However, many women get infections without any symptoms. Often the only treatment needed is a short course of vaginal suppositories or creams. For stubborn infections, your doctor can prescribe oral medications.

REMEMBER

Yeast infections usually don't cause problems for the fetus or newborn.

Handling Pre-Pregnancy Conditions

The following sections detail conditions that you may have before you get pregnant and how those conditions may affect your pregnancy and vice versa.

Asthma

Predicting how pregnancy can affect a woman's asthma is difficult. Some women find that their condition improves when they're expecting. Some find it gets worse, and about half notice no difference at all.

The main concern that women with asthma have is whether they can safely continue taking their medications during pregnancy. Remember, the biggest problem with asthma isn't the medications; it's the possibility of pregnant women with asthma under-treating themselves. If you're having trouble breathing, you may not be getting enough oxygen to the baby. Most commonly used asthma treatments are quite safe for the baby, including the following:

>> Beta-agonists (Serevent, albuterol [Proventil], metaproterenol, terbutaline, Alupent)

>> Corticosteroids (prednisone)

>> Cromolyn sodium

>> Theophylline (Theo-Dur)

>> Inhaled steroids (Flovent, Vanceril, Beclovent, Azmacort, and so on)

You can take preventive measures to control acute attacks. Predicting attacks by self-monitoring is useful for asthmatic patients with peak expiratory flow rates (most asthma patients know what these are — if you don't, ask your lung specialist). Naturally, it helps to avoid situations that trigger attacks.

Chronic hypertension

Chronic hypertension refers to high blood pressure that occurs independently of pregnancy. Although many women who have this condition are aware that they have it before they conceive, doctors occasionally diagnose it during pregnancy. If you have mild or moderate chronic hypertension, chances are good that you'll have an uneventful pregnancy. However, your doctor will be on the lookout for certain conditions that can affect you or the baby.

TECHNICAL
STUFF

Women with chronic hypertension stand an increased risk of developing pre-eclampsia, so your doctor will look for any signs that you're developing this condition. The main risk for the baby is intrauterine growth restriction (IUGR) or placental abruption (see Book 6, Chapter 2). Your doctor may use repeated sonograms to check on the baby's growth and to make sure that you have adequate amniotic fluid. She may also suggest that you undergo some tests later during your pregnancy for fetal well-being, such as non-stress tests (NSTs; see Book 2, Chapter 3). The overall management of your pregnancy depends on how well-controlled your blood pressure is, your overall health, and how the baby grows.

EXPECTANT MOTHERS ASK . . .

Q: "Are blood pressure medications safe?"

A: Most medications are safe, but many haven't been well-studied during pregnancy. Discuss this important question with your doctor. Certain medications, however, should be avoided. Angiotensin converting enzyme inhibitors (known as ACE inhibitors) pose some risk for kidney problems in the fetus. Beta-blockers and certain calcium channel blockers are generally considered safe in pregnancy. Commonly used anti-hypertensive medications include labetalol, nifedipine, and Aldomet (methyldopa). Also, diuretics are best avoided, unless they're the only way of treating the high blood pressure.

Deep vein thrombosis and pulmonary embolus

A *deep vein thrombosis* (DVT) is a blood clot that develops within a deep vein, most commonly in the leg. A *pulmonary embolus* is a blood clot within the lung, often a clot that has dislodged itself from one of the deep veins of the leg and made its way to the lung. Both of these conditions are rare, affecting far less than 1 percent of pregnant women.

Symptoms of a DVT include pain, swelling, and tenderness, usually in the calf, and a rope–like hardness running down the back of the lower leg. Diagnosing DVT before it has the chance to lead to a pulmonary embolus is important.

REMEMBER

Keep in mind that muscle pain, cramping, and swelling are common symptoms of a normal pregnancy, and a DVT is quite unusual. Let your doctor know when you're experiencing the sudden onset of these symptoms, but don't panic about them.

Diabetes

Diabetes comes up as a problem in pregnancy in two ways:

>> You already have the condition before you become pregnant.

>> You develop what's called *gestational diabetes,* which is unique to pregnancy and usually goes away after pregnancy.

Diabetes before pregnancy

If you have a history of diabetes, talk to your doctor about it before you get pregnant. If you have your blood sugar level under good control before you conceive, your pregnancy is more likely to proceed smoothly. Women with pregestational diabetes stand a higher-than-average risk of having a fetus with certain birth defects, but you can reduce this risk down to the normal range if you achieve excellent glucose control.

Some doctors suggest that you have a blood test called a *hemoglobin A1C* to check how well your sugar has been controlled over the past few months. Your doctor may also suggest that you have a special sonogram called a *fetal echocardiogram* (see Book 2, Chapter 2) to make sure that the baby's heart is okay. If you take an oral medication to control your blood sugar, your practitioner may suggest you switch to insulin injections for better control. Some women with diabetes suffer kidney complications, but this kind of problem isn't likely to worsen during pregnancy. If you have eye problems related to diabetes (proliferative retinopathy), have your doctor closely monitor and possibly treat your eyes during pregnancy.

REMEMBER

The vast majority of diabetic women proceed through pregnancy without a hitch. However, your doctor may need to adjust your insulin dose. Your doctor will also be on the lookout for high blood pressure and follow the baby's growth with periodic ultrasound exams. In the third trimester, your doctor will probably begin to monitor the fetus closely, performing certain tests for fetal well-being (periodic NSTs, for example — see Book 2, Chapter 3).

When you're in labor, your doctor will keep a close eye on your glucose level and may give you insulin. With optimal glucose control and close monitoring of the baby and mother-to-be, most women with diabetes have an excellent outlook for pregnancy.

Gestational diabetes

Gestational diabetes is one of the most common medical complications in pregnancy, occurring in 2 to 3 percent of all pregnant women. Your practitioner can diagnose gestational diabetes by giving you a special blood test. (See Book 2, Chapter 2 for information on this test.)

If you have gestational diabetes and you don't control your glucose levels, your baby may be at higher risk for certain problems. If your blood sugar levels are high, the fetus's are, too. And high blood sugar levels cause the fetus to produce certain hormones that stimulate fetal growth, which may cause her to grow too large (see Book 6, Chapter 2). Furthermore, if the fetus has high blood sugar levels while still in the uterus, she may have temporary problems with sugar regulation after birth. If the mother's (and fetus's) glucose levels are controlled during pregnancy, the risk of these complications drops dramatically.

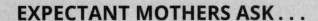

EXPECTANT MOTHERS ASK...

Q: "If I develop gestational diabetes, will I recover when my pregnancy ends?"

A: Most women do recover completely, but a minority remains diabetic. In these cases, pregnancy itself didn't cause the diabetes. Instead, the women were already at risk for developing the condition. If you develop gestational diabetes, being tested for diabetes within a few months after you deliver is important. Also, keep in mind that your risk for developing diabetes at some point later in your life increases.

TIP

You need to control your sugar levels if you have gestational diabetes. Most of the time, altering your diet is enough. (Most women have a consultation with a nurse and/or a nutritionist to come up with a specific diet plan.) Exercise also helps. Only in rare cases do women need to resort to taking medication to keep their sugar levels under control.

Traditionally, doctors prescribed insulin injections to control blood glucose levels, but recent research suggests that an oral agent called *glyburide* is safe and effective. If you develop gestational diabetes, your doctor will ask you to check your sugar level several times during the day or on a weekly basis. You do this by pricking your finger (called a *fingerstick*) and placing the drop of blood onto a test strip, which you then insert into a small meter that gives immediate results.

Fibroids

Fibroids (also called *uterine myomas*) are benign growths of the muscle cells that make up the uterus. They're extremely common, and your practitioner often diagnoses them during routine sonograms. The high levels of estrogen in a pregnant woman's bloodstream can encourage fibroids to grow larger. However, predicting whether any woman's fibroids will grow, stay the same, or shrink during pregnancy is difficult. Most of the time, fibroids cause no problems for a pregnancy.

In extreme cases, fibroids can cause difficulties, such as the following:

>> Fibroids may grow so fast that they outgrow their blood supply and begin to degenerate, which sometimes causes pain, uterine contractions, and even preterm labor. Symptoms of degeneration include pain and tenderness directly over the fibroid (in the lower abdomen). Short-term treatment with anti-inflammatory medications (Motrin or Indocin, for example) may help.

Pregnancy from Sickness to Health

>> Very large fibroids in the lower portion of the uterus or near the cervix may interfere with the baby's ability to make her way through the birth canal. Thus, they may increase the risk for cesarean delivery, although this situation is quite unusual.

>> Large fibroids within the uterus can sometimes increase the likelihood that the baby will be in the breech or transverse position. But this possibility, too, is rare.

Most commonly, fibroids cause no problem at all. And most often, they shrink after delivery.

Immunological problems

Immunological problems are conditions in which a person's immune system produces atypical antibodies, which can lead to a variety of problems. In most cases, women who have immunological problems already know they have them before they become pregnant. If you're one of those women, discuss your problem with your doctor before you become pregnant or as early in your pregnancy as possible.

Antiphospholipid antibodies

Antiphospholipid antibodies are a class of antibodies that circulate in some women's blood. The two most common kinds are lupus anticoagulant and anti-cardiolipin antibodies. They may be found in some women with collagen vascular diseases (such as lupus), in women who have had blood clots, and in some women with no known medical problems. They're significant in pregnancy because they've been associated with recurrent miscarriages, unexplained fetal death, early onset of preeclampsia, and intrauterine growth restriction.

Doctors don't routinely screen for these antibodies because many women who have them experience no resulting problems. But if you have one of the following conditions, your doctor will probably want to test you:

>> Autoimmune platelet conditions

>> A false positive test for syphilis

>> A history of spontaneous blood clots in the legs or lungs

>> A history of stroke or transient ischemic attacks (a "temporary" kind of stroke)

>> Lupus (or other collagen vascular disease)

Your doctor may also want to test you if you've had any of the following obstetrical problems in the past:

>> Early-onset preeclampsia

>> Problems with fetal growth (intrauterine growth restriction)

>> Recurrent miscarriages

>> Unexplained stillbirth or fetal death

Antiphospholipid antibody syndrome is diagnosed when a woman has antiphospholipid antibodies in her bloodstream plus one of the listed risk factors. If you have the syndrome, depending on its severity, your doctor may recommend that you take baby aspirin, heparin, oral steroids, or some combination of these medications. She probably will also recommend that you have periodic ultrasound exams to make sure the baby is growing appropriately and that you undergo tests for fetal well-being (see Book 2, Chapter 3).

REMEMBER

This syndrome may sound scary, but the good news is that most women who receive adequate medical care have normal pregnancies and healthy babies.

Lupus

Systemic lupus erythematosus (SLE), or lupus, is one of several so-called *collagen vascular diseases.* Pregnancy doesn't make the disease worse, but some women do experience more flare-ups during pregnancy.

On the other hand, lupus can affect pregnancy in some cases, depending on the problem's severity going into pregnancy. If you have a mild form of lupus, chances are it will have little effect on your pregnancy. Some women with more severe lupus stand an increased risk of miscarriage, problems with fetal growth, and preeclampsia (see Book 6, Chapter 2). Depending on your medical history, your doctor may recommend certain medications such as heparin, baby aspirin, or oral steroids. She may also recommend more frequent sonograms and other measures of fetal well-being. Your best bet for a successful pregnancy is to have the disorder under control as much as possible before you become pregnant.

Inflammatory bowel disease

The two kinds of inflammatory bowel disease are Crohn's disease and ulcerative colitis. Fortunately, pregnancy does nothing to exacerbate either condition. If you have inflammatory bowel disease but your symptoms were minor or nonexistent during the months before you became pregnant, chances are good that they'll remain at bay during your pregnancy. Doctors often recommend that women whose symptoms are frequent and severe postpone pregnancy until the disease abates or is brought under control. Most medications to control symptoms are considered to be safe and effective during pregnancy.

Seizure disorders (epilepsy)

Most women who have epilepsy can have an uneventful pregnancy and give birth to a perfectly healthy baby. However, epilepsy does require that a woman's obstetrician and her neurologist work together to come up with the right strategy for controlling seizures.

Studies show that women whose seizures are well-controlled on a minimal dose of a single medication before they get pregnant have the best pregnancy outcomes. So by all means, consult your neurologist before you get pregnant, and don't stop taking your medications unless your doctor advises you to.

All medications used to treat seizures pose some risk of birth defects. The problems they can cause vary, depending on the particular medication, but they include facial abnormalities, cleft lip and cleft palate, congenital heart defects, and neural tube defects. For this reason, women who take seizure medications need to have an ultrasound to evaluate fetal anatomy and a fetal echocardiogram (see Book 2, Chapter 2) to look for abnormalities in the baby's heart.

TIP

Women with seizure disorders should begin taking extra folic acid about three months before trying to conceive, because some seizure medications can affect folic acid levels.

WARNING

Don't adjust or stop your medications on your own, especially after you become pregnant. Your seizure activity could increase, which would probably be worse for the developing baby than the medications themselves.

Thyroid problems

Problems with thyroid function are relatively common in women of reproductive age. Although these conditions require extra testing, they usually don't cause significant problems for pregnancy.

Hyperthyroidism (overactive thyroid)

There are many causes of hyperthyroidism, but the most common by far is Grave's disease, which is associated with its own special set of antibodies (thyroid-stimulating immunoglobulins, or TSIs) in the blood. These antibodies cause the thyroid to make too much thyroid hormone. Women with an overactive thyroid must receive adequate treatment during pregnancy (ideally, beginning before conception) in order to reduce their risk of complications such as miscarriage, preterm delivery, and low birth weight.

If you have an overactive thyroid, unless your condition is extremely mild, your doctor is most likely to recommend that you take certain medications to lower the amount of thyroid hormone circulating in your blood. Some of these medications may cross the placenta, so your doctor will watch the fetus closely, usually by performing regular sonograms, to look for any evidence that the medications are lowering the baby's thyroid levels too much. Specifically, she'll monitor the baby's growth and heart rate to see that they're normal and check for any evidence that the fetus has developed a goiter (an enlarged thyroid).

Your doctor probably also will monitor the levels of thyroid-stimulating antibodies in your blood because these antibodies may, in some rare cases, cross the placenta and stimulate the baby's thyroid. After delivery, your baby's pediatrician will watch the baby carefully for any evidence of thyroid problems.

Some women develop hyperthyroidism in the first trimester due to high levels of the pregnancy hormone hCG. This is usually self-limited and resolves without treatment.

Hypothyroidism (underactive thyroid)

A woman with an underactive thyroid (hypothyroidism) can have a healthy pregnancy as long as her condition is adequately treated. If it's not, she stands a higher risk of developing certain complications, such as a low birth-weight baby. The condition is treated with a thyroid replacement hormone (Synthroid, for example). This medication is safe for the baby because very little of it crosses the placenta. If you have an underactive thyroid, your doctor may want to periodically check your hormone levels to see whether your medication needs to be adjusted. Although some doctors recommend routine testing (and possibly treatment) for hypothyroidism in the first trimester in women *without* a history of thyroid disease, this isn't actually recommended by major obstetrical organizations such as the American Congress of Obstetricians and Gynecologists (ACOG).

Chapter 4

Coping with the Unexpected

We wish we had no reason to include this chapter. We wish every pregnant couple could end up delivering a healthy baby. Most do, but not everyone is so fortunate. Those who suffer the loss of a fetus or discover that their baby has a significant abnormality need to understand what happens and figure out how to respond when things go wrong. If you're experiencing any of the problems covered in this chapter, we hope you find some of this information helpful.

Perhaps you're drawn to this chapter because you've had an unsuccessful pregnancy in the past. If so, you may be anxious about your current pregnancy. That's entirely normal. For many women who've had poor outcomes in the past, the only thing that can truly alleviate their anxiety is to hold a healthy baby.

TIP

One way to at least minimize your worry is to sit down with your doctor and discuss the situation. Ask him to map out a plan for your current pregnancy that maximizes your chances of a favorable outcome and helps you cope with your concerns. When you feel certain you're doing everything you possibly can do to avoid a recurring problem, you may rest a little easier. Your worry probably won't disappear, but remember that although a certain part of the process is in Mother Nature's hands, you can take medical steps to maximize your chances of having a healthy baby.

Surviving Recurrent Miscarriages

Unfortunately, a first-trimester miscarriage is a fairly common occurrence. Doctors estimate that about 15 to 20 percent of recognized pregnancies — those that have yielded a positive pregnancy test — end up in miscarriage. Still more early embryos (also called *conceptuses*) are lost before they're actually known to exist — that is, before a woman takes a pregnancy test. More than half the time, the cause of first-trimester miscarriage is the presence of some chromosomal abnormality in the embryo or fetus. Another 20 percent of early miscarriages are due to structural abnormalities in the embryo. Usually they're spontaneous events with low chances of recurrence.

REMEMBER

Fortunately, 80 to 90 percent of women who experience a single early miscarriage subsequently deliver a normal baby.

Recurrent miscarriage — technically, the loss of three consecutive pregnancies — is far less common. This problem occurs in only 0.5 to 1 percent of women. A variety of causes contribute to recurrent miscarriage, including the following:

>> Genetic causes

>> Uterine abnormalities

>> Immunologic causes (though not all physicians agree that this is a factor)

>> Inadequate progesterone secretion

>> Certain infections (although this cause is also controversial)

>> Antiphospholipid antibody syndrome (lupus anticoagulant or anticardiolipin antibodies; see Book 6, Chapter 3)

>> Certain environmental toxins or drugs (such as antimalarials and some anesthetic agents)

Most doctors suggest that women undergo certain tests after having three miscarriages; some begin testing even sooner. Because chromosomal abnormalities are the most common cause of miscarriage, an important first diagnostic step is to run tests on the chromosomes of the fetal tissue, when possible.

Various strategies for treating recurrent miscarriage are available, but doctors may disagree about which one, if any, is best. Choosing a strategy is easier if you know what the problem is. For example, your doctor may be able to surgically repair an abnormally shaped uterus. If doctors can't find a cause for recurrent miscarriage, knowing which treatment is best may be difficult. Note, however, that even if no treatment is attempted, women who have had three consecutive miscarriages still have a greater than 50 percent chance of having a normal, successful pregnancy.

Coping with Late-Pregnancy Loss

Late-pregnancy loss refers to a fetal death, a stillbirth, or the death of an infant in the immediate newborn period. Fortunately, these losses are infrequent and rarely occur more than once. Some causes of late losses include

>> Chromosomal abnormalities

>> Other genetic syndromes

>> Structural defects

>> A massive placental abruption or separation (see Book 2, Chapter 2)

>> Antiphospholipid antibodies or clotting disorders (see Book 2, Chapter 3)

>> Umbilical cord compression

>> Unexplained reasons, which are very common

REMEMBER

Women who suffer a loss of pregnancy often ask, "Did I do something to cause this?" The answer is almost always *no*, so you have no reason to add to your grief by mixing in guilt. Many patients find it helpful, after the initial hurt has begun to subside, to gather all their pregnancy records, including any pathology reports, and consult with their doctor or a specialist. Sometimes your doctor can identify a cause, and sometimes not. Either way, most patients benefit from sitting down with their doctor and mapping out a strategy for trying to prevent a loss in future pregnancies. Having a plan to focus on makes many patients feel less helpless. Support groups are also very helpful (see the "Finding Help" section later in this chapter).

In subsequent pregnancies, your doctor may recommend that you undergo blood tests to check for certain abnormalities that have been associated with fetal loss. Often, if you've experienced a prior late-pregnancy loss, doctors follow your progress with regular ultrasound examinations and tests of fetal well-being. Your doctor may recommend that you deliver somewhat early, before you go into labor. You're likely to feel anxious during subsequent pregnancies, which is completely normal. But keep in mind that suffering a pregnancy loss a second time is quite unlikely.

TIP

A good online source of support and information on pregnancy loss is `www.marchofdimes.org/complications/loss-and-grief.aspx`.

Dealing with Fetal Abnormalities

All prospective parents wonder whether their baby will be "normal." And for most, the answer is *yes*. Still, 2 to 3 percent of babies end up having a significant abnormality. Some of these abnormalities can be repaired and have very little impact on the baby's overall quality of life. Occasionally, however, the condition can have a bigger impact, whether it's a structural, chromosomal, or genetic abnormality.

REMEMBER

When an abnormality occurs, the first question many women ask is "Is this my fault?" And the answer, most often, is *no*. From what is known about fetal abnormalities, most are what are called *sporadic*, meaning they occur randomly and have no identifiable cause. If your doctor can't identify a cause, chances are low that the same kind of abnormality will recur in a subsequent pregnancy. (If the cause is genetic, there may be some chance that the abnormality could occur again.)

If your fetus is diagnosed with a birth defect or genetic disorder by ultrasound or some other test, your doctor may recommend that you have additional tests to look for other factors that have been associated with that particular problem. He may recommend that you see a genetic counselor to discuss the implications of the abnormality. If the condition is a structural defect that can be surgically repaired or treated, your doctor may recommend that you meet with a specialist who can treat the baby after she is born. These discussions help you prepare for what lies ahead during the newborn period and also later on in your child's life.

Nobody wants to get the news that a fetus has an abnormality, but having this information is helpful for several reasons:

>> If you're aware of some disorders, such as fetal anemia or obstructions in the urinary tract, doctors may be able to treat them.

>> The knowledge helps to prepare you for what happens after the baby is born.

>> This information helps you manage your pregnancy and consider all possible options.

>> The information can give you important insights into the management of future pregnancies.

Finding Help

If your pregnancy didn't turn out as you had hoped, the first and most obvious place to look for support is from your partner. Family members, friends, and clergy can also be very helpful. Professional advice or treatment from a psychotherapist or social worker may be useful for many couples. Support groups also can provide understanding and expert insight into your problem — you can find hundreds of support groups on the Internet. Dozens of helpful books are also available, including the following:

- **»** *How to Go on Living after the Death of a Baby,* by Larry G. Peppers and Ronald J. Knapp (Peachtree Publishers)

- **»** *Loss during Pregnancy or in the Newborn Period,* by James Woods, Jr., and Jenifer Esposito Woods (Jannetti Publications, Inc.)

- **»** *Roses in December: Comfort for the Grieving Heart,* by Marilyn Willett Heavilin (Harvest House Publishers)

- **»** *When Mourning Breaks: Coping with Miscarriage,* by Melissa Sexson Hanson (Morehouse Publishing Co.)

Beginning to Heal

Couples naturally feel a strong emotional attachment to their unborn child, beginning as early as the first trimester. As a result, many couples experience the same grief after the loss of a fetus as they would after the loss of another family member or a close friend. The loss of a fetus is no less significant than the loss of another child. Parents who decide to terminate a pregnancy because of an abnormality also go through tremendous grief.

Both parents should acknowledge their need — and their right — to grieve after a pregnancy loss. The emotional response takes time and typically goes through a number of stages, beginning with shock and denial, progressing to anger, and eventually reaching acceptance and the ability to carry on with life. Understand that each of you will grieve in a different way.

After you go through the stages of grief and feel you're physically and emotionally strong, you'll probably be ready to start trying to conceive again. In some couples, one person progresses through the grieving process faster than the other. Make sure both of you are ready before you begin trying to get pregnant again. And remember that a successful pregnancy, although joyful, doesn't replace a lost one, so the grieving process is necessary.

From a medical perspective, make sure that you finish looking into possible causes for the loss and have a plan of action for the next pregnancy. Realize that your next pregnancy will be somewhat stressful and that you'll need extra attention and compassion from your family, friends, and healthcare professionals.

Index

deli meats, 298, 302

delivery. *See also* labor; vaginal delivery

about, 199

babysitting arrangements for, 463

cesarean, 209–213

early, 470

for multiples, 452, 453

operative vaginal, 208–209

placenta, 207

post-, 214–218

preparing body for, 320

vaginal, 200–207

without anesthesia, 86

dental care, 77–78

determining

pregnancy, 8–10

whether multiples are identical or fraternal, 447–449

developing flexibility and muscle tone, 319

DHA (docosahexaenoic acid), 49, 284–285, 292

DHM omega-3, 281

diabetes

about, 501–503

birth weight and, 41

gestational, 292–293, 318, 502–503

for multiples, 455

before pregnancy, 502

diagnosing preeclampsia, 472

diagnostic test, 111–112

diamniotic/dichorionic, 447

diamniotic/monochorionic, 447–448

diarrhea, as a sign of labor, 174

diastasis test, 372

Dick-Read, Grantley (obstetrician), 161

diet and exercise

about, 39, 335, 347

activities for bed rest, 342–346

activities to avoid, 341–342

additional activities, 339–341

aerobic exercise, 53, 337

breast milk production and exercise, 367

caloric intake, 42–46

diet for multiples, 451

exercise after delivery, 254–255

exercise for competitive athletes, 354–359

exercise for constipation, 65, 99–100

exercise for fitness buffs, 354–359

exercise for post-delivery, 371–372

exercise programs, 49–54

fatigue and exercise, 329

gestational diabetes and exercise, 293

healthy weight gain, 39–42

maintaining diet during breastfeeding, 389–391

novice exerciser, 348–353

post-pregnancy exercise, 269–270

safety of foods, 46–48

special dietary needs, 48–49

staying fit, 336–339

dietary supplements, 45–46, 281–287

Dieting For Dummies (Kirby), 372

digestive system

of baby, 400–401

of newborns, 228

digestive tract, changes with, 62–67

dilation, 94, 177

dilation and curettage (D&C), 117, 214–215

dilutional anemia, 45

dioxins, 310

diphtheria, 32

dirty diapers, counting, 424

diuretic, 98

dizygotic twins, 446–447

dizziness, as a symptom of overdoing exercise, 332

DNA, 111–112

docosahexaenoic acid (DHA), 49, 284–285, 292

doctor visits

baby's first, 230–232

first postpartum, 252

DONA (Doulas of North America), 165

Doppler studies, during second trimester, 138

doppler velocimetry, during third trimester, 159

shots, 86

shoulder dystocia, 206

shoulder raise, 343–344

shrimp, 311

"Siamese twins," 448

Sickle-cell anemia, 105

sickness. *See also* foodborne illnesses

    about, 58–61, 487

    during first trimester, 97–98

    infections, 487–499

    pre-pregnancy conditions, 499–507

silent (symptom-free) bladder infections, 487–488

sitz baths, 237

six-days-per-week workout plan, 353

size

    of newborns, 225

    of undergarments, 334

skiing, 339, 340, 341–342, 357

skim milk, drinking, 268

skin changes, during second trimester, 125–126

skin tags, 126

SLE (systemic lupus erythematosus), 505

sleep

    for baby, 86

    for baby blues, 250

    improving, 318–319

SMA (Spinal Muscular Atrophy), 104

smaller-than-average babies, 479–480

smallpox, 34

smoked meat/fish, 47

smoking, 34–35, 41, 467

soccer, 340, 357

sodium, hemorrhoids and, 66

sore nipples, 393

soy, allergy to, 296

space, arranging for breastfeeding, 405–408

Spanish mackerel, 310

special considerations

    about, 441

    age, 442–445

for multiples, 445–456, 453–456

nontraditional family, 461–462

preparing other children for a new baby, 462–464

subsequent pregnancies, 457–461

special dietary needs

    vegan, 49

    vegetarian, 48

spider angiomas, 125

spina bifida, 128

spinal anesthesia, 195

Spinal Muscular Atrophy (SMA), 104

spontaneous vaginal delivery, 200

spotting, as a side effect of amniocentesis, 135

sprouts

    during pregnancy, 298

    salmonella and, 303

squatting position, for pushing, 202

SSRIs (selective serotonin reuptake inhibitors), 30

standard tests, first prenatal appointment and, 107–111

standing up straight, 363–364

starchy vegetables, in MyPlate, 43

station, checking, 178

staying fit, 336–339

steam rooms, 75–76

step-down area, 230

stethoscope, in hospital room, 180

stevia, 308

stevia leaf extract sweeteners (Truvia/Stevia), 48

stomach viruses (gastroenteritis), 497

stool softener, for constipation, 65, 99–100

stopping

    milk production, 397

    preterm labor, 469–470

stork bites, on newborns, 223

strengthening muscles, 53–54, 343–345

stress, 58

stretch marks, during third trimester, 153

stretching, 342–343, 349, 350

stroller
  lifting baby from, 364–366
  pushing a, 370–371
structural changes, 50
stuffing, during pregnancy, 299
subchorionic hemorrhage, 116
subcutaneous ring block, 229
sucralose (Splenda), 48, 309
suitcase, packing your, 164–165
superficial thrombophlebitis, 155
supine hypotension syndrome, 49
supplements, 281–287
supplies, gathering for breastfeeding, 405–408
surfactant, 120
sushi, 47, 277
sweating, postpartum, 248
sweeteners
  about, 48, 306
  acesulfame K, 306
  agave nectar, 307
  aspartame, 307
  high-fructose corn syrup (HFCS), 307
  honey, 308
  saccharin, 308
  stevia, 308
  sucralose, 309
swelling
  about, 70
  after delivery, 239–240
  as a symptom of overdoing exercise, 332
  during third trimester, 154
swimming, 337, 348
swordfish, 310
symptoms
  of altitude sickness, 340
  of campylobacter, 300
  of colic, 431–432
  of emotional changes, 57
  of mercury poisoning, 304–305
  of overdoing exercise, 332–333
  of salmonella, 303

systemic lupus erythematosus (SLE), 505
systemic medications, 192
systemically, 192

T

tachycardia, 181
Tay-Sachs, 105, 106
Technical Stuff icon, 3
temperature, body, 328
TENS (Transcutaneous Electrical Nerve Stimulation), for labor pain, 196
terbutaline, 500
term, 50
term PROM, 477–478
tests and testing
  about, 86
  for Down syndrome, 129–130
  during pregnancy, 19–20
tetanus, diphtheria, and pertussis (Tdap), 32, 34
tetracycline, 30
Theo-Dur (theophylline), 500
theophylline (Theo-Dur), 500
thermal reconditioning, 74
third stage, of labor, 191
third trimester
  about, 143
  baby development during, 143–146
  body changes during, 146–156
  calories needed during, 275–276
  causes for concern during, 167–171
  fitness program during, 331
  gauging lung maturity during, 157
  infant CPR, 162
  partner support during, 151, 155, 160, 172
  prenatal visits during, 156–159
  preparing for breastfeeding, 152
  preparing for labor, 159–163
  preparing for the hospital, 164–167
three Ps, of labor, 187
3D ultrasounds, 133
thrush, 427, 430

V

vaccinations, 32–34, 228

vacuum extractor, 208–209

vaginal birth after cesarean (VBAC), 460

vaginal delivery. *See also* delivery

  about, 200–201

  delivering the baby, 206–207

  delivering the placenta, 207

  episiotomy, 204–205

  prolonged second-stage labor, 205

  pushing, 201–203

  repairing perineum, 207

  watching, 203

vaginal discharge, 72

vaginal infections, 498–499

valsava maneuver, 54

Vanceril, 500

vanishing twin, 446

varicella (chickenpox), 34, 108

varicella-zoster immune globulin (VZIG), 489

varicose veins, during third trimester, 154–156

VBAC (vaginal birth after cesarean), 460

VDRL, 107–108

vegans, 49

vegetables

  eating, 267

  in MyPlate, 43

vegetarians, 48, 291–292

Verifi, 20

vernix caseosa, 220

vertex presentation, 144

very young moms, 445

viable, 16, 120

videos, 86

visualizing ideal births, 82–83

vitamin A, 29, 286

vitamin B12, 49, 292

vitamin C, 473

vitamin D, 45–46, 109, 281, 285–286, 292

vitamin E, 473

vitamin K, 227

vitamins

  after delivery, 256

  prenatal, 12, 29, 46, 97

volleyball, 340

vomiting, 58–61, 101

VZIG (varicella-zoster immune globulin), 489

W

walking, 255, 337

walking epidurals, 193, 194

warming up, 349

Warning icon, 3

watching the delivery, 203

water

  for constipation, 65, 99–100

  drinking, 268

water aerobics, 337

water birth, 88

water-skiing, 341–342

waxing, 74

weakened cervix, sex and, 142

websites. *See specific websites*

weeks, 93

weeks 0 to 4, 12

weeks 5 to 8, 12–13

weeks 9 to 12, 13–14

weeks 13 to 16, 14–15

weeks 17 to 20, 15

weeks 21 to 24, 15–16

weeks 25 to 28, 16–17

weeks 29 to 32, 17–18

weeks 33 to 36, 18

weeks 37 to 40, 18–19

weeks 40 to 42, 19

weepiness, during third trimester, 155

weight

  avoiding an obsession over, 40

  of baby, 41–42, 422, 437

  checking, 26, 232

About the Authors

Joanne Stone, MD, is a professor in the internationally renowned Department of Obstetrics and Gynecology at The Icahn School of Medicine at Mount Sinai in New York City. She is the director of the Division of Maternal–Fetal Medicine and also cares for patients with problem pregnancies. She has lectured throughout the country, is widely published in medical journals, and has been interviewed frequently for television and magazines on topics related to pregnancy, with a special emphasis on the management of multi-fetal pregnancies. Away from the hospital, she loves to spend time with her husband, George, and her two wonderful girls, Chloe and Sabrina.

Keith Eddleman, MD, works with Joanne Stone at Mount Sinai. He is a professor in the medical school and the Director of Obstetrics at the hospital. He teaches medical students, residents, and fellows; lectures throughout the world; and appears often on television to discuss issues concerning the care of pregnant women. His areas of special expertise are ultrasound and reproductive genetics. His free time, when he has any, is spent with his family at their apartment in Manhattan and at their country house in upstate New York.

Catherine Cram, MS, is an exercise physiologist who specializes in pre- and postnatal fitness certificate trainings and information for health/wellness organizations and the military. She is the co-author of the 2012 edition of *Exercising through Your Pregnancy* (Addicus Books) with Dr. James Clapp and is a contributing author of *Women's Health in Physical Therapy* (Lippincott Williams & Wilkins). She is a maternal fitness expert for Babycenter.com and has been featured in prenatal fitness articles for *Fit Pregnancy, Parenting, Glamour, Babytalk,* and *The American Journal of Medicine and Sports.*

Tara Gidus Collingwood, MS, RDN, CSSD, is a registered dietitian nutritionist (RDN), a Board Certified Specialist in Sports Dietetics (CSSD), and a recognized expert in nutrition and health promotion. Tara co-authored *Flat Belly Cookbook For Dummies* (Wiley). Along with being an expert in pregnancy nutrition, Tara specializes in performance nutrition for athletes and busy professionals. She is the team dietitian for the NBA's Orlando Magic and a sports nutrition consultant to the athletes at the University of Central Florida and runDisney. Tara runs her own nutrition consulting business in Orlando, Florida, and is wife to husband, John; mother to two boys, Basil and Levi; and stepmother to two more boys, Maxim and Samuel. She loves to run and does numerous races, from 5K to marathon, each year.

Rachel Gurevich is a freelance health writer and author, most notably of *The Doula Advantage: Your Complete Guide to Having an Empowered and Positive Birth with the Help of a Professional Childbirth Assistant* (Three Rivers Press). Rachel also writes about fertility for About.com. Originally from the United States, she currently lives in Israel with her husband and four children, including a set of twins. Her website is www.rachelgurevich.com.

Matthew M. F. Miller was a member of the University of Iowa undergraduate writer's workshops in poetry, fiction, and nonfiction and is a graduate of the University of Southern California's Master of Professional Writing program. His infertility blog, Maybe Baby, was the catalyst for a book of the same name. Matthew currently lives in Tennessee with his wife and two daughters.

Sharon Perkins has been an RN for more than 25 years, mostly in maternal–child health, and has spent her fair share of time on the maternity floor, both while at work and while having five children, although one arrived via plane from Korea. She has authored or co-authored multiple *For Dummies* books. She lives in New Jersey but visits Disney World frequently and loves spending time with her three grandchildren.

Tere Stouffer is the author or co-author of 20 books on topics as diverse as travel, finance, fitness, and cooking. She's also an award-winning digital-content strategist who guides nonprofits, associations, and small businesses on budget-friendly content strategy, social-media management, and branded campaigns. Find out more at terestouffer.com.

Carol Vannais, RN, has been an RN for 33 years. She is currently a staff nurse at Cooper Center for In Vitro Fertilization in Marlton, New Jersey. Prior to Cooper Center, she worked in labor and delivery for 18 years as an RN and a Certified Childbirth Instructor. Prior to working in maternal–child health, she worked in critical care. She lives in New Jersey with her husband, Leon, and has four sons.

Publisher's Acknowledgments

Senior Acquisitions Editor: Tracy Boggier

Compilation Editor: Tracy L. Barr

Project Manager: Michelle Hacker

Development Editor: Georgette Beatty

Copy Editor: Danielle Voirol

Technical Editor: Anne McCartney

Art Coordinator: Alicia B. South

Production Editor: Selvakumaran Rajendiran

Illustrator: Kathryn Born, MA

Cover Image: ©Yarkovoy/Shutterstock

Apple & Mac

iPad For Dummies,
5th Edition
978-1-118-72306-7

iPhone For Dummies,
7th Edition
978-1-118-69083-3

Macs All-in-One
For Dummies, 4th Edition
978-1-118-82210-4

OS X Mavericks
For Dummies
978-1-118-69188-5

Blogging & Social Media

Facebook For Dummies,
5th Edition
978-1-118-63312-0

Social Media Engagement
For Dummies
978-1-118-53019-1

WordPress For Dummies,
6th Edition
978-1-118-79161-5

Business

Stock Investing
For Dummies, 4th Edition
978-1-118-37678-2

Investing For Dummies,
6th Edition
978-0-470-90545-6

Personal Finance
For Dummies, 7th Edition
978-1-118-11785-9

QuickBooks 2014
For Dummies
978-1-118-72005-9

Small Business Marketing
Kit For Dummies,
3rd Edition
978-1-118-31183-7

Careers

Job Interviews
For Dummies, 4th Edition
978-1-118-11290-8

Job Searching with Social
Media For Dummies,
2nd Edition
978-1-118-67856-5

Personal Branding
For Dummies
978-1-118-11792-7

Resumes For Dummies,
6th Edition
978-0-470-87361-8

Starting an Etsy Business
For Dummies, 2nd Edition
978-1-118-59024-9

Diet & Nutrition

Belly Fat Diet For Dummies
978-1-118-34585-6

Mediterranean Diet
For Dummies
978-1-118-71525-3

Nutrition For Dummies,
5th Edition
978-0-470-93231-5

Digital Photography

Digital SLR Photography
All-in-One For Dummies,
2nd Edition
978-1-118-59082-9

Digital SLR Video &
Filmmaking For Dummies
978-1-118-36598-4

Photoshop Elements 12
For Dummies
978-1-118-72714-0

Gardening

Herb Gardening
For Dummies, 2nd Edition
978-0-470-61778-6

Gardening with Free-Range
Chickens For Dummies
978-1-118-54754-0

Health

Boosting Your Immunity
For Dummies
978-1-118-40200-9

Diabetes For Dummies,
4th Edition
978-1-118-29447-5

Living Paleo For Dummies
978-1-118-29405-5

Big Data

Big Data For Dummies
978-1-118-50422-2

Data Visualization
For Dummies
978-1-118-50289-1

Hadoop For Dummies
978-1-118-60755-8

Language & Foreign Language

500 Spanish Verbs
For Dummies
978-1-118-02382-2

English Grammar
For Dummies, 2nd Edition
978-0-470-54664-2

French All-in-One
For Dummies
978-1-118-22815-9

German Essentials
For Dummies
978-1-118-18422-6

Italian For Dummies,
2nd Edition
978-1-118-00465-4

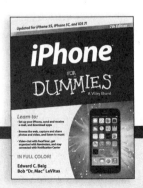

Available in print and e-book formats.

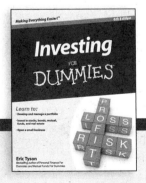
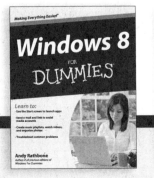
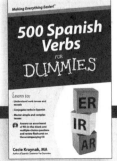
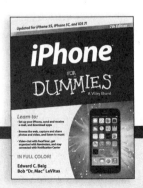

Available wherever books are sold. **For more information or to order direct visit www.dummies.com**

Math & Science

Algebra I For Dummies,
2nd Edition
978-0-470-55964-2

Anatomy and Physiology
For Dummies, 2nd Edition
978-0-470-92326-9

Astronomy For Dummies,
3rd Edition
978-1-118-37697-3

Biology For Dummies,
2nd Edition
978-0-470-59875-7

Chemistry For Dummies,
2nd Edition
978-1-118-00730-3

1001 Algebra II Practice
Problems For Dummies
978-1-118-44662-1

Microsoft Office

Excel 2013 For Dummies
978-1-118-51012-4

Office 2013 All-in-One
For Dummies
978-1-118-51636-2

PowerPoint 2013
For Dummies
978-1-118-50253-2

Word 2013 For Dummies
978-1-118-49123-2

Music

Blues Harmonica
For Dummies
978-1-118-25269-7

Guitar For Dummies,
3rd Edition
978-1-118-11554-1

iPod & iTunes
For Dummies, 10th Edition
978-1-118-50864-0

Programming

Beginning Programming
with C For Dummies
978-1-118-73763-7

Excel VBA Programming
For Dummies, 3rd Edition
978-1-118-49037-2

Java For Dummies,
6th Edition
978-1-118-40780-6

Religion & Inspiration

The Bible For Dummies
978-0-7645-5296-0

Buddhism For Dummies,
2nd Edition
978-1-118-02379-2

Catholicism For Dummies,
2nd Edition
978-1-118-07778-8

Self-Help & Relationships

Beating Sugar Addiction
For Dummies
978-1-118-54645-1

Meditation For Dummies,
3rd Edition
978-1-118-29144-3

Seniors

Laptops For Seniors
For Dummies, 3rd Edition
978-1-118-71105-7

Computers For Seniors
For Dummies, 3rd Edition
978-1-118-11553-4

iPad For Seniors
For Dummies, 6th Edition
978-1-118-72826-0

Social Security
For Dummies
978-1-118-20573-0

Smartphones & Tablets

Android Phones
For Dummies, 2nd Edition
978-1-118-72030-1

Nexus Tablets
For Dummies
978-1-118-77243-0

Samsung Galaxy S 4
For Dummies
978-1-118-64222-1

Samsung Galaxy Tabs
For Dummies
978-1-118-77294-2

Test Prep

ACT For Dummies,
5th Edition
978-1-118-01259-8

ASVAB For Dummies,
3rd Edition
978-0-470-63760-9

GRE For Dummies,
7th Edition
978-0-470-88921-3

Officer Candidate Tests
For Dummies
978-0-470-59876-4

Physician's Assistant Exam
For Dummies
978-1-118-11556-5

Series 7 Exam For Dummies
978-0-470-09932-2

Windows 8

Windows 8.1 All-in-One
For Dummies
978-1-118-82087-2

Windows 8.1 For Dummies
978-1-118-82121-3

Windows 8.1 For Dummies,
Book + DVD Bundle
978-1-118-82107-7

Available in print and e-book formats.

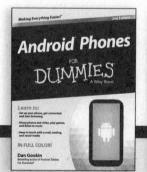

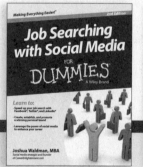

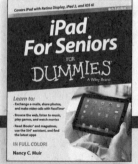

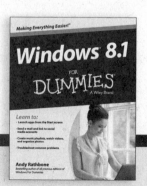

Available wherever books are sold. **For more information or to order direct visit www.dummies.com**

Take Dummies with you everywhere you go!

Whether you are excited about e-books, want more from the web, must have your mobile apps, or are swept up in social media, Dummies makes everything easier.

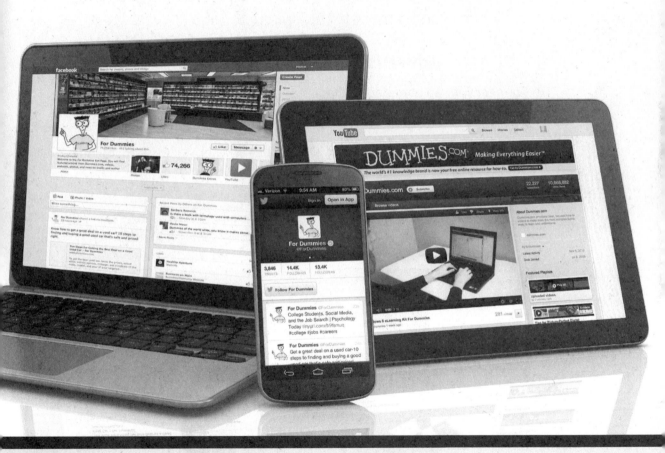

For Dummies is the global leader in the reference category and one of the most trusted and highly regarded brands in the world. No longer just focused on books, customers now have access to the For Dummies content they need in the format they want. Let us help you develop a solution that will fit your brand and help you connect with your customers.

Advertising & Sponsorships

Connect with an engaged audience on a powerful multimedia site, and position your message alongside expert how-to content.

Targeted ads • Video • Email marketing • Microsites • Sweepstakes sponsorship

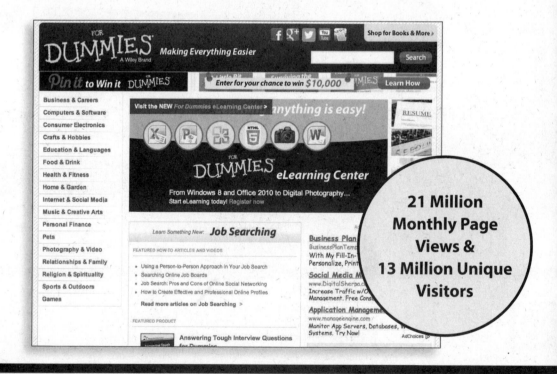

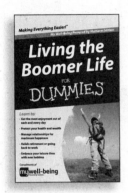
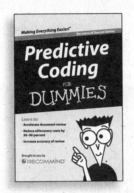
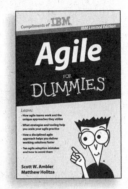
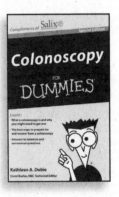
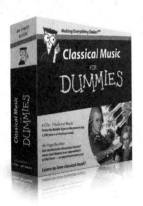
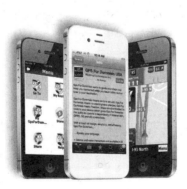
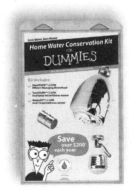
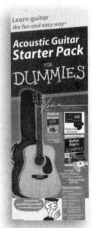
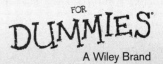

Dummies products make life easier!

- DIY
- Consumer Electronics
- Crafts

- Software
- Cookware
- Hobbies

- Videos
- Music
- Games
- and More!

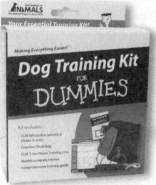

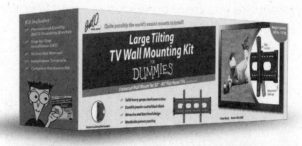

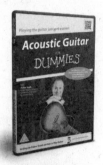

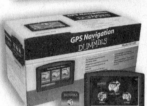

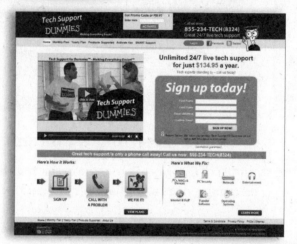

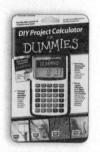

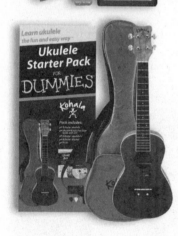

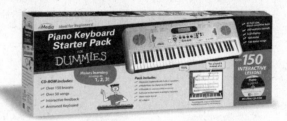

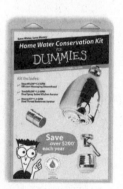

For more information, go to **Dummies.com** and search the store by category.

FOR
DUMMIES
A Wiley Brand